Group Wellness Programs

for Chronic Pain and Disease Management

Group Wellness Programs

for Chronic Pain and Disease Management

Carolyn A. McManus, PT, MA, MS

Clinical Coordinator for Wellness Services
Rehabilitation Services
Swedish Medical Center
Seattle, Washington

Foreword by Jon Kabat-Zinn, PhD

Professor of Medicine Emeritus
University of Massachusetts Medical School

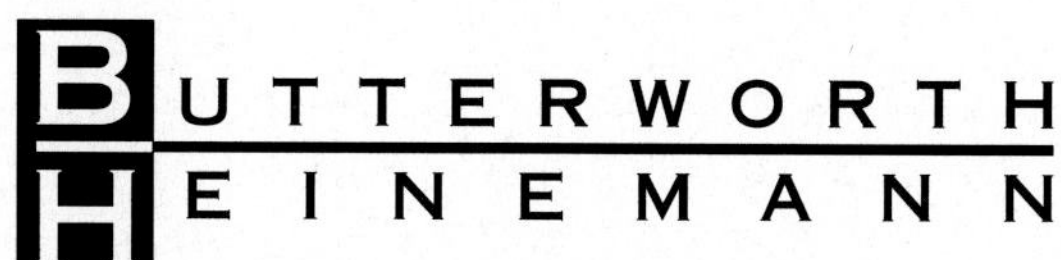

An Imprint of Elsevier Science

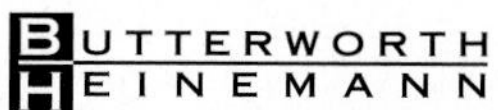

An Imprint of Elsevier Science

11830 Westline Industrial Drive
St. Louis, Missouri 63146

GROUP WELLNESS PROGRAMS FOR CHRONIC PAIN AND DISEASE MANAGEMENT 0-7506-7397-4

NOTICE

Physical Therapy is an ever-changing field. Standard safety precautions must be followed, but as new research and clinical experience broaden our knowledge, changes in treatment and drug therapy may become necessary or appropriate. Readers are advised to check the most current product information provided by the manufacturer of each drug to be administered to verify the recommended dose, the method and duration of administration, and contraindications. It is the responsibility of the licensed health care provider, relying on experience and knowledge of the patient, to determine dosages and the best treatment for each individual patient. Neither the publisher nor the editor assumes any liability for any injury and/or damage to persons or property arising from this publication.

International Standard Book Number 0-7506-7397-4

Publishing Director: Andrew Allen
Executive Editor: Marion S. Waldman
Editorial Assistant: Louise Bierig
Publishing Services Manager: Pat Joiner
Project Manager: Keri O'Brien
Designer: Studio Montage
Senior Designer: Mark A. Oberkrom

Printed in China
Last digit is the print number: 9 8 7 6 5 4 3 2 1

To Eleanor and Richard McManus

About the Author

Carolyn McManus holds a Bachelor's Degree of Science in Zoology from the University of Massachusetts (1977), a Master's Degree of Science in Physical Therapy from Duke University (1980), and a Master's Degree of Arts in Psychology from Antioch University (1991). In her clinical practice, she has specialized in a whole person approach to the care of people with chronic pain and disease. She designed and is the instructor for The Wellness Program, a mindfulness-based wellness, exercise, and stress reduction program for individuals with chronic pain and disease at Swedish Medical Center in Seattle. She has served as a consultant and instructor in research examining the effectiveness of mindfulness-based stress reduction and other self-management approaches in the treatment of individuals with chronic pain and disease. She is national consultant and speaker on the topics of wellness and the role of mindfulness in health care.

About the Contributor

Kathleen Putnam holds a Bachelor's Degree of Science in Dietetics from Oregon State University (1992) and a Master's Degree of Science in Nutrition Science from Bastyr University (2000). She is a nutrition counselor in private practice in Seattle and a local and national consultant and speaker on the topics of healthy nutrition and a whole person approach to dietary changes. She has served as a nutrition educator in the Cardiac Rehabilitation Program at Swedish Medical Center (SMC) and as a nutrition consultant and educator in The Dean Ornish Program for Reversing Heart Disease. She developed and teaches the Healthy Weighs Program, a comprehensive lifestyle approach to weight management at SMC. She has served as a clinical nutrition supervisor at Bastyr University Health Clinic and nutrition instructor at Seattle community colleges.

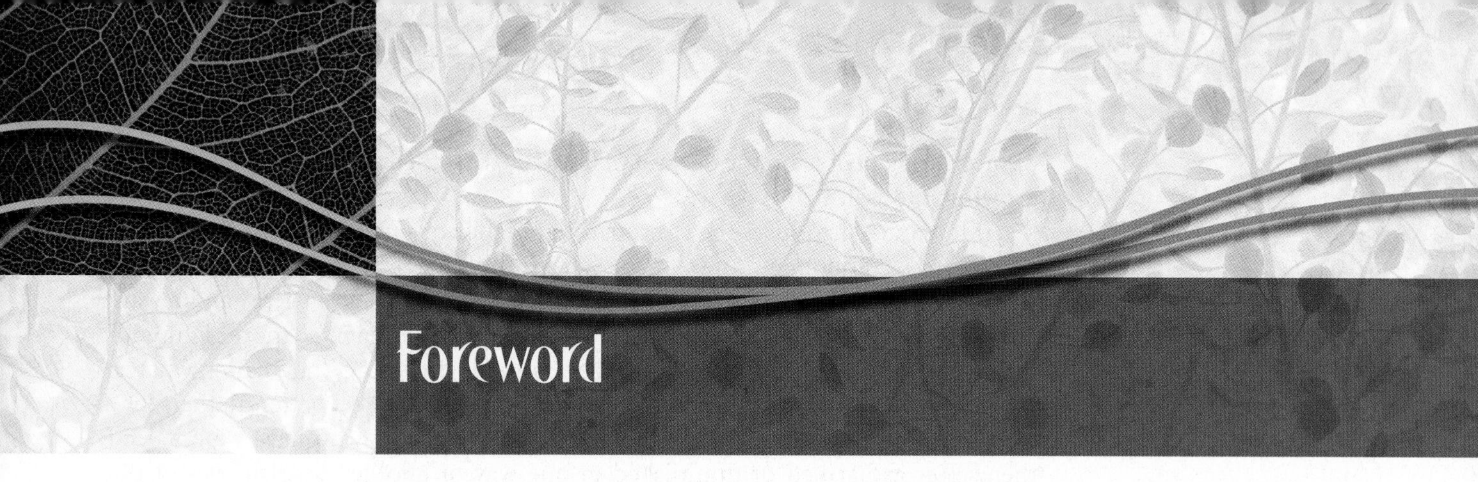

Foreword

This pioneering textbook addresses a major challenge within health care today, namely how to effectively bring people suffering with chronic medical conditions and lifestyle-related health problems to actively investigate and develop their potential for optimizing their health and well-being across the lifespan as a vital complement to the efforts of their health care providers. It advocates an approach that differs significantly from other programs in that its aim is not "fixing" people who are seen as "broken," but rather engaging people who are seen as fundamentally whole. It encourages people to embark on a lifetime adventure of learning and growing, based on connecting in new ways with their own experience and on discovering and then mobilizing their own deep inner resources for healing and transformation to whatever degree healing and transformation may be possible, always unknown. The transformation I am referring to is nothing less than a new way of seeing oneself and a new way of being within oneself and embracing the realities of one's life situation in the present moment. These life realities sometimes include varying degrees of stress, pain, disability, and disease that one may have to come to terms with and learn to live with. The challenge is to engage in that learning. It is usually a lifetime's work. But such active engagement has the potential to give a person's life back to him or herself.

Too often, sadly, health care providers merely tell people who do not respond well to available treatments that they will have to learn to live with their chronic medical conditions. This book instructs clinicians in *how* to engage people in that learning, rather than just sending them off at that point to fend for themselves without support, information, or ongoing guidance. McManus offers health professionals interested in wellness and rehabilitation a practical, detailed, and highly structured way to ignite energy and enthusiasm in people for that very process of learning, using the powerful vehicle of a group intervention that can, in short order, grow into a community of common affliction and common purpose and, in so doing, set the stage for significant and sometimes dramatic shifts in insight and understanding to occur in the participants.

The outcome? Rather than exercise being one more "should" to squeeze into one's day, a person who has been through a group wellness program of this kind might be more likely to simply say: "This is now who I am" rather than "this is what I have to do." In this shift in orientation, there is less burden and less forcing the issue, less striving to be some other way, and more acceptance and embodiment of the new way itself. The same would be true of a new way of eating (not so much "I am on a new diet," with all its attendant pitfalls and conflicts, but "this is the way I eat"), or of being more in touch with sensations in the body (perhaps less "Oh my God, my back is killing me" and more "how am I going to relate to what I am experiencing in this moment?"). The numerous case examples of Wellness Program participants and reports of their insights and lifestyle changes tell the tale quite eloquently and attest to the transformative potential of such work and the possibility of motivating people on the deepest of levels to trust their own inner capacities for growing into well-being.

McManus introduces the concept and practice of *mindfulness*[1] as a necessary and central component of wellness. The mindfulness approach meets people wherever they are and works with them there, which is always "here" and always "now." It sees people as "already whole and complete," as having "more right with them than wrong with them while they are still breathing" no matter what is "wrong." Such statements are not clichés to make people feel better. Rather, they represent a profound and respectful way to invite people who have experienced themselves as harmed or diminished in one way or another, as casualties of the human condition so to speak, for whatever reason, to participate in their own movement toward greater levels of health and well-being in collaboration with all the members of their health care team, and in this case, in collaboration with their group wellness instructor and fellow program participants. This approach is intrinsically motivating, honoring the powerful potential latent within all of us if we are willing to suspend judgment for a time and simply engage openheartedly in these wellness-enhancing practices based on cultivating attention and awareness. The McManus approach could easily be called "mindfulness-based wellness" because it is so firmly grounded in practices of both body awareness and mind awareness, and because it is equally grounded in a generosity of spirit that sees people as miraculous beings, as geniuses who are capable of just the kinds of transformations of view and action and ways of living that such programs invite. It shares a great deal with the approach known as mindfulness-based stress reduction (MBSR)[2,3] developed in the late 1970s at the University of Massachusetts Medical Center, and can be thought of as a highly cost-effective way to engage people as active participants in their own health care,[4] in what has been called "participatory medicine."[5]

McManus' program and MBSR both hark back to the concept of "high level wellness" described by Ardell.[6] This concept provides a framework for orienting people to the importance of doing something for themselves as a complement to what the medical system can do for them, an approach that was strongly advocated by the 1979 Surgeon General's report on health promotion and disease prevention.[7] In it, Joseph Califano, Jr., then Secretary of Health, Education, and Welfare who commissioned the report, stated: "You the individual, can do more for your own health and well-being than any doctor, any hospital, any drug, any exotic medical device." In emphasizing prevention and health promotion, the report augmented a movement known as "self-care"[8] which stressed the role of individual responsibility for participating in one's own health and well-being as a complement to, not a substitute for, more traditional health care modalities. In this era of fiscal crisis in health care and with the need for clinically effective and cost-effective evidence-based group interventions to promote positive health attitudes and behaviors in a rapidly aging demographic, such an approach is more important than ever. McManus' book, and the program it encapsulates, is a welcome extension and deepening of this movement at a critical moment. The climate for the widespread acceptance and implementation of its approach has never been better.

Ardell emphasized that health could be thought of as a continuum from premature death to what he called high level wellness, rather than merely to a point where disease and dysphoric symptoms are absent. One could begin anywhere along the continuum, wherever one found oneself, and then move toward greater degrees of wellness by taking personal responsibility for one's own health regardless of one's diagnosis (without any implication that one is blaming oneself for one's condition, but rather experimenting to see if now, from this point on, one can actively participate in doing something about it), rather than passively being carried in the opposite direction, through signs and symptoms to increasingly severe or chronic disease and greater degrees of disability. The neutral point, where nothing was particularly bothersome, the absence of disease, was not seen as the end of the health continuum, as it so frequently is, but rather the middle. This was the most important point. For "health," although not as simple and linear as this model suggested, is a mysterious gift. In many ways, health is still only poorly understood because almost all the funding for research is devoted to studying disease. Very little was or is going to the investigation of health or prevention. For the most part, we still have a disease-care system rather than a health-care system.

Health can be thought of as a dynamic, nonlinear process that is continually readjusting itself along the lifespan from infancy to old age and from conception to death.[9] It is possible to be healthy and well at any age, the wellness orientation asserts, but at the same time, it is important to keep in mind that the health of a 20-month-old baby is not the same as the health of a 20-year-old person, is not the same as the health of a 40-, 60-, 80-, or 90-year old. Nor is health exclusively found in the mere absence of disease or signs or symptoms, for one can be healthy in the face of disease. One can be healthy even in approaching one's death, or in living with a severe disability, or both.[10] And since the biology of men and women differ in fundamental ways, men's health and women's heath need to be understood differently, a conclusion that was finally reached in Congress and the NIH with the development of the Women's Health Initiative and in increased funding for breast cancer research.

So health should not be thought of, as it commonly is, as a commodity that one can store up and keep hold of. Rather, it is a dynamic condition much like balance, that can be compromised if the organism tips too much in one direction or another. It is the condition of homeostasis that keeps us continually regulating and adjusting to both external and internal conditions of body and mind, soul and spirit.

Although health cannot be stored in any conventional sense, the more robust one is, the greater one's chances of "bouncing back" from an illness or injury, of mobilizing all of one's inner and outer resources, of rallying to reestablish balance and regain momentum in the direction of high level well-being or wellness. This requires taking responsibility for one's own health, and not just leaving it to the experts. It requires having some awareness of lifestyle factors, of attitudes, habits, and behaviors that over time can erode well-being or strengthen it. For this reason, it is critical that people learn how such maladaptive responses to stress and pressure as smoking, excessive alcohol consumption, overeating, a sedentary lifestyle, chronic anger, hostility and cynicism, social isolation and the like can lead to disease and the erosion of homeostasis and health. It is equally critical that they come to understand and to "taste" directly through their own successful efforts, that adaptive ways of dealing with the stress of life, including the burden of chronic pain, disease, and disability, can generate movement toward greater levels of health and well-being, and that no one on the planet can to this work for them. It has to be shouldered by their own efforts, in collaboration with skilled clinicians who can support them in the effort and give them powerful tools to work with, along with training in how to use them. That is the foundation of all efforts at high-level wellness and a key element in all mindfulness-based stress reduction programs.[11,12] For medical patients with chronic disorders, this is nothing less than rehabilitation at its best, whether we are speaking of people with chronic low back pain, headache, other musculoskeletal problems, or with cardiac disease or chronic obstructive pulmonary disease.

The deep meaning of the word *rehabilitation* is to learn to live inside again.[13] That, when all is said and done, is the fundamental curriculum McManus' approach offers patients through the group wellness intervention paradigm. Creating such a learning environment and shepherding participants through it with gentleness and skill takes a high degree of mindfulness on the part of the clinician, whether he or she be trained as a nurse, social worker, physician, physical therapist, occupational therapist, exercise physiologist, psychologist, dietitian, or wellness-instructor. McManus has provided a framework for continuing with one's own professional development as one enters the waters of sharing this profound orientation with those who need a helping hand in learning to trust and deepen their own capacity for growing toward greater health and well-being and inhabiting their bodies with awareness and loving kindness, nourishing themselves on multiple levels through mobilizing body and mind, soul and spirit. The life of the instructor is, in many ways, the first life to benefit from the program, and that benefit tends to sustain itself and deepen as one delves deeper into the process and into the practice of mindfulness.

In the physical therapy department at the University of Massachusetts Medical Center (which graciously provided the original home for MBSR and the nascent Stress Reduction Clinic before it moved into the Department of Medicine), I came to appreciate deeply the attention physical therapists pay to mobilizing the body's capacity for movement and for expanding what they so beautifully term the "degrees of freedom" of the body. Physical therapists employ two wonderful slogans that convey profound truths that are applicable across all health care disciplines dealing with chronic pain and disease management. One is "If you don't use it, you lose it." The other is "If it's physical, it's therapy." The first is as true for the mind as it is for the body. The second statement is even truer if the mind is present along with the body during the somatic engagement, whatever it happens to be, from relearning to walk to weight training for rehabilitation, from water exercises to cutting vegetables, from mindful movement practices to practicing the body scan, from opening a window ergometrically to hugging a child. The program presented here will go far toward enlivening those truths for health care providers in all specialties, and for the people they serve.

The present volume is grounded in the author's personal experience healing from an injury and in her own enduring quest for wellness, in her training in physical therapy and psychology, in her experience working in private practice, home care, and hospital settings, and in her extensive training in and commitment to mindfulness. These elements combine to bring a compelling power and authenticity to this comprehensive and inspiring treatment of both the clinical and organizational domains of group wellness programs for chronic pain and disease management. It is clear, concise, and masterful in its presentation, and of great value to health professionals and students alike. If health care practitioners in various fields, from medicine to nursing and from physical therapy to occupational therapy, from dietitians to medical social workers were to adopt and implement the broad outlines of the McManus program, modulated to the specific needs of their patient populations, it would signal a profoundly positive, indeed, a revolutionary improvement in the delivery of health care.

Jon Kabat-Zinn, PhD
Professor of Medicine Emeritus
University of Massachusetts Medical School

References

1. Kabat-Zinn J. *Wherever You Go, There You Are: Mindfulness Meditation in Everyday Life.* New York: Hyperion, 1994.
2. Kabat-Zinn J. *Full Catastrophe Living: Using the Wisdom of Your Body and Mind to Face Stress, Pain, and Illness.* New York: Delacorte Press, 1990.
3. Santorelli S. *Heal Thy Self: Lessons on Mindfulness in Medicine.* New York: Bell Tower, 1999.
4. Kabat-Zinn J. Six-month hospital visit cost reductions in medical patients following self-regulatory training. Poster presented at SBM, Washington, DC, March 22, 1987.
5. Kabat-Zinn J. Participatory medicine. *Journal of the European Academy of Dermatology and Venereology* 2000;14:239-240.
6. Ardell DB. *High Level Wellness: An Alternative to Doctors, Drugs, and Disease.* New York: Bantam, 1979.
7. *Healthy People: The Surgeon General's Report on Health Promotion and Disease Prevention - 1979.* U.S. Department of Health, Education, and Welfare, Public Health Service Publication No. 79-55071.
8. Travis JW. *Wellness Workbook for Health Professionals.* Mill Valley, Calif: Wellness Resource Center, 1977.
9. Edelman CL, Mandle CL. *Health Promotion Throughout the Lifespan* 5th ed. St Louis: Mosby, 2002.
10. Simmons P. *Learning to Fall: The Blessings of an Imperfect Life.* New York: Bantam, 2000.
11. Kabat-Zinn J. An out-patient program in Behavioral Medicine for chronic pain patients based on the practice of mindfulness meditation: Theoretical considerations and preliminary results. *Gen Hosp Psychiatry* 1982;4:33–47.
12. Kabat-Zinn J. Mindfulness meditation: health benefits of an ancient Buddhist practice. In Goleman D, Gurin J (eds), *Mind/Body Medicine.* Yonkers, NY: Consumer Reports Books, 1993, pp. 259-275.
13. Kabat-Zinn J. Mindfulness: The heart of rehabilitation. In Leskowitz E (ed), *Complementary and Alternative Medicine in Rehabilitation.* St Louis: Churchill Livingstone, 2003, pp. xi–xiv.

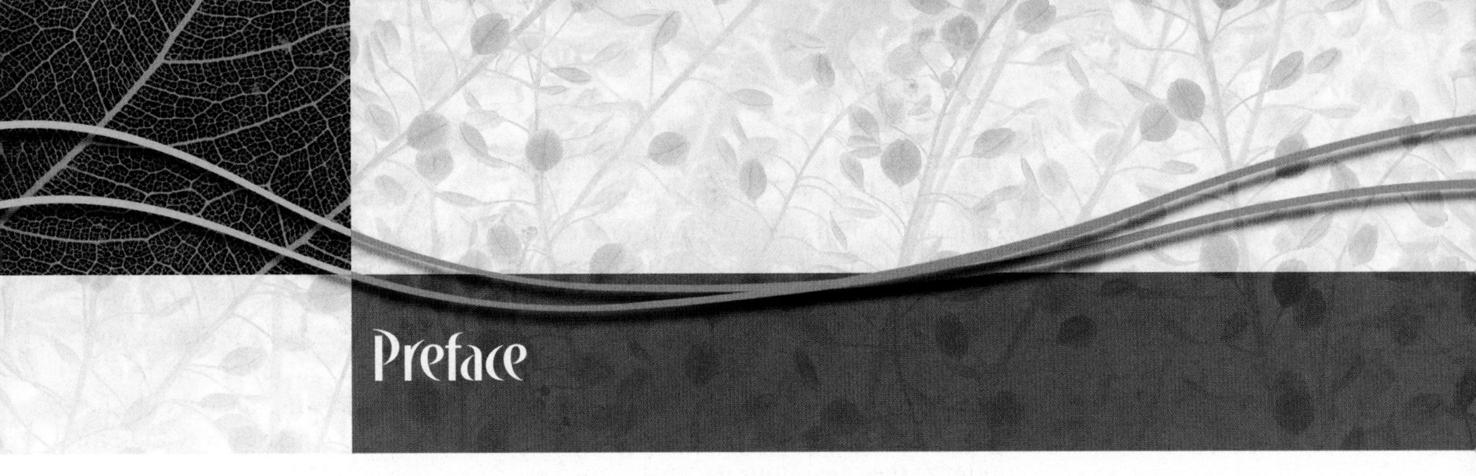

Preface

The intent of this book is to provide health care professionals with a framework to develop group wellness programs for people living with chronic pain and disease. This group wellness model advocates helping people identify and maximize what they can do for themselves to optimize their health, well-being, and function. It is a model applicable to health care services for people with cardiovascular disease, diabetes, chronic pain, osteoporosis, cancer, fibromyalgia, arthritis, HIV/AIDS, and other chronic conditions. This book is based on my interests in wellness and experience teaching an 8-week group program for people with chronic medical conditions since 1996 called The Wellness Program. The many case examples presented in this text are the true stories of people who participated in this program.

It is my hope that this book will be useful in several areas. First, our health care system is better equipped to meet the needs of people with acute physical medical problems than at addressing the complex physical and psychosocial concerns of the chronically ill. People are told they have to learn to live with their problems, but are often left with little or no guidance on how to manage the multiple challenges they face. This text can serve as one resource for clinicians to address these often-neglected concerns.

Second, it is well known that the senior segment of our population is rapidly growing. The number of people over 65 years of age is projected to increase from 35 million in 2000 to 53 million by the year 2020 and to 70 million by the year 2030.[1] Because chronic disease commonly accompanies the aging process, adequately caring for this large number of seniors will pose a huge challenge to our health care system. Providing cost-effective interventions that promote healthy lifestyle behaviors will be essential to prevent, delay the onset, or slow the progression of chronic disease and promote functional independence among these older adults. This book contributes to the resources available to assist in the development of these programs.

Third, I hope this book will contribute to the dialogue on wellness and how we, as health care providers, can effectively support and promote health and wellness in our communities. The vast majority of the American public knows they need to exercise and eat right for health benefits, yet 40% remain inactive and the number of obese Americans has been on a steady rise. There are no simple answers to the problem of the dismal health habits of the American public. We must keep examining how to effectively respond to this major health problem.

In addition, there is increasing interest and use of complementary and alternative medical services by the general public. Because mainstream medical interventions cannot offer cures to those with chronic conditions, many people turn to complementary and alternative medicine for additional treatment. In my own case, I began studying mindfulness meditation and yoga in the early 1980s following a back injury I sustained while transferring a patient. I believe had I not been drawn to a whole-person approach that engaged the mind and the body,

I might have become another patient with chronic back pain running from physician to physician seeking a cure that ultimately had to come from within me. Mindfulness is a main theme in The Wellness Program that I teach at Swedish Medical Center in Seattle. In this text I introduce mindfulness meditation and discuss its direct applications to living well with chronic medical problems. I also examine how principles of mindfulness can be integrated with traditional exercise programs and describe movement disciplines from both the East and West that emphasize mind-body awareness. I hope this book will contribute to the growing dialogue in the mainstream community on how we can creatively bridge these two worlds to optimize the care of our patients.

Finally, this is a book for health care clinicians across disciplines including medicine, nursing, physical therapy, occupational therapy, nutrition, exercise physiology, and psychology engaged in an exploration of wellness. If we are going to offer group wellness programs, we must continually ask ourselves, "What is wellness? What is wellness in the context of living with a chronic illness or life-threatening medical condition? What is healing in these circumstances?" It is my hope this text will inspire an examination of these questions and serve as a catalyst for clinicians to develop wellness programs that address their depth and breadth. It is also my hope that this text will help clinicians bring their strengths and gifts to their communities, create work they love, and bring benefit to those they serve.

Carolyn A. McManus

Reference

1. U.S. Health and Human Services Web Site: www.aoa.gov/aoa/stats/AgePop2050.html.

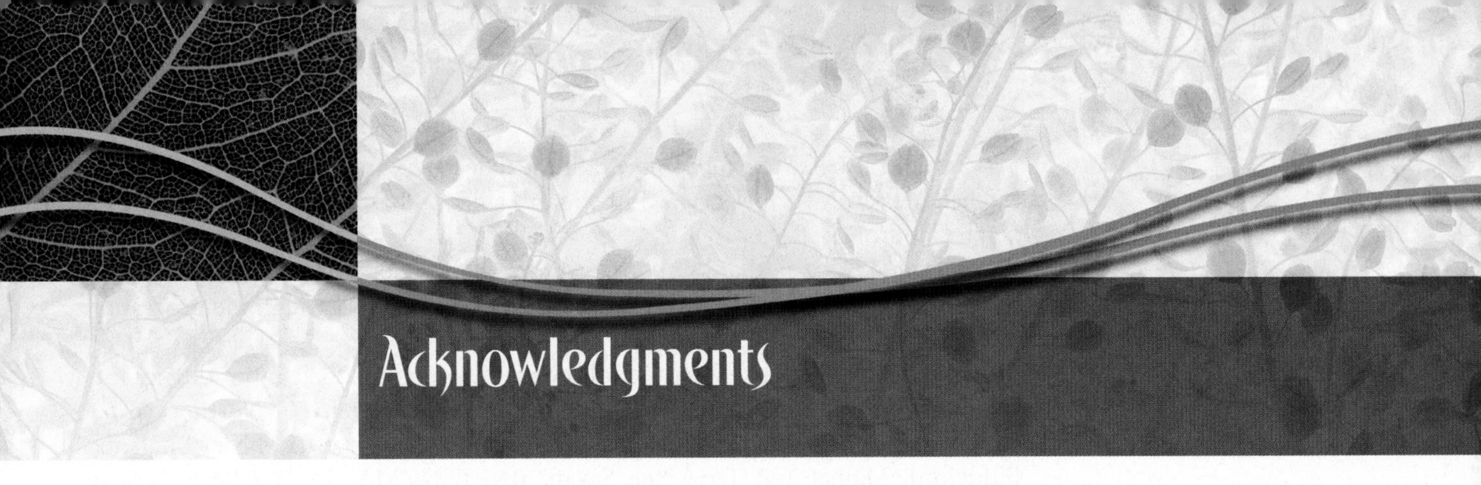

Acknowledgments

I feel tremendous gratitude toward the many people who so generously offered their support for this project. I would like to especially thank all those who have been participants in The Wellness Program. They have been a constant source of inspiration throughout the writing of this text.

I would like to thank David Clawson, MD, Medical Director of Rehabilitation Services and Flossie Bergum, PT, Director of Rehabilitation Services at Swedish Medical Center (SMC), for inviting for me to join an outstanding team of clinicians and offer The Wellness Program at a major medical center. I would like to thank my direct supervisor, colleague, and friend, Rich Bettesworth, PT, for his boundless support for my work and this book and his careful review of the initial manuscript. I would also like to thank friend, colleague, and teacher of The Wellness Program, Peggy Maas, PT, for offering her encouragement, wit, and wisdom throughout this project.

I am deeply grateful to Kathleen Putnam, RD, MS, for the generous contribution she made of her time, talent, and energy writing the chapter on nutrition.

I extend my gratitude to Jon Kabat-Zinn, PhD, and his colleagues associated with The Center for Mindfulness in Medicine, Health Care and Society at the University of Massachusetts Medical School: Saki Santorelli, EdD, Melissa Blacker, MA, Elana Rosenbaum, MSW, and Ferris Urbanowski, MA. Their inspiring work in mindfulness-based stress reduction served as a springboard for The Wellness Program and, ultimately, this book. I am grateful for the support of colleagues and friends. Many read sections of the text and offered suggestions. They include: Mary Lynn Pulley, EdD, Howard Schubiner, MD, Sandy Levy, MD, Cora Trujillo, PT, Steve Overman, MD, David Zucker, MD, Kristi Kujawski, MPH, Judy Ellis, PT, Carol Beber, PT, Diane Kurth, PT, Karen Sziel, OT, John Wynn, MD, Julia Smith, MD, Barbara Young, PT, Wolf Brolley, PT, Lisa Morishige, MS, Chris Pamp, MS, Mary Francis Kennedy, RN, Cate Brummett, PT, Pam Burnell, RN, Bev Ricker, PT, Leslie Pickett, PT, Marion Zuk, PT, Jim Walsh, PT, Elizabeth Tomeres, PT, and Laurie Pepin, PT. I would like to thank Ester Sternberg, MD, for her bibliography suggestions and Kim Ivy for sharing her expertise on T'ai Chi and Qigong. I would also like to thank Cheryl Nelson, LCSW, for her thoughts on wellness and wholeness. I am grateful for the friendship and computer assistance given throughout this project by Jeff Holdsworth. I feel tremendous appreciation for the librarians at the SMC medical library, Cheryl Goodwin, MLS, Bob Hollowell, MLS, and Mike Scully.

I would like to especially thank John Mazzarella, MD, for his early support for my work and his enthusiasm for its role in the care of people with heart disease. I am grateful to the many physicians who have been strong supporters of The Wellness Program. They include Peter Mohai, MD, Sylvia Lucas, MD, Sheena Aurora, MD, Gordon Irving, MD, David Sinclair, MD, Robbie Sherman, MD, Julie Carkin, MD, Paul Brown, MD, and Henk Dawson, MD.

I would also like to express my gratitude to teachers and sources of inspiration, Michelle Levey, MA, Joel Levey, PhD, Joan Halifax, PhD, Thich Nhat Hanh, and Pema Chodron.

I extend special thanks to my editors at Elsevier, Marion Waldman, Jill Rembetski, and Louise Bierig, for gracefully navigating me through the process of publication.

I would also like to thank the following reviewers for their input during the writing process: Cindy Flom-Meland, MPT, NCS, University of North Dakota, Grand Forks, ND; Nancy MacRae, MS, OTR/L, FAOTA, University of New England, Biddeford, Maine; and Terry Sue Savan, RN, BSN, MA, PA-C, CRNP, Lehigh University, Bethlehem, Penn.

Carolyn A. McManus

Contents

I The Group Wellness Model

Chapter 1 Wellness

This chapter identifies current trends underlying the growing interest within the health care community in group wellness programs for people with chronic medical conditions. Studies highlighting the benefits of several group wellness models are reviewed. A vision of wellness is introduced that incorporates the physical, mental, emotional, and spiritual dimensions of the human experience and recognizes the fundamental wholeness of each individual. Health care practitioners shifting from disease treatment to wellness promotion are encouraged to recognize how their own personal perceptions and understanding of wellness will influence this developing field.

A Context for Wellness Programs in Health Care

Wellness services are those health services that promote health and prevent disease. They provide people with education, skills, experiences, and resources that enable them to maximize what they can do for themselves to improve, maintain, or slow the decline of their health and function. They have an important role to play in promoting health and function in people with chronic medical conditions, such as cardiovascular disease, chronic pain, diabetes, obesity, arthritis, fibromyalgia, multiple sclerosis, and HIV/AIDS.

The demand for wellness services in health care is rapidly increasing. Several trends are fueling this development. These include aging baby boomers seeking to maximize their health, businesses wanting to lower health care costs, and hospitals in search of new sources of revenue. In addition, the U.S. Department of Health and Human Services has established an ambitious health promotion agenda for the nation. Under the leadership of the Office of Disease Prevention and Health Promotion, the Healthy People 2010 Initiative sets national health goals and objectives that include establishing wellness services in school, the workplace, health care, and community-based settings.[1]

Medical insurance providers are also showing interest in wellness services as a means to contain costs and provide competitive insurance plans. Studies demonstrating reduced health care utilization following participation in health promotion and wellness programs offer insurance providers incentives to include these services in their plans.[2-8] Also individuals who are offered health promotion programs are more satisfied with their health plans than those who are not offered these programs.[9] In a highly competitive market, consumer satisfaction with health promotion coverage is an attractive benefit to insurance purchasers.

The prevalence of chronic medical conditions in the population is also catalyzing the interest in health promotion and wellness services. Thirty-two million Americans have some form of activity limitation due to a chronic medical condition.[10] Although chronic disease is commonly associated with the elderly, it is prevalent in all age groups. More than one third of young adults 18 to 44 years of age and two thirds of adults 45 to 64 years of age have at least one chronic condition. Rates of chronic disease are highest in the elderly, in which 88% have at least one chronic medical condition. In 1990, the elderly comprised 1 in 8 persons in the United States; by 2030, 1 in 5 persons will be 65 years of age or older. This increase in the numbers of elderly persons, combined with healthier lifestyles, advances in medical science and technology, and improved medical services, will result in a continued increase in the number of people living with chronic conditions.

The financial cost of caring for people with chronic conditions is another factor motivating interest in wellness programs. It is estimated that noninstitutionalized Americans with one or more chronic conditions account for three fourths of U.S. health care expenditures.[10] As our health care system is organized to address acute illness, it is not well designed to meet the ongoing and complex needs of the chronically ill and aging population. Public and private medical service payers as well as policy makers recognize the growing costs of caring for the chronically ill and the need to develop effective services that address the complex problems of this population.[11-13]

Health Promotion and Wellness Research

Research demonstrates health improvements and medical cost reductions among participants in a range of health promotion and wellness programs.[3-9] Studies specifically involving the chronically ill also demonstrate these improvements. Lorig et al evaluated the effectiveness of a self-management program for people with chronic diseases.[6] In this study, 952 people 40 years of age or older, with a physician-confirmed diagnosis of heart disease, lung disease, stroke, or arthritis participated in a program of seven weekly 2.5-hour training sessions. Each group consisted of 10 to 15 participants. Program facilitation was provided by trained laypeople. Participants were provided with instruction in a range of self-management strategies that included exercise, symptom management techniques, nutrition, sleep and fatigue management, use of community resources, communication with others including health professionals, and problem solving strategies. As compared with the controls, the treatment group increased the number of minutes per week of stretching, strengthening, and aerobic exercise; increased the practice of cognitive symptom management; and improved their communication with their physicians. The treatment group also showed significant improvement in their self-rated health and increased their social/role activities. They decreased fatigue, disability, and health distress. The intervention group also had fewer hospitalizations and fewer total days spent in the hospital.

Barlow et al examined the effects of Lorig's self-management program on perceived control and self-management ability of patients with osteoarthritis and rheumatoid arthritis.[14] A total of 89 participants attended a health education program that covered self-help principles, exercise, information on the disease, communication with health professionals, and realistic goal setting. After 4 months, participants demonstrated increases in arthritis self-efficacy. They felt more confident in their ability to manage pain and fatigue. They demonstrated a significant, although moderate, improvement in pain. They also increased their practice of stretching and strengthening exercise programs and relaxation exercises.

Using a randomized, wait-list controlled study design, Speca et al examined the effectiveness of a mindfulness-based stress-reduction program on mood and symptoms of stress in cancer outpatients.[15] Participants included both men and women with a wide variety of cancer diagnoses, stages of illness, and ages. Treatment involved instruction in mindfulness meditation, gentle yoga, visualization, and cognitive restructuring. Following the intervention, the treatment group had significantly lower scores on total mood disturbance and subscales of depression, anxiety, anger, and confusion and higher scores on vigor compared to control subjects. In addition, the treatment group had fewer symptoms of stress, including fewer cardiopulmonary and gastrointestinal symptoms than control subjects.

Frost et al examined the effectiveness of a fitness program for patients with chronic low back pain.[16] Seventy-one people with chronic low back pain were randomly assigned to a supervised fitness program or a control group. Both groups were taught four specific exercises to be carried out at home and were referred to a back school for education in back care. Additionally, participants allocated to the fitness program attended eight 1-hour exercise classes supervised by a physical therapist over 4 weeks. The fitness program included stretching and light aerobic exercise. As compared with the controls, the fitness group demonstrated significant improvements on the Oswestry low back pain and disability index, in reports of pain, self-efficacy, and in walking distance after treatment and at 6-months follow-up.

Ferrell et al evaluated a walking program for elderly people with chronic musculoskeletal pain.[17] Thirty-three patients were randomly assigned to one of three groups. Group 1 received a 6-week supervised walking program. Group 2 received a pain education program that included instruction and demonstration in the use of heat, cold, massage, relaxation, and distraction. Group 3 received usual care. Both intervention groups demonstrated significant improvements in pain and functional status. No changes were observed in the control group.

These studies demonstrate wellness programs provided to people with chronic pain and disease result in improved health measures and, when examined, decreased health care use. This research shows that a range of interventions, from a comprehensive disease management program to a walking program can be effective in achieving identified health goals.

A wellness program is more than just patient education and exercise. It involves helping people change behaviors and live fully. It requires coaching people to access inner resources for well-being and adopt health-enhancing activities, not as a short-term solution, but as a way of life. At an individual level, these programs can make a profound difference in people's lives as the following three stories of participants in my class demonstrate.

Case Example 1.1.

Lisa was a 38-year-old woman diagnosed with systemic lupus erythematosus and fibromyalgia. She experienced constant musculoskeletal pain and fatigue that varied in intensity. A successful accountant in a large corporate accounting firm, she found it increasingly difficult to meet the demands of long work hours, deadlines, and impatient clients. She had recently retired on disability when she enrolled in The Wellness Program. Lisa was highly critical of her physical limits and had lost the self-worth she gained from her work. Her goals for The Wellness Program were to (1) learn to relax; (2) be consistent with self-management strategies, including regular exercise and appropriate pacing of activity; (3) decrease pain and fatigue; and (4) learn skills to cope with her limitations and her life without her work. During the last class, I ask participants what they learned in the program. Lisa touched everyone in the group when she answered "Compassion." She said listening to other people's stories, the class material, and exercises had taught her to meet herself with understanding, acceptance, and kindness. Less self-critical and more self-confident, she found it easier to remain motivated and consistent with her home program of walking, stretching, and mindfulness meditation. She recognized how her constant self-criticism had, in part, contributed to anxiety and her increased muscle tension. Learning to be kind to herself, along with breathing exercises, strategies for body awareness, and mindfulness meditation, helped Lisa achieve the relaxation she sought. She experienced a decrease in the intensity of her pain and fatigue. Rather than finding meaning in her work as an accountant, she was finding new depth and meaning in her relationships with family and friends and value and joy in maintaining her home. She still had challenges to face to create a full life without her work, but she now realized it was possible.

Case Example 1.2.

Martha was a 48-year-old woman who had a 20-year history of chronic severe migraine headaches and multiple food allergies. She had moderate success controlling her pain with medication for many years; however, her neurologist had recently informed her she needed to decrease her drug use because of adverse effects on her liver. She enrolled in The Wellness Program to learn alternative strategies for pain management that would help decrease her medication use. Toward the end of the program, a close childhood friend of Martha's, now living in a different state, asked Martha to care for her after a planned surgery. Martha was torn between her desire to help her friend and her own concerns about coping with headache pain and dietary needs while away from home. In the past, her fear and turmoil would have triggered a severe headache and prevented her from traveling. Instead, Martha chose to apply wellness tools from the class. These tools included diaphragmatic breathing, gentle yoga, and mindfulness meditation. Instead of falling into her old habit of fantasizing a negative outcome, she repeatedly returned her focus to the present moment. Rather than ruminate on her headache and food history, she affirmed her strengths and abilities. She made the trip and, to her own surprise, had a wonderful time. Before the surgery, Martha and her friend shared many memories and laughs. After surgery, Martha felt useful and experienced an increased closeness with her friend as she provided her care. Through a wellness approach, Martha's self-confidence increased, headache frequency decreased, and she was able to manage her dietary needs away from the structure and routine of her home setting. She was able to identify her strengths and abilities and prioritize the application of self-care skills to maximize her function and realize her goal of caring for her friend. At the end of the 8-week program, her medication use was unchanged; however, 1 year after completing the program, she had cut her medication use by half.

Case Example 1.3.

Beth, a 38-year-old woman diagnosed with fibromyalgia, attended The Wellness Program to learn skills to manage pain, fatigue, and anxiety. A very successful sales representative for a medical equipment supplier,

Beth was on a 3-month medical leave. She described what she learned in the final class: "I came to this program believing my body and symptoms were my enemy. A lot of my energy went into that battle. There was never a winner. Learning to be more accepting of my body and listen without always judging myself was a huge change. I'm not so hard on myself. I am more accepting of my physical limits when I have bad days. I also don't let how I physically feel define me. I am taking better care of myself. My symptoms are less because I don't constantly push myself to do more and more. I rest when I need to. For me, this has been an experience about love. I am finally learning to love myself enough to do what is good for me."

Wellness and Wholeness

Bert is someone I recently met in the gym at my local YMCA. At 75 years of age, Bert has suffered two heart attacks, a stroke, and has undergone heart surgery. After his first heart attack, he made changes in his lifestyle, became a regular at the YMCA, and subsequently lost 60 pounds. He once told me he has exercise equipment at home, but chooses to go to the gym because he loves the people. On his way to the treadmill, he stops to greet his many friends. I am among the new ones. One day, after a brief conversation in which he beamed as he spoke of his granddaughter's college graduation, I said to him, "Have a great day." He burst into laughter and replied, "Carolyn, any day I am above ground is a great day." I laughed with him and stood in awe of the aliveness and joy he radiated in spite of his medical history and physical limitations.

Two thousand years ago Plato observed: "The great error in the treatment of the human body is that physicians are ignorant of the whole. For the part can never be well unless the whole is well."[18] The same could be said today. Often when we health care professionals think of wellness, we reduce our focus to the clinical indicators of a person's physical condition. Aerobic capacity, body mass index, and the absence of disease may come to mind as components of wellness. This view excludes the depth and complexities of the human experience and the multiple factors that impact well-being. It does not begin to capture Bert's aliveness. It seriously limits our understanding of the chronically ill person who may live with varied physical symptoms, restrictions in activity, and weight fluctuations. It fails to account for the roles that belief and attitude, stress, social support, spirituality, and the environment play in well-being.

Wellness is a general term that has different meanings to different people. In my classes, I frequently ask participants what wellness means to them. The responses vary and the most common ones include the following:

1. I feel content with my life and experience inner peace.
2. I have a sense of purpose and meaning.
3. I am connected with an inner experience of myself and my values. In the midst of chaos and change, this connection provides stability and "meaning to the madness."
4. How I use my time and energy is in balance and consistent with what I value. I avoid losing perspective and going to extremes by obsessively putting my energy into one aspect of my life at the expense of others.
5. I am in control of how I use my time and energy. Rather than being dictated by the needs, wants, and expectations of others, I make my own choices. I can say "no" to the things that drain me and make time for what is most important.

6. I am able to do most of the things I like to do.
7. I feel connected with my family and friends and am involved in my community.
8. I can laugh, lighten up, and not take myself so seriously.

In defining wellness, no one has ever answered, "being fit" or "eating right." If health care practitioners are to adequately meet the needs and interests of the public, we must develop concepts of wellness that reach beyond medical indicators of physical function to embrace the whole person and the varied dimensions of the human experience. We must articulate and promote the elements of physical health within a larger framework that addresses a definition of wellness and the needs and goals meaningful to the people we serve. The World Health Organization defines health, within the context of health promotion, as "a resource for everyday life that permits people to lead individually, socially and economically productive lives. It is a positive concept emphasizing social and personal resources as well as physical capabilities."[19] In the medical literature, wellness is conceptualized in holistic terms, highlighting the fundamental wholeness of each individual and the capacity of each person to maximize his or her unique potential.[20] It is identified as an individual's ability to realize aspirations, satisfy needs, and respond positively to the challenges of the environment.[21]

A wellness approach requires this broader vision of health. It incorporates physical function into a larger model that embraces the dynamic integration of the physical, mental, emotional, and spiritual components of the human experience. This multidimensional experience of wellness is never fixed or isolated, but is always in a constant state of change, growth, and renewal and in a ceaseless interaction with a larger environment and community.

The word *health* is derived from the Anglo-Saxon word *haelen*, which means "to make whole." The experience of wholeness is an important theme in wellness programs for the chronically ill and has a major impact on an individual's ability to cope and live fully. Many people living with a chronic condition feel impaired and inadequate rather than whole. The energy and effort required to meet daily challenges often leads people to believe their disease is their identity. Many people take on a sick-role, defining themselves by their symptoms and limitations and emphasizing their isolation from others. Compared with the ideal body promoted by the media, they may perceive theirs as damaged and unlovable. With this outlook, they attempt to respond to their circumstances from their limitations and weaknesses. This is not true of everyone. There are individuals like Bert who radiate resilience and inspire everyone around them.

An understanding and experience of wholeness provides people with a new perspective and enables them to respond to their circumstances from their strengths. People need to know themselves as whole human beings who happen to also have a medical condition. This is not to diminish the challenges they face, but rather to recognize the disease is not their identity. This is an astonishing insight for many. It does not change their disease process in any way; however, it offers a shift in their *relationship to* their disease process. Rather than navigate life from a perspective of feeling broken and inadequate, people are empowered to meet their world from a position of wholeness and draw on their abilities and strengths.

If people can experience themselves as somehow bigger than their disease, they are in a much better position to cope. The following two stories address this perspective. Thich Nhat Hanh, a monk who witnessed tremendous human suffering, worked tirelessly for peace and was nominated by Martin Luther King, Jr. for the Nobel Peace Prize during the Vietnam War, was asked, "How do you transform great suffering?" He responded, "To transform great suffering, you must become great like a great river. If I had a glass of water and put into the glass, a handful of dirt or compost, you would think that the water was no longer good. However if I threw that same handful of dirt or compost into a great, great river, the river could receive it, incorporate and transform it. This is what you must do. You must come to recognize you are this great, great river."[22] This image points to something within a person that is greater than the suffering they experience.

The second story is told by Rachel Naomi Remen, MD, a physician and author who works with people with chronic and life-threatening medical conditions. She speaks from experiences both as a physician and as a patient with Crohn's disease. In her book, *My Grandfather's Blessings,* she writes of a 17-year-old person who was diagnosed with juvenile onset diabetes.[23] Angered and in despair over his diagnosis and its complications, he refused to follow his prescribed treatment. He was sent to Rachel with hopes she could somehow help. Several months went by without improvement. Then he had a dream. In the dream, he was sitting in a room with a small statue of a Buddha. He was not a religious or spiritual person and recognized the figure only because he was from California where pictures of Buddha are common. As he sat in company with this small statue, he experienced a feeling of peace and calm. Then suddenly, a dagger flew from over his shoulder and landed in the center of the statue's chest. He felt immense distress and anger. "Why is life like this?" was his cry. As he sat in despair and rage, he noticed something about the statue was changing. It was growing. It grew and grew and grew until the dagger was but a small speck on the chest of the statue. As he recounted the dream to Rachel, he began to recognize its meaning. He understood that perhaps he too could respond to his suffering by growing, such that his life, though not an easy one, could be a large, full, and meaningful one. After this experience, he followed his physician's treatment recommendations.

The previous two stories often help people glimpse the larger wholeness and wisdom that is within them and, although not a cure, can catalyze new insight and understanding. As there are no cures for chronic disease, it is useful to distinguish a difference between curing and healing. To cure is to completely restore the body to a condition free of disease. Although considerable medical research is devoted to finding cures for many diseases, these solutions often remain years away. A broader concept of healing is practical in the care of the chronically ill. Healing can be considered as an experience that restores a person to wholeness. It is an insight or shift in understanding and enables people to adopt a new attitude toward their circumstances. People discover, within themselves, the wisdom, courage, and capacity to meet the challenges of life in a manner consistent with their deepest beliefs, values, and desires. This fresh outlook enhances a person's quality of life and frequently results in behavioral changes.

One component of this larger understanding of wellness is the recognition of an individual's connection with other people and experience of community. The perception of being separate, isolated, and alone is very common and compounds the suffering of people with chronic medical conditions. Giving people a place to be themselves and candidly share their thoughts and feelings often relieves the distress they feel resulting from isolation. They realize firsthand that they are not alone. Others share their same fears and concerns, joys, and sorrows. Rather than experience their problems as something that separates them from others, they learn to approach their problems in a way that connects them to others. They recognize something the media does not acknowledge or advertise: Illness is a part of life. The group format is an ideal and powerful setting to help people make this profound shift.

Developing the Wellness Model

Health care professionals making the change from disease treatment to wellness are pioneering a new paradigm in medical care. Ultimately, how we personally understand wellness will have a powerful impact on how this field develops. We must examine how we create or fail to create an experience of wellness in our own lives. If we attempt to promote the health of others on a foundation of failure to promote our own, we will never be successful. If we neglect our own wellness, we will lack the understanding and insight needed to truly help others value their health and overcome obstacles to achieving well-being. From the efforts to discover wellness in our own lives, we bring the wisdom and skill derived from lived experience to helping others.

What does wellness mean? What is wellness in the context of living with a chronic illness? The contemplation of these questions invites us toward a model of wellness that recognizes the whole person and the multidimensions of the human experience. As we develop this new model, movement schools that are already rooted in an understanding of and respect for the interrelationship of mind and body and emphasize awareness are a valuable resource. These schools include Feldenkrais, the Alexander Method, yoga, and tai chi. Also valuable in this exploration is mindfulness meditation, a disciplined training in present moment awareness that recognizes the capacities within each individual to live fully, experience profound insight, relieve suffering, and cultivate inner peace. These practices are gaining attention among health care providers and are playing a growing role in medical care. They are discussed in greater detail in Chapters 3 and 8. The philosophies and practices taught in these schools provide avenues to move beyond the narrow examination of an impaired body part or disease process to embrace and develop the strengths of the whole person. They identify awareness as central to promoting well-being. Although the ability to teach any of these practices requires intensive training and dedicated practice, their fundamental tenets provide all practitioners with a rich framework for contemplating a whole person approach to the care of people with chronic pain and disease.

Summary

The demand for wellness and health promotion programs is rapidly growing due to a number of trends. Among these trends are the prevalence of chronic medical conditions in the general population and the increasing costs of caring for an aging population. Research demonstrates health benefits and cost reductions among participants in a range of wellness and health promotion programs. Health care providers have an opportunity to develop wellness programs for people with chronic medical conditions that acknowledge the fundamental wholeness of each individual and help people recognize their own inner strengths and wisdom. These programs help people maximize what they can do for themselves to achieve optimal function, minimize limitations, improve or maintain health, and enhance quality of life.

References

1. Healthy People 2010. (Referenced from the Web) www.health.gov/healthypeople.

2. Fries J, Bloch D, Harrington H et al. Two-year results of a randomized controlled trial of a health promotion program in a retiree population: the Bank of America study. *Am J Med* 1993 May;94(5):455-462.
3. Fries J, Harrington H, Edwards R et al. Randomized controlled trial of cost reductions from a health education program: the California Public Employees' Retirement System (PERS) study. *Am J Health Promot* 1994 Jan-Feb;8(3):216-223.
4. Leigh P, Richardson N, Beck R et al. Randomized controlled trial of a retiree health promotion program: the Bank of America study. *Arch Int Med* 1992 June;152:1201-1206.
5. Lorig K, Mazonson P, Holman H. Evidence suggests that health education for self-management in patients with chronic arthritis has sustained health benefits while reducing costs. *Arthritis Rheum* 1993 Apr;36(4):439-446.
6. Lorig K, Sobel D, Stewart A et al. Evidence suggesting that a chronic disease self-management program can improve health status while reducing hospitalization. *Med Care* 1999;37(1):5-14.
7. Sevick M, Dunn A, Murrow M et al. Cost-effectiveness of lifestyle and structured exercise interventions in sedentary adults: results of project ACTIVE. *Am J Prev Med* 2000 Jul;19(1):1-8.
8. Pruitt RA. Effectiveness and cost efficiency of interventions in health promotion. *J of Adv Nursing* 1992;7:926-932.
9. Schauffler H, Rodriguez T. Availability and utilization of health promotion programs and satisfaction with health plan. *Med Care* 1994 Dec;32(12):1182-1196.
10. Hoffman C, Rice D, Sung H. Persons with chronic conditions: their prevalence and costs. *JAMA* 1996 Nov;276(18):1473-1479.
11. Fries J, Koop E, Beadle E et al. Reducing health care costs by reducing the need and demand for medical services. *N Eng J Med* 1993 Jul;329(5): 321-325.
12. Wagner E, Austin B, Von Korff M. Organizing care for patients with chronic illness. *Milbank Q* 1996;74(4):511-543.
13. Gordon C, Harris RA. Health promotion for seniors: what is over the horizon? *Manag Care Q* 1997 Autumn; 5(4):34-42.
14. Barlow J, Williams B, Wright C. "Instilling the strength to fight the pain and get on with life": learning to become an arthritis self-manager through an adult education program. *Health Educ Res* 1999;14(4):533-544.
15. Speca M, Carlson L, Goodey E. A randomized, wait-list controlled clinical trial: The effect of a mindfulness-based stress reduction program on mood and symptoms of stress in cancer outpatients. *Psychosom Med* 2000;63:613-622.
16. Frost H, Moffett J, Moser J et al. Randomized controlled trial for evaluation of fitness programme for patients with chronic low back pain. *BMJ* 1995 Jan;310:151-154.
17. Ferrell B, Josephson K, Pollan et al. A randomized trial of walking versus physical methods for chronic pain management. *Aging Clin Exp Res* 1997;9(1-2):99-105.
18. Jaffe DJ. *Healing from Within.* New York: Simon & Schuster; 1980, p. 4.
19. World Health Organization. Health Promotion Glossary (Referenced from the Web) www.who.org.

20. Davidhizar R, Shearer R. Helping the client with chronic disability achieve high-level wellness. *Rehabilitation Nursing* 1997 May/June;22(3): 131-134.
21. McWilliams CL, Stewart M, Brown JB et al. Creating health with chronic illness. *ANS Adv Nurs Sci* 1996 Mar;18(3):1-15.
22. Story shared in a discussion by Thich Nhat Hanh during a meditation retreat in the Fall of 1998 at Plum Village in France.
23. Remen RN. *My Grandfather's Blessings: Stories of Strength, Refuge and Belonging.* New York: Riverhead Books, 2000, pp. 141-143.

Annotated Bibliography

Edelman CL, Mandle CL (eds). *Health Promotion Throughout the Lifespan* 5th ed. St. Louis: Mosby, 2002. This comprehensive text provides an exceptionally thorough foundation for developing wellness and health promotion services. Drawing primarily on the expertise of leading nurses in the field, it examines principles central to promoting and protecting health and preventing disease; identifies factors influencing individual, family, and community health; offers specific interventions for health promotion; and examines the application of health promotion to human development. It includes current research in health promotion and disease prevention, discusses multicultural perspectives, and provides clinical case examples and care plans. This gem of a text offers a wealth of practical information and is a valuable resource to any clinician providing wellness and health promotion services.

Gorin SS, Arnold J. *Health Promotion Handbook*. St. Louis: Mosby, 1998. This text broadly examines the field of health promotion. The authors explore the many ways health is defined and understood. They offer a theoretical framework for designing health promotion programs and provide guidance to apply this framework to specific behavior change. In addition, Gorin and Arnold discuss the political and economic factors shaping this emerging field.

Kabat-Zinn J. *Full Catastrophe Living: Using the Wisdom of Your Body and Mind to Face Stress, Pain and Illness.* New York: Delacorte Press, 1990. This book describes in detail a nationally recognized mindfulness-based stress reduction group program founded and taught at the University of Massachusetts Medical Center and School since 1979. Kabat-Zinn offers a thorough examination of mindfulness and its practical application to the circumstances of people living with chronic medical conditions. The many experiences of participants in the program described in this text offer a rich perspective and valuable insight into a whole person approach to wellness.

Ornish D. *Love and Survival.* New York: Harper Collins, 1998. Dean Ornish is a physician nationally recognized for his innovative approach to the treatment of heart disease through diet, exercise, yoga, and group support. In this text he shares personal experiences, patient stories, and scientific research to describe the powerful roles social support, the experience of connectedness and community, love, and intimacy play in health and illness. He invites leaders from the fields of medicine, scientific research, psychology, and theology to share their thoughts on science and the mystery of life, healing and love.

Remen, RN. *My Grandfather's Blessings: Stories of Strength, Refuge and Belonging.* New York: Riverhead Books, 2000. Rachel Naomi Remen is a physician, clinical professor of family and community medicine, and a counselor to people with chronic and life-threatening illness. She is also a master storyteller and gifted writer. Through stories about her relationship with her grandfather, her work as a physician and counselor, and her clients' experiences, she continually reveals to the reader the capacities of the human spirit to face adversity with dignity, grace, wisdom, and love. This is an inspiring book for any clinician.

Chapter 2 Group Leadership

This chapter examines the advantages of offering wellness services in a group format. The characteristics of an effective group leader are identified. Teaching styles and introductory guidelines for facilitating group discussions are presented. Recommendations for dealing with participants who present challenging behaviors are discussed.

The Advantages of Groups

For health care professionals with experience treating people only on an individual basis, facilitating groups brings new challenges and rewards. Groups create a lively and engaging setting for exploring the many dimensions of wellness.

The general benefits of providing services in a group format include the following:

1. *Cost-effective strategy*. Groups offer clinicians the opportunity to provide information and instruction to more people in a cost-effective manner.
2. *Feedback and reinforcement*. Groups, meeting at regular intervals for an established time period, provide participants with the opportunity to receive feedback and reinforcement that is helpful in making behavior changes. Participants experiment with class material and return to the group to discuss what worked and what did not. They examine what was helpful in being consistent with dietary changes, exercise and other self-management strategies and identify what were obstacles to success. People receive positive feedback for healthy choices and problem solve with the group to effectively address the challenges they face.
3. *Modeling opportunities*. Groups offer an ideal opportunity for participants to increase self-efficacy through modeling. An individual, observing peers make healthy choices, can find the inspiration and confidence to do the same. Modeling also enables participants to see themselves as experienced experts. They recognize their own strengths and the valuable role they have in helping others. They often provide ideas and inspiration to each other that a health care professional cannot offer. As a participant in one of my classes commented to the group, "The flier for this program indicates Carolyn is the teacher, but the truth is, everyone in this group is my teacher."
4. *Decrease isolation*. Groups help people learn they are not alone in facing adversity. In an atmosphere of learning together, people share information, experiences, and insights and build an experience of community. By sharing their own stories and listening to the stories of other group members, isolation is diminished and bonds of friendship are established. People learn that their problems need not isolate them from others, but can provide avenues for experiencing compassion and connection with

others. This interaction can help people maintain a positive attitude and feel greater confidence when facing the challenges associated with a disease or injury.[1]

5. *Improved community relations.* In an era when physician visits can be as brief as 10 minutes, providing people with support, education, and exercise instruction in a group setting is a valued and needed service. A group program offering wellness strategies and addressing otherwise unmet needs provides people with a positive experience of the sponsoring health organization. During the program, participants can become familiar with the health organization and the range of additional services it offers. They may choose to seek further services with this organization or refer others for services.

Promoting Social Support

Because social support is consistently associated with a range of positive health behaviors, it is important for clinicians to recognize its value and promote social support in health promotion and wellness programs. The importance of supportive relationships in health has been demonstrated by several studies. Both the quality and quantity of supportive social relationships have been reliably related to morbidity and mortality.[2-4] Increases in various measures of social support are associated with improvements in medication compliance, participation in physical activity, weight loss, lower blood pressure, and successful smoking cessation.[4] Higher social support is also associated with better immune system function.[2]

There are probably multiple physiological pathways by which social support influences disease status. Social support may act as a buffer to stress and protect an individual under stress by minimizing maladaptive physiological responses.[2] Social support provides people with the opportunity to share feelings and may decrease loneliness, depression, and anxiety. By sharing information and encouragement, people may learn alternative ways to deal with the limitations imposed by their condition and increase participation in health-promoting activities.[1]

Within the group setting of a wellness program, clinicians can create a comfortable atmosphere in which mutual support develops among participants. By providing this positive social experience in which participants learn about disease management and participate in physical activity, clinicians may increase the likelihood that participants will maintain newly learned health behaviors beyond the program.

Selecting a Group Size

There is no magic number of participants for an optimal group size. In several research studies, class size is generally 10 to 15 participants.[5-10] One program enrolls 30 participants.[11] A group should not be so large that the clinician has difficulty addressing the needs and health goals of individual group members. Too large a group may prevent a clinician from effectively answering questions and providing education and encouragement in the time allowed. Conversely, a group should not be so small that the group dynamic significantly suffers if members are absent.

The severity of health problems of participants plays a role when selecting a group size. It is feasible to work with a larger group whose members are in overall good general health. It is appropriate to work with a smaller group of people diagnosed with complex medical conditions requiring more attention.

Financial considerations also influence a group size. A certain number of participants are required to cover the cost of providing services. Pricing your program is covered in Chapter 12.

When I began my program, my initial classes had eight participants. This small group size was ideal for the experimentation and adjusting processes that go along with starting any new program. As I grew more comfortable with running the group and referrals increased, class size grew to 14 to 18 participants.

Personal Characteristics of an Effective Group Leader

The outcome of any group directly depends on the skills and effectiveness of the group leader. Corey and Corey, leaders in the field of group work, have identified characteristics of an effective group leader.[12] These characteristics include the following:

1. *Ability to model.* Skilled group leaders walk the talk. They teach by example. They understand the role their behavior plays in influencing the members of a group. They do what they ask group participants to do. Their credibility is enhanced by their own practice of the healthy lifestyle activities they promote. The person who is overweight and sedentary is not going to be an effective instructor in a weight management program. In contrast, a person who has overcome personal obstacles and poor health habits to achieve greater well-being and who continues to explore adopting healthy behaviors brings the insight gained from personal experience to helping others.
2. *Presence.* A key quality of effective leaders is the ability to bring their full attention to group members. It includes the willingness to be interested in and touched by people's stories, struggles, and joys, and to feel compassion and empathy. By bringing this quality of presence to a group, leaders can respond effectively to the questions and concerns of participants.
3. *Goodwill and caring.* Effective group leaders maintain sincere interest in the health and well-being of all group participants. They genuinely value and respect each individual. They make an effort to meet group members with compassion, kindness, and understanding. When leaders find it challenging to experience caring toward a participant, they examine their own feelings, attempt to gain insight, and find ways to understand and value that individual.
4. *Belief in the value of groups.* Effective group leaders believe in the individual's ability to change and in the role of a group to support that change. They have confidence in the individual's capacity to learn, grow, and adopt positive health behaviors. They value the role a group plays in helping members find their own strengths and abilities needed to meet life's challenges.
5. *Self-knowledge and awareness.* Effective leaders value self-knowledge and awareness. They reflect on their own goals, motivations, values, strengths, and limitations. Insight into their own health behaviors provides a foundation for facilitating the health behaviors of group participants. This exploration of self is recognized as a lifelong process.

6. *Sense of humor.* Although medical problems present people with serious challenges, humor can play a role in coping and in easing distress. The ability to laugh at oneself and find humor in the human predicament can keep problems in perspective and decrease tensions. Effective leaders bring a lightness to a situation when appropriate through the use of humor.
7. *Inventive.* Effective leaders are creative. They cultivate a fresh perspective and maintain a quality of aliveness and spontaneity in teaching. Effective leaders avoid presenting programmed techniques or canned presentations that are drained of inspiration.
8. *Knowledgeable.* Effective leaders are knowledgeable and skilled in their field. They bring both professional training and experience to their leadership roles. They participate in continuing education programs that advance their professional knowledge and skill level. They are also open to learning from group members.
9. *Endurance.* Providing group services can be demanding. Many pieces and responsibilities are required to create a successful group. From developing handouts to marketing the program to leading the group, a leader is extended in multiple directions. An effective leader has the sustained motivation and energy to meet these varied demands.

I would like to add to this list: acknowledges wholeness in self and others. Effective leaders recognize and respect the innate wholeness in themselves and others. They do not see group members as being "broken" and in need of being "fixed." Nor do they see themselves as life's expert and group members as being inadequate or incapable of meeting life's challenges. If facilitators view those in a group as "broken" or lacking, they create feelings of distance and separation between themselves and group members. They are more likely to adopt an authoritarian role or show themselves to be smarter than or ahead of group members. Under these circumstances it is less likely that the true strengths of group members will develop. If leaders view group members as whole human beings with the personal capacities to respond to whatever difficulties they face, those group members are supported to recognize and develop their inner strengths and resources. The leader is not separate or distant from group members, but rather participates in a process of collaboration and mutual exploration of program themes.

Co-leadership

There are circumstances in which the co-leadership of a group may be of benefit in achieving program goals. Because there are multiple dimensions to the subject of wellness, collaboration among health care professionals across disciplines can be necessary to achieve program goals. For example, a physical therapist and a nutritionist may combine their skills to offer a successful weight management program. To work effectively, co-leaders must have a relationship based on trust, respect, and cooperation. They must be able to work out differences and conflicts in a constructive manner.

The advantages of co-leadership include the following[12]:

1. Co-leaders learn from each other.
2. If one leader is absent because of illness or vacation, the group continues under the guidance of the other leader.
3. By sharing responsibilities for the group program, leader "burnout" is reduced.

4. The group benefits from the expertise of two professionals.
5. Co-leaders can confer with each other on the progress of group members and develop strategies together to enhance participant success.

A disadvantage of the co-leadership model is the added costs of services of a second professional. In addition, conflict between co-leaders can occur because of differences in philosophy, teaching styles, and agendas. Co-leaders can become competitive instead of collaborative. Sometimes these conflicts can lead to a broader understanding and richer experience for both professionals. Other times conflicts result in constant tension and resentment that can diminish the effectiveness of a group program.

Teaching Styles

Different teaching styles can be employed by an instructor to achieve desired outcomes. An effective instructor remains flexible and is able to apply appropriate teaching styles to meet the needs of the group and program goals.[13,14] Teaching styles include the expert instructor and the supportive facilitator.

The Expert Instructor

In the role of the expert instructor, the clinician provides participants with educational information based on his or her professional training and experience. For example, a physical therapist would assume this role when teaching principles of proper posture, body mechanics, or the physiology of stress. A dietitian assumes this role when providing information on the fundamentals of good nutrition.

The Supportive Facilitator

In the role of supportive facilitator, the clinician supports and reinforces the strengths, abilities, and insights of the participants. The focus is not on instructor expertise, but on the participants' skills, inner resources, and capacities. The instructor may present questions, but the participants explore possibilities, produce ideas, and identify solutions on their own. An answer to a question becomes secondary to teaching a process of inquiry, discovery, and problem solving.

For example, in a group in which participants are having difficulties adhering to a home program, the clinician might ask, "What gets in the way of following through with a regular exercise program and other self-care activities?" After participants generate a list of obstacles, the clinician invites the group to brainstorm ways to overcome these obstacles. Answers come from participants, not the instructor.

Sometimes the facilitator does not model a process of finding solutions, but rather ways to explore and experience life's questions. For example, a participant in my class, Pat, stated that instead of doing his home program he went straight to the computer or TV when he got home. He had plenty of time but avoided the mindful body scan (see Chapter 3) because it brought up unpleasant feelings. He recently retired on disability and moved from a large home to a small condominium. He said he got his identity from his work and from owning a beautiful home. The body scan required him to stop and become aware of how he was feeling. It reminded him that he no longer knew who he was.

I asked if other members of the group could relate to Pat's story. All heads nodded yes. I explained that this happens to all of us. We attach our sense of self to something that is impermanent. It may be a job, a house, or a role we play such as parent or employee. Then one day, what we anchored ourselves to changes or is gone altogether. It brings up this question, "Who am I?" It is a good question. I asked Pat if he were feeling those uncomfortable feelings as he described his situation. He responded, "Yes." After Pat agreed to explore this situation more closely in the group, I invited him to bring his attention to his breathing.

Drawing from my personal experience in mindfulness meditation (see Chapter 3), I guided, "First notice the story you tell yourself about this situation, and then observe what physical sensations you experience." I continued, reminding Pat to breathe from time to time, and asking that he observe his physical sensations and his feelings. There was no need on his part to attempt to change anything or to try to make anything happen. I coached him to observe his present moment experience and, if he felt comfortable to do so, to share what he noticed with the group. The question, "Who am I?" is not a problem resolved with a simple answer or a quick solution, but a mystery of life to be explored and experienced. With complete trust that the answer was within him, I could participate with him in an exploration of the question. I could model a *process* to examine a question that he and other group members could adopt.

Sometimes during the course of group discussions, participants recognize complex problems and strong feelings that are not appropriate for processing in a support group setting. It is necessary for a clinician to have psychological services available for referral for these situations.

Although people may begin a wellness program perceiving the instructor as an expert, by the end of a program, they should experience themselves as the experts and authorities in their own lives. This recognition by participants of their own authority occurs as the instructor repeatedly guides a process of inquiry and discovery. People recognize that many answers come from within themselves. The wisdom in this approach is revealed in the well-known adage: Give a man a fish and he will eat today. Teach a man to fish and he will eat for the rest of his life.

Facilitating Group Discussion

Promoting health behavior changes among participants in a group requires much more than lecturing. Specific concepts can be learned from a book, but the art of successful group facilitation comes with experience. It is common to feel nervous when you are leading a group for the first time. Many clinicians have little or no training in group instruction and process. If you have never led a group or feel uncertain of your ability to facilitate one, participating in established support, wellness, or exercise groups is a good place to begin. Many hospitals and national organizations sponsor ongoing groups. By participating in an ongoing group you can contribute your expertise to the group while learning the skills of group facilitation. I recommend participating in several groups to observe the teaching styles of different instructors and to gain a range of experiences in group process.

Participation in a more thorough training program in group facilitation and process may be required depending on your present skill level and the goals of your program. Once your program is underway, consulting a clinician who is trained and experienced in group process can alleviate anxiety, assure your competent management of a group, and advance your skill level.

A thorough examination of group facilitation and process is beyond the scope of this book. Initial guidelines and suggestions are presented here. Additional references are provided at the end of this chapter.

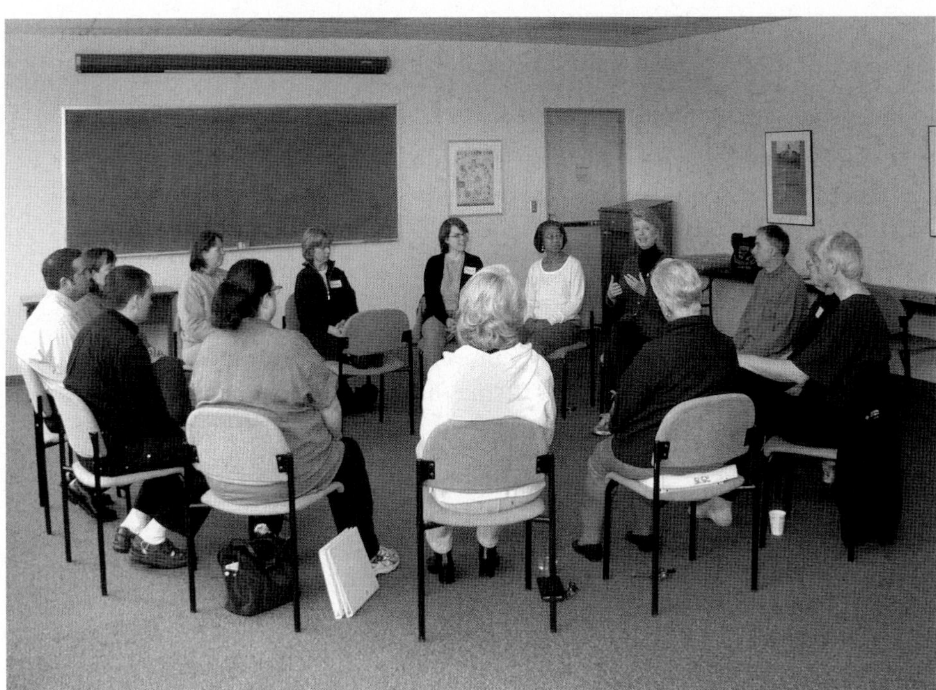

Figure 2-1 A clinician facilitates a discussion.

The amount of time allowed for formal group discussion will depend on the goals, needs, and size of the group and intentions and training of the instructor. This period can be as short as 15 minutes or as long as an hour. In my program, I allow approximately 45 minutes for group discussion of class themes and experiences with class homework. Class participants appreciate this opportunity to have questions answered and receive support and learn from one another.

Guidelines for Group Discussion

When offering a formal period of group discussion in a wellness program, provide participants with basic guidelines for the discussion by introducing the importance of group confidentiality, staying focused on topic, and sharing from personal experiences. Participants should be asked to avoid giving advice (Figure 2-1).

Developing the skills and confidence to effectively facilitate a group requires practice, experience, and feedback. There is no one formula for effective group facilitation. One of the most exciting parts of leading a group is its unpredictability and aliveness. A leader needs to respond in the moment to each situation as it arises. Recognizing this fundamental element of group facilitation, the following guidelines are helpful:

1. *Use reflective listening.*
   Reflective listening is repeating in your own words what you have heard someone say.[15] You paraphrase in a nonjudging way what the other person has expressed. It does not include your own feelings, judgments, attitudes, or reactions. This skill involves simply saying in your own words only what you have heard.

Example

Participant Mary: Initially when I took 30 minutes to myself for exercise, my kids or husband would frequently interrupt me. Because I've always been on call for them, responding to their every request, they did not know how to handle my new behavior. They seemed resentful. Now they are used to my routine and leave me alone.

Facilitator: So, when you first took time for the exercises, your family members interrupted you, but you stuck to your plan and with time, they accepted your new routine.

2. *Identify and respond to the universal theme in an individual comment.*
   a. Universalize participant comment.
   Universalizing a comment requires identifying in an individual's statement an experience or theme that other group members can easily relate to. This adds to the experience of connectedness in the group and enables the facilitator to address the entire group as well as the individual who made the comment.

Example

Facilitator: I think this is a common experience. We make a change in our behavior, and family or friends sometimes resist or take time to adjust to the new behavior. This might involve any change in health behavior. For example, adopting an exercise program, changing our diet, choosing to stop smoking, or saying "no" to activities that deplete us. Do other people relate to Mary's experience?

   b. Respond to the universal theme or experience.
   Once a facilitator has identified the common experience or theme in a participant's comment, he or she can respond to this universal element.

Example

Facilitator: Sometimes family and friends are supportive of our new health behaviors. Other times they may experience a period of disorientation or feel resentful or resistant to our changes. We always have control over how we want to respond to this resistance when it occurs. It can sometimes require courage and determination to maintain the new healthy behavior until friends and family members accept and adjust to the change.

3. *Allow for peer feedback and reinforcement.*
   Because peers inspire and encourage one another in ways a health care provider cannot, it is helpful to create opportunities for participants to provide feedback and support.

Example

Facilitator: I'm wondering if Mary's story triggered any thoughts or feelings in others?

4. *Provide positive feedback for participant contributions.*[16]
   A simple response such as "You bring up an important subject," helps create an open atmosphere in which participants feel comfortable and

confident asking questions and sharing experiences. Other positive phrases include the following:

That's a good question.

I'm glad you brought that up.

That's an important point you make.

I appreciate that you brought this to our attention.

Positive feedback can also be provided nonverbally with a smile or nod of your head.

5. *Summarize and repeat important themes.*
   To avoid getting lost in the details of a participant's story or sidetracked by a tangential comment, clarify the core point you want to emphasize by summarizing the central theme exemplified by the participant's story. This approach keeps the discussion on subject and helps reinforce important topics. Because repetition promotes retention of material, state core themes and repeat them in different ways at various times during the program.
6. *Ask open-ended questions.*[16]
   Avoid asking questions that can be answered "yes" or "no." Open-ended questions stimulate discussion. For example, an instructor might ask, "What experiences did you have this past week as you integrated the home program into your schedule?" This would generate more discussion than the question, "Did you follow through on the home program?"

The Challenging Participant

A wellness program attracts people with various personalities. I worked with one group in which most participants were very shy, and it was only with great effort on my part that any discussion took place. In another group, everyone talked at once and it was my job to bring order and sometimes limit the discussion. Although each group is unique, the challenging personality types are consistent. Experts in the field of group process have identified several types of challenging participants.[16,17] Those I have found in my classes include the talker, the quiet type, and the belligerent type.

1. *The Talker.* Sometimes one person in a group has ideas on everything and shares them with endlessly long monologues. Although occasionally these comments are relevant, often they consume precious time. A facilitator must be direct with these people and not allow them to dominate a discussion. There is an art to quieting or redirecting the talker. You might find a pause in the monologue and interrupt, saying, "Thank you, Kathy. In the interest of time, I would like to hear from some other group members." If the person has gone off topic, you might intervene by saying, "Your story is interesting, but I would like to keep comments focused on how the class material helps you manage symptoms." Or, paraphrase a relevant point you heard the person make, and ask for another group member's opinion on the subject.

   When one person in a group dominates, everyone loses. Even if it feels slightly awkward or uncomfortable to interrupt someone, it is sometimes necessary for the optimum experience of all group members. Practice and experience managing this situation are helpful.
2. *The Quiet Type.* Some people are shy and find it very difficult to speak in groups. It is helpful to draw them out by asking for their thoughts on a

subject or experience of an exercise. Keep it simple. Avoid asking a complex question that they might have difficulty answering. Follow up their answer with positive feedback to reinforce their participation.

3. *The Belligerent Type.* Occasionally someone shows up in a class who is not ready to learn the skills covered in a program. He or she may be there only because a physician or family member insisted on his or her attendance. Whatever the instructor may say or try, the response is a variation of: "This does not work for me and I cannot imagine that it ever will." Frequently the best solution is for this person to leave the program. Often he or she will drop the class after the first or second session. Occasionally, after hearing the stories of other group members, this person opens up to the class material; however, sometimes the clinician needs to guide the person to withdraw. An instructor might comment, "What I'm hearing is these exercises are not working for you. They are not meeting your needs at this time. I do not want to take class time to discuss this now, but I would like to meet with you after class to talk about what would be best for your situation." In this situation it is often easy to recommend that the person choose a course of individual treatment rather than the group format.

Summary

Providing group services to people offers new challenges and opportunities for clinicians. The group setting enables clinicians to (1) provide education, instruction, and support to a number of people cost-effectively; (2) provide participants with feedback and reinforcement needed to establish and maintain new health behaviors; (3) promote self-efficacy through modeling; and (4) improve community relations. The clinician can also create an atmosphere of social support in a group that decreases isolation among participants and is associated with a range of positive health behaviors, including diet and exercise adherence. The clinician can select the group size that is consistent with the needs and goals of group participants and with financial requirements. He or she can develop effective leadership qualities and apply different teaching styles and group facilitation strategies to successfully promote wellness principles and practices.

References

1. Lewis DJ, Frain KA, Donnelly MH. Chronic pain management support group: a program designed to facilitate coping. *Rehab Nsg* 1993 Sept/Oct;18(5):319.
2. Undreno BN, Cacioppo JT, Kielcolt-Glaser JK. The relationship between social support and physiological processes: a review with emphasis on underlying mechanisms and implications for health. *Psychol Bull* 1996;119(3):488.
3. Berkman L. The role of social relations in health promotion. *Psychosom Med* 1995;57:246.
4. Ford ES, Ahluwalia IB, Galuska DA. Social relationships and cardiac disease risk factors: findings from the third national health and nutrition examination study. *Preventive Med* 2000;30:83.

5. Lorig K, Mazonson P, Holman H. Evidence suggests that health education for self-management in patients with chronic arthritis has sustained health benefits while reducing costs. *Arthritis Rheum* 1993 Apr;36(4): 439-446.
6. Lorig K, Sobel D, Stewart A et al. Evidence suggesting that a chronic disease self-management program can improve health status while reducing hospitalization. *Med Care* 1999;37(1):5-14.
7. Sevick M, Dunn A, Murrow M et al. Cost-effectiveness of lifestyle and structured exercise interventions in sedentary adults: results of project ACTIVE. *Am J Prev Med* 2000 Jul;19(1):1-8.
8. Barlow J, Williams B, Wright C. "Instilling the strength to fight the pain and get on with life": learning to become an arthritis self-manager through an adult education program. *Health Educ Res* 1999;14(4): 533-544.
9. Frost H, Moffett J, Moser J et al. Randomized controlled trial for evaluation of fitness programme for patients with chronic low back pain. *BMJ* 1995 Jan;310:151-154.
10. Ferrell B, Josephson K, Pollan A et al. A randomized trial of walking versus physical methods for chronic pain management. *Aging Clin Exp Res* 1997;9(1-2):99-105.
11. Kabat-Zinn J. An out patient program in behavioral medicine for chronic pain patients based on the practice of mindfulness meditation: theoretical considerations and preliminary results. *Gen Hosp Psychiatry* 1982;4:33-47.
12. Corey MS, Corey G. *Groups: Process and Practice.* Pacific Grove, Calif: Brooks/Cole Publishing Co.; 2002, pp. 14-20.
13. Toropainen E, Rinne M. What are groups all about?—basic principles of group work for health-related physical activity. *Patient Educ and Counsel* 1998;33:S107.
14. Rinne M, Toropainen E. How to lead a group—practical principles and experiences of conducting a promotional group in health-related physical activity. *Patient Educ and Counsel* 1998;33:S71.
15. McKay M, Davis M & Fanning P. *Messages: The Communication Skills Handbook*. Oakland, Calif: New Harbinger Publications, 1983.
16. Lorig K. *Patient Education: A Practical Approach*. Thousand Oaks, Calif: SAGE Publications, 1996.
17. Corey MS, Corey G. *Groups: Process and Practice* 6th ed. Pacific Grove, Calif: Brooks/Cole Publishing Co.; 2002, pp. 184-188.

Annotated Bibliography

Corey MS Corey G. *Groups: Process and Practice.* Pacific Grove, Calif: Brooks/Cole Publishing Co., 2002. Drawing on extensive clinical experience working with groups, Marianne and Gerald Corey define basic concepts of group process and provide specific guidelines for leading groups. They use case examples and sample dialogues to clarify important themes. Although this text primarily addresses a psychotherapeutic group model, sections of the book offer valuable perspectives on group leadership and are applicable to facilitating group support.

Lee RJ, King SN. *Discovering the Leader in You: A Guide to Realizing Your Personal Leadership Potential.* San Francisco: Josey-Bass, 2001. What better world would you like to imagine? Who inspires you? What gives you energy? Drawing from their experience at the nationally recognized Center for Creative Leadership, Robert Lee and Sara King ask these questions and more as they guide the reader on a worthwhile self-exploration to identify a personal vision, core values, personal strengths, and leadership styles. Based on the understanding that your effectiveness as a leader is founded on who you are, they offer a step-by-step process to comprehensively examine the fundamental issues that create the foundation for leadership. Although this text draws from the authors' experience in business leadership, it is a great book for the clinician interested in assuming any leadership role.

Lorig K. *Patient Education: A Practical Approach.* Thousand Oaks, Calif: SAGE Publications, 1996. Kate Lorig is an Associate Professor at Stanford University School of Medicine, Director of the Stanford Patient Education Research Center, and leader in the field of group education programs for people with chronic medical conditions. In this text, she provides specific and practical guidelines to conduct a needs assessment and develop a group program. She offers advice on group process strategies, responding to challenging participants, promoting program adherence, and working with culturally diverse populations. This well-written text by an inspiring leader in the field is an outstanding resource for clinicians developing group programs.

Santorelli S. *Heal Thy Self: Lessons on Mindfulness in Medicine.* New York: Bell Tower, 1999. Saki Santorelli, Ed.D., is the director of the Stress Reduction Clinic at the University of Massachusetts Medical School. Santorelli shares his personal experiences with teaching as well as the transformation that occurs for participants in an 8-week group mindfulness-based stress reduction program. He provides rich insight into group process and into the personal and professional challenges that come with group leadership. Acknowledging the wound in every healer and the inner healer in every patient, he examines the clinician-patient relationship with refreshing sensitivity, insight, and wisdom. This is an inspiring and informative text for any group leader.

II Wellness Program Subjects

Chapter 3 Mindfulness

Mindfulness means present moment awareness or paying attention. Mindfulness meditation is the deliberate training of the mind in present moment awareness and is the foundation for the information, examples, and exercises presented in this chapter. The roles of present moment awareness in injury prevention, rehabilitation, medical treatment, coping, and enhancing quality of life are examined. Exercises in mindful awareness and key attitudes that are central to mindfulness are presented. For the clinician who is new to mindfulness, this chapter offers an introduction to mindfulness and a rationale for its integration into the care of the chronically ill. It provides suggestions for presenting introductory concepts and exercises to a group. For the clinician with experience in mindfulness meditation, this chapter offers specific ideas and exercises for the practical application of mindfulness to wellness services.

Applications of Mindful Awareness

When I trained in physical therapy in the late 1970s, no one mentioned awareness as a necessary ingredient for health. Only after my own back injury and years of patient care experience did I begin to fully appreciate how central awareness is to well-being. Mindful awareness has important and practical applications to the broad and multiple challenges faced by people living with chronic medical conditions. From a framework for body awareness that is key in injury prevention to a practice for developing insight, wisdom, and peace in difficult circumstances, mindful awareness is a powerful resource for people. The following descriptions and examples examine several applications of mindful awareness to the circumstances of people living with chronic medical conditions and offer a basis for including mindful awareness in a group wellness program.

Prevention of Injury

Awareness is key to the prevention of injury. Awareness enables people to make choices throughout the day to ensure physical comfort and well-being. When they are unaware of the body's signals, people place themselves at risk for injury, as the following case example illustrates:

Case Example 3.1.

When Kate enrolled in The Wellness Program, she had bilateral forearm pain that began after weeks of long workdays spent typing. She commented, "I had a vague feeling something was wrong, but I didn't pay attention. I'm dedicated to my job, so I focused on my work, not my body. Then one morning, I couldn't hold a pen, turn a doorknob, or tie my shoe without excruciating pain."

As this example demonstrates, a lack of awareness can put a person's health at risk. If Kate had paid more attention to her body, she could have recognized the discomfort in her arms early in its onset and assessed her options. These options would have included adjusting her chair and workstation for optimal upper extremity comfort, taking scheduled breaks for stretching and forearm relaxation, discussing with her supervisor opportunities to vary her work tasks, and seeking professional advice. The ability to listen to her body and make adjustments based on awareness could have prevented her repetitive strain injury.

With mindfulness, we make such adjustments throughout our day. Awareness allows a person sitting in a chair with poor back support to recognize low back discomfort and change chairs. Lacking awareness, he or she only recognizes a problem an hour later when experiencing pain and stiffness with standing from the chair. A person with the ability to listen to his or her body experiences mild chest and left arm pain and goes immediately to an emergency room for evaluation. Without awareness a person fails to recognize or minimizes these sensations, continues with activity, and suffers a severe myocardial infarction.

Many clinicians can take body awareness for granted or assume that it is an innate ability. We overlook that people often have no understanding of how to listen to the body or pay no attention to the body until something goes wrong. Exercises that teach the skill of *how* to listen to the body are an important part of any wellness program. Mindfulness, however, is much more than body awareness.

Rehabilitation

The skill of awareness enhances a person's rehabilitation. People often have physical, mental, and emotional reactions to symptoms that exacerbate their condition or limit their healing process. By becoming aware of these reactions and their influence on symptoms, a person can recognize options and make health-enhancing choices. This is demonstrated in the following case example:

Case Example 3.2.

Lisa was a 50-year-old woman with a 10-year history of chronic low back pain. Her pain worsened at the end of the day and would intermittently worsen when she increased her activity level. Her primary goal for her participation in The Wellness Program was to learn what she could do to manage her pain. As she became familiar with mindfulness, she observed the role her reaction played in contributing to her pain. With the onset of pain, she recognized the physical sensation of pain and the components of her reaction that included increased muscle tension, shallow breathing, fear, and negative self-talk. By applying diaphragmatic breathing, relaxation exercises, and compassionate self-talk, she was able to decrease her back pain intensity and duration and increase her tolerance of reconditioning exercises. Awareness was the first step in developing this ability to choose a skillful response to pain that decreased her symptoms and increased her exercise tolerance.

Mindfulness plays an important role in preventing symptom exacerbation that results from stressful circumstances, as demonstrated by the following example:

Case Example 3.3.

Pat was a 30-year-old woman who participated in The Wellness Program while also receiving physical therapy for a neck injury sustained in a motor vehicle accident. Five weeks into the class, her mother fractured her hip and Pat found herself in the busy emergency room of a major medical center waiting for her mother to receive care. She later told the group, "Without awareness and the skills to breathe and relax, I would have been eating muscle relaxants and tranquilizers. I noticed when tension began building in my neck and shoulders and I held my breath and started to panic. I applied mindfulness and observed my breathing. Gradually my breath became more calm and steady. I was able to relax my shoulders. I felt more clear-headed and was able to comfort my mother. I surprised everyone, including myself, with how well I handled it." Awareness was the first step in Pat's ability to choose a skillful response to a stressful situation and prevent a flareup of symptoms.

In addition, awareness is necessary to maximize reconditioning. Whereas no movement leads to decreased strength, flexibility, and endurance, overdoing activity puts a person at risk for symptom exacerbation or injury. Awareness is what enables a person to train his or her body at the boundary between these two behaviors to maximize the benefit of an exercise program.

Medical Treatment

People with chronic medical problems frequently endure procedures and treatments that are uncomfortable or have unpleasant side effects. Mindfulness helps people manage these difficult situations and minimize their discomfort with greater skill. People are able to observe their reactions *to* the procedure or treatment and consciously choose responses that decrease their distress. The value of this ability is reflected in the following story:

Case Example 3.4.

Patrice was a 35-year-old woman diagnosed with osteomyelitis. Following her participation in The Wellness Program, she underwent hyperbaric oxygen therapy. Hyperbaric oxygen therapy is administrated in a chamber in which patients breathe 100% oxygen at greater than one atmosphere of pressure using a mask or hood. This increases the amount of oxygen delivered to tissues, encourages the rebuilding of capillaries, and promotes wound healing. A period of 15 to 20 minutes is required to bring the chamber to the necessary therapeutic pressure. Patients remain at this increased pressure condition for 90 to 120 minutes. Another 15 to 20 minutes is required to return the chamber to normal surface pressure. Although newly constructed chambers are designed to maximize patient comfort and include TV and audio systems, older models have none of these amenities. Patrice was treated in an older chamber. Forty sessions were prescribed. Although they became easier to tolerate with time, her first treatment session was quite unpleasant.

She described her experience: "The chamber was small and circular. With the nurse, three other patients, and me, it was a cramped situation and I was sitting knee to knee with the others. I am not usually an anxious person, but I found myself feeling very anxious. I had been offered anti-anxiety medication but declined it because I knew I could handle whatever happened with the tools I learned in The Wellness Program. I became hypersensitive to my breathing because the hood would expand and contract with each breath. It was disconcerting and I found myself frequently holding my breath. The nurse's instructions were to relax and breathe normally, but this became more difficult as I became more anxious. It was very hot, so sweat constantly trickled down my face, only to accumulate where the hood was tightly secured to my neck. There was a constant loud sound of hissing air, making it impossible to have a conversation. I wanted to listen to my meditation tape during the treatment, but could not bring a Walkman into the chamber because, under the high-pressure conditions, the batteries would be flammable. I brought a book, but was unable to read because I felt nauseous and dizzy. I was miserable. I did not want to be there.

"I wanted to close my eyes and meditate. I knew it would help, but I felt very self-conscious closing my eyes in front of these other people. They would have no idea what I was doing and might think I was sleeping or in distress. I became aware of my breathing with my eyes open. I assessed the situation and made the decision to just do what was going to help me through this. Making this choice was the most significant moment for me in the whole process. I closed my eyes and observed my breathing. I told myself to meditate and that the treatment was impermanent and would end soon. I brought my awareness to my abdomen and began breathing more deeply. I stared counting my out breaths. I tried to keep my focus in the present moment. I felt my muscles relax. My breathing pattern became more calm and natural. What a relief that was! The heat, noise, dizziness, and nausea were all still there, but I was becoming increasingly calm in the midst of it all. Then I began to imagine my breath to be a healing river carrying lots of oxygen through my body to promote my healing. Eventually the treatment session ended. I did it! Focusing on the present moment and my breath was the only thing that got me through this."

Coping with Chronic Pain and Illness

Mindfulness helps people cope more effectively with chronic pain and illness. In addition to those avenues already stated, awareness helps people experience greater understanding and insight into themselves and their circumstances.

People with chronic illness often become identified with their pain or disease process. They falsely conclude that their medical condition is their identity. Mindfulness enables people to recognize themselves as whole human beings who also happen to have medical conditions. Physical and cognitive problems are just that; they are physical sensations and cognitive events, but these symptoms are not a person's identity. Awareness enables people to experience this realization directly for themselves. They are then empowered to respond to life's challenges from a foundation of wholeness rather than from an attitude of impairment. This attitude is demonstrated by the following case example:

Case Example 3.5.

David was a 22-year-old man diagnosed with Crohn's disease. He entered The Wellness Program depressed and discouraged by the life he faced coping with a chronic disease. He felt that mindfulness enabled him to move beyond an excessive focus on what was wrong with his body. During one mindfulness exercise that required paying attention to different body parts, he recognized there was much more functioning right in his body than was problematic. His disease still presented personal challenges, but it was not the whole story of his body, his health, or his sense of self.

When we experience something unpleasant or unwanted, one response is for our awareness to become very narrow. We focus exclusively on the negative situation to the exclusion of everything else. Using the analogy of a camera, our awareness becomes stuck in a zoom lens focus. As a way of life, this zoom lens focus on any symptom or medical condition grossly distorts a situation and can severely limit a person's function. Mindfulness offers people the opportunity to discover a wide-angle lens view and greater flexibility and control of their mental attention. People explore a broader field of experience and sense of self in which a physical sensation, medical condition, or any situation occurs. They can closely examine a physical sensation, emotion, or thought in a deliberate manner but with an open and unwavering quality of awareness. People often experience an innate quality of wholeness and recognize that they have choices. They frequently gain the insight that there is more right with their bodies than is malfunctioning. They know their symptoms are not who they are. These insights can profoundly influence a person's ability to manage their situation, as the following example illustrates:

Case Example 3.6.

Elizabeth was a 38-year-old woman with signs and symptoms of an autoimmune disorder. Although her rheumatologist believed she might have systemic lupus erythematosus, she was not typical in her clinical presentation and was undergoing additional diagnostic tests when she enrolled in The Wellness Program. Despite a course of treatment of methotrexate and other medications, her symptoms, including a significant decrease in cognitive function, continued to worsen. In her own words, "I do not know how much of my cognitive problems were due to the disease or the medications, but the end result was I felt like I was losing my mind and, to my way of thinking, losing myself. I was very frightened. So much of who I was, including my college achievements, graduate studies, and running my own business, had been based on my intellectual abilities. Now I was losing the ability that had defined so much of my life and that I mistakenly believed defined me as a human being. I felt like a failure. Not only could I not keep track of what day it was or whether I had taken my medications, I had difficulty doing the reading for the program and following discussions during the class. I was too embarrassed to tell anyone this was happening.

"After the fourth class, I finally found the courage to talk to Carolyn. I poured out everything that was wrong, how I could not read the book or follow class discussions, how I kept forgetting and losing things, and most importantly, how I felt like I was losing me. After a comforting and encouraging discussion with Carolyn, I decided to keep with the program and to practice being kind to myself. That night, I really listened to the words on the mindful mediation tape and took them to heart. I experienced the unpleasant feeling that I was losing the cognitive abilities that I believed defined who I was as a human being; however, as I focused on my breath and listened to the guided instructions, I recognized the qualities of wisdom, compassion, and understanding were also within me. I realized that my cognitive abilities did not define who I was, but rather they were just another quality in the presence of these larger qualities and dimensions of my being. At that moment, I quit being scared. This insight has not changed my problems, but it has made a huge change in how I am dealing with them. I feel more confident and calm and can handle my problems without falling into a paralyzing panic and fear of losing me."

Mindfulness also helps people recognize how attitudes, emotions, behaviors, and situations influence their medical condition. They become more skillful managers of their lives and their symptoms, as demonstrated by the following example:

Case Example 3.7.

Joanne was a 52-year-old woman who suffered from severe migraines that were unresponsive to medication management. On learning to practice mindfulness, she realized that with the onset of a migraine she would spiral into increasing despair and feel totally out of control. When she was headache free, she would spiral into frantic activity and also feel totally out of control. Before the program, she was completely unaware of this pattern. The class provided her with the skills of mindfulness, breathing, and relaxation that she applied with the onset of a headache. She became calm and felt in control. She described her experience to be like that of a sailor guiding her ship through a storm. She no longer went spiraling downward. When she was headache free, she did not overschedule her day with multiple activities, but rather she prioritized, paced herself, and remembered to enjoy what she was doing. She felt this change dramatically improved her ability to cope with her pain. Although she continued to have migraines, they decreased in frequency and she felt in greater control of her pain and her life.

Quality of Life

Mindfulness enhances a person's quality of life not only through the previously described applications, but also through the invitation to live in the present moment. When we are mindful, our full attention is in the here and now. The present moment is the only moment we have to experience life, yet often our attention is everywhere but here. It is so easy to spend hours ruminating over the past, worrying about the future, or simply lost in thought. Perhaps you have had the experience of driving from point A to point B only to find yourself arriving at point B with no memory of the journey in between. This is an instance of unawareness. If we are not careful, we can spend large amounts of our life in this condition.

Mindfulness does not mean never thinking about the past or the future. It means not *living* in the past or future. I like to tell people, "Plan for the future, but don't spend your life there." When we are mindful, we experience the present moment fully. We touch life in a deep and rich way. Sometimes this choice of focus reveals experiences of aliveness, conditions for happiness, and opportunities for meaning that are previously unnoticed. Paying attention in the present moment to sensory input, physical sensations, thoughts, and emotions opens opportunities for insight, understanding, and transformation that are otherwise unavailable, as illustrated by the following examples:

Case Example 3.8.

Martha was a 63-year-old breast cancer survivor with severe rheumatoid arthritis. She participated in a morning warm-water pool program for arthritis patients that always ended with a period of floating. Before being introduced to mindfulness, she spent this period worrying about how the rest of her day would go, how much pain she might have, wondering if she would be able to do the activities she had planned, and so on. Practicing mindfulness, she let her full attention be with the experience of floating. Sharing what it was like with the class, she described the water as warm and soft, and the sensation of being buoyed by the water was very pleasant and comforting. She noticed how the sunlight filtered through the windows to reflect on the rippling water and was moved by this simple beauty. She experienced a feeling of community and connection with the other people in her class. She held her focus, moment to moment, on her experience of floating and experienced ease and comfort. She found this experience to be deeply restful. Her pain diminished during this period and she felt content and peaceful. Applying mindfulness, she successfully shifted from anxious thinking about the future to what was a positive experience in the present. She now considers this closing period of floating to be an important element of her exercise program, one that provides her with a feeling of renewal, peace, and well-being.

Case Example 3.9.

Rich, a 48-year-old physician who attended The Wellness Program to learn skills to help manage chronic neck pain, described the following experience: "The most profound experience with mindfulness to date happened simply driving to work on Friday. The trip from my house to the hospital is 2 miles. During the drive along Smith Street at 6:30 AM I am usually thinking about the upcoming surgeries, hassles at work, and so on. I often drive mindlessly as I check my voicemail via cell phone. On this day, I decided to approach the drive more mindfully, first getting in touch with my breathing, then with the sound of the gentle rainfall, then with the trees, the birds, and the people. I looked into the eyes of each pedestrian and driver heading in my direction. I was amazed at the number of people who looked back. I felt a kind of connection with them. This trip takes 10 minutes. It affected me for the remainder of the day. I felt more relaxed and at peace. I felt a closer connection with the people that I interacted with at the hospital."

Case Example 3.10.

Alicia was a 60-year-old woman who was diagnosed with high blood pressure and had experienced a mild stroke. Halfway through the program, her elderly mother with whom she had a difficult relationship began to fail and move toward death. Alicia made a deliberate decision to practice mindfulness as often as she could when in her mother's company. She described sitting by her bedside and letting go of her concepts about her mother, past grievances, and negative feelings. Instead, she chose to be open to the present moment. She thought of the image of an empty cup, not filled with the conflicted history of their relationship, but empty and open, choosing a beginner's mind and an attitude of not knowing. She described a level of communication, understanding, and healing taking place between the two of them that she never dreamed possible. She found she had the capacity to listen to her mother with new insight, appreciation, and understanding. Rather than feel isolated from her mother, she experienced a deep sense of love and connection. She believed that without the practice of mindfulness, she never would have been open to such a possibility.

Alicia commented that a story I shared about my father had inspired her to try this approach with her mother. In my situation, my father was not dying. He was just eager to share with me the computer program he created to play bridge. I do not play bridge, know absolutely nothing about the game, and have no interest in computers and computer programming. Out of respect, however, I sat beside him as he began to describe the details of his bridge program. Was I frustrated! I had so many other things I wanted to do, and I knew my father could carry on for quite some time about his project. As I was going over and over in my mind all the places I would rather be, I suddenly stopped myself and observed what I was doing. I made the choice to bring my mind back to the present moment and to be with things just as they were. I let go of the mental chatter about preferring to be somewhere else and opened myself to the present moment. Much to my amazement, I suddenly found myself embraced with an experience of my father's love for me. There was a powerful warmth and radiance flowing from him. I was deeply touched and could have sat next to him for hours. Without mindfulness, this moment of connection had been a moment of isolation. I wondered how many other moments like this one I had missed because my mind was elsewhere.

An Introductory Exercise in Mindful Awareness

In The Wellness Program, I introduce mindfulness through a mindful eating exercise described in the book *Full Catastrophe Living* by Jon Kabat-Zinn, Ph.D. It simply requires eating three raisins, one at a time, with full awareness. The first time I presented this activity to a group, I had no idea how people would respond and felt I was taking a risk. Would I meet skepticism or curiosity? Experience taught me that people generally respond positively to this exercise, gain insight into what mindfulness is, and glimpse how awareness influences their experience. It is a simple, but powerful exercise. If you have no previous experience in mindfulness, it is a wonderful introduction.

Mindful Eating Exercise

1. Hold one raisin in an open palm and observe it as if you were seeing a raisin for the first time.
2. Pay attention to the color, texture, and the reflection of light on the ridges of the raisin. Observe the sensation of the raisin resting against the skin of your palm and fingers. Also, smell the raisin.
3. Observe the difference between your direct sensory experience of this object in your hand and the story you create about it. We use terms such as "raisin," "small," "brown," and "rough surface."
4. In addition, if you like raisins, you might be experiencing a positive feeling as you examine the raisin. If you don't like raisins, you might be experiencing a negative feeling toward the raisin. Or perhaps you feel neutral toward raisins. Whatever your experience is, simply observe this feeling.
5. As you examine the raisin, reflect on the fact that this raisin did not just drop out of thin air to land in your hand, but certain conditions contributed to this arrival of the raisin in your hand. A seed was planted in the earth (that seed, of course, has its own conditions), which required certain nutrients in the soil, rain, and sunlight. Someone harvested and dried the grape. People were involved in the packaging and distributing process. As you bring your awareness to the raisin, can you begin to look into the raisin and see the multitude of conditions and connections that brought this raisin to be here, resting in your hand?
6. Observe your motivation or intention to eat the raisin. You might notice the release of salivary fluids in your mouth in anticipation of eating.
7. With awareness, raise the raisin toward your mouth. Feel your arm move through space.
8. Place the raisin in your mouth and let it simply rest on your tongue. Roll the raisin around in your mouth and simply observe your experience.
9. When you are ready, with full awareness, bite into the raisin and very slowly chew the raisin. You might notice your jaw movement, the release of salivary fluids, even the different textures of the skin of the raisin and the inner body of the raisin. Take your time.
10. Experience the taste of the raisin.
11. When you feel ready, mindfully swallow the raisin. For a moment, reflect on the fact that the raisin will now be broken down in a process that is both routine and miraculous, into elements that can be used by your cells.
12. Repeat the same process with the remaining two raisins.

If you choose to include this exercise in a class, when participants have finished eating the three raisins, initiate a discussion of what people experienced. Invite people to share with the group what it was like to eat a raisin with this much attention and awareness.

Participants' responses are generally positive and insightful. Often they report that if they ate this way, they would eat less and enjoy their food more. With awareness, people describe a much richer and stronger flavor in one raisin than they have ever experienced in the handfuls they usually eat without attention. This is an important metaphor for experiencing life. Also, people begin to recognize the difference between a situation—in this case, a raisin—and their reactions *to* a situation. They observe the physical sensations, thoughts, and feelings they experience in reaction to the raisin. Understanding this distinction between a situation and one's reaction to it is an important step in helping people recognize the choices they have when responding to their symptoms.

Qualities of Mindful Awareness

Mindfulness involves learning *how* to pay attention to any experience in a wise and skillful manner. Often people pay no attention to their bodies until something goes wrong. Then all they know to do is focus on the problem. For other people, their ability to listen to their bodies is clouded by feelings of shame about being sick. Others cannot pay attention without getting stuck in anger toward themselves or imagining the worst possible outcome. Still others fear what is happening to them and are constantly trying to avoid or deny their experience. The fundamental struggles people have about their bodies and symptoms create stumbling blocks to well-being. For people with chronic pain, the conflict they experience about their pain may increase their risk of depression.[1] Teaching people a more constructive, practical, and effective way to listen to their bodies and experiences makes a significant difference in their ability to cope and manage symptoms.

How we look at something influences what we see. The quality of attention we bring to something directly impacts our perception of it. The truth of this concept came home to me when I was remodeling my bathroom and found myself paying attention to the details of every bathroom I went into during this time. I could accurately describe the bathroom colors, tiles, tubs, and shower curtains in the homes of family, friends, and even hotels! Certainly I had been in these rooms many times before, but I now experienced them in a completely new way. The rooms themselves had not changed, however the quality of my attention had shifted.

Often we hear people say, "I didn't feel the exercise irritate my symptoms at the time, but later that night, I couldn't move." I sometimes wonder if these people aren't encountering something similar to my experience of bathrooms before my remodel. Perhaps the information was there, but they did not know how to tune in. Helping people cultivate a skillful way to listen to their experience has a positive impact on their sense of self and their ability to cope with chronic conditions and make healthy choices. The question becomes, "How do we develop a way of listening that best serves our well-being?" Mindfulness offers guidelines. The following specific qualities of attention, based on the work of Kabat-Zinn and Gunaratana, are keys to this skillful way of listening[2,3]:

1. *Present moment.* When mindful, our awareness is in the here and now. Life itself can only be experienced in the present moment. The past exists in the mind only as a memory, an idea, or an image. So too the future exists as a dream, a fantasy, or a concept. Mindfulness invites us to wake up to the experience of life itself in the present.

   Many people perceive the present moment as not enough. They believe themselves and life as it is to be insufficient. Out of fear of this perceived insufficiency, they constantly drive themselves to do more and more. There is an underlying tension and anxiety to their efforts, and an abiding happiness and well-being remains elusive. In contrast, mindful awareness offers the opportunity to experience peace and well-being here and now. We still dream, plan, and work to achieve personal goals; however, these aspirations and efforts are not obstacles to the peace and well-being available in the present moment.

2. *Fundamental kindness.* This attitude is expressed in the adage, "Be on your side, not on your case." As we observe our experience, whatever it is, we are friendly toward ourselves. We meet ourselves with kindness.
3. *Nonjudging.* Our common habit is to judge our experiences as something we like or dislike or are neutral toward. We can be especially hard on ourselves, finding fault for our common human flaws and shortcomings. We are like puppets being jerked by the strings of our likes, dislikes, and by what we find neutral or dull. These judgments trigger automatic behaviors and lock us into a limited understanding of ourselves and life. Our capacity to see reality clearly and to respond effectively is compromised.

   Mindfulness frees us from the distortions of our judgments and the automatic behaviors they trigger. When we are mindful, we observe our experience from the position of being an impartial witness. All experiences are treated equally. Whether the experience is pleasant, unpleasant, or neutral, we observe it with an unchanging quality of nonjudging attention.
4. *Acceptance.* When we are mindful, we accept our thoughts, feelings, and physical sensations just as they are. Even ones we do not like. If a person experiences pain, muscle tension, or paresthesias, he or she observes and accepts the sensation, just as it is. This may be especially important for people who are living with chronic pain. Preliminary research exploring the role of acceptance of pain in pain adjustment found that greater acceptance of pain was associated with less anxiety and depression and less physical and psychosocial disability related to pain.[4]

   Sometimes people confuse acceptance with defeat. This is a misunderstanding of acceptance. Acceptance does not mean giving up or taking a passive stance in response to life. Acceptance requires the courage to see things as they are in the present moment. Acceptance does not negate actively choosing a course of action. For a sailor caught in a storm, to deny that the storm exists or to struggle with the reality of the storm would put the ship and lives at risk. A sailor acknowledges and accepts the storm and makes choices to safely navigate the turbulent sea.

   We can expend a lot of energy fighting and denying the truth. We often make poor choices when fear or anger clouds our perception. Acceptance requires that we see things just as they are. It creates the possibility for insight and understanding and enables us to make choices based on a clear picture of what is true at a particular time. When facing major losses and changes, coming to acceptance can require time. This process can include moving through stages of fear, anger, and grief until we are finally able to acknowledge the truth.
5. *Nonstriving.* This attitude is reflected in the saying, "Don't push the river." Our effort is directed toward being fully aware of our experience, just as it is, without trying to force or change our experience. We are not trying to get somewhere or make anything happen. Sometimes it is when we try hard that we create obstacles to a natural ability to change and grow.

   My first experience with the benefit of a nonstriving attitude was when I was a high school gymnast. Not particularly talented, I rarely was in competition and participated in the sport for the fun and friendships. One afternoon another gymnast was sick and my coach asked me to compete on the balance beam. I was delighted. The coach just needed one more body in the lineup. The rules called for throwing out the lowest score, which surely would be mine. I remember the joy of competing and the ease with which I performed each movement. Much to everyone's surprise I performed very well and my score was included in the team tally. My coach then assigned me to compete in the next competition. I worked very hard in the following week and felt well prepared; however, I was a disaster in competition. I could not relax or find the rhythm of my routine. I was trying too hard and fell several times. When I later reflected on the two different experiences, I realized that trying hard became an obstacle to my natural physical ability. When I did not try so hard, my body naturally flowed through the different elements of my routine and performed at a far higher level of mastery.

It might seem like a paradox to think that we can achieve something by not pushing or forcing it to happen, but just like a gardener does not need to force the arrival of spring, there are dimensions of life and aspects of our growth that do not need to be forced. When we choose a nonstriving attitude, like a good gardener, we listen to this intrinsic process and the inner timing of life. We do not force the agenda of our preconceived ideas and concepts.

6. *Not knowing.* What we think we know can be the biggest obstacle to learning anything new. A full cup has no room for fresh water. When we are mindful, we temporarily suspend preconceived ideas, concepts, and expectations. We allow life to be revealed to us as it is rather than dictated and distorted by our predetermined agenda. We let go of expectations. We meet the world with a "beginner's mind," a willingness to see things as if for the first time.
7. *Letting go.* Life is change. Seeking happiness and security, we tend to grasp at pleasant experiences, trying to make them last while pushing away unpleasant experiences. Because everything changes, this effort does not bring us the lasting relief we seek. Consider pleasant experiences to be one type of cloud and unpleasant ones to be another. Mindful awareness is like the sky. The sky does not push away storm clouds while grasping at fair weather ones. Practicing mindfulness, we develop this open, nonattached quality of awareness.

Introducing these qualities of attention empowers people to listen to themselves in a healthy and healing manner and has multiple beneficial consequences, as demonstrated by the examples cited in this chapter.

Mindful Breathing

When participants in the classes I teach are asked to identify what was the most valuable thing they learned in the program, many of them respond: "Mindful breathing." Breathe. It sounds so simple, yet people often hold their breath when they are in pain, exercising, and under stress. Breathing is essential for life, and a healthy breathing pattern is necessary for optimal physical function. Although breathing exercises are commonly taught to people with respiratory disorders, these exercises are often overlooked in the treatment of other medical conditions. *Every wellness program should include some type of instruction in diaphragmatic breathing and its applications to pain and stress management.*

Mindful breathing exercises help people develop the skill of observing their automatic physical, mental, and emotional habit reactions. They can gain an understanding of how their reactions to situations contribute to their symptom severity and overall distress. This new awareness makes it possible for them to choose alternative responses. In addition, breathing exercises enable people to glimpse the experience of living in the present moment—the only moment available for living.

This instruction to observe your breathing and take a deep breath sounds simple, but it is not always easy to do, especially when stress and pain levels are high. Encouraging people to develop the habit of observing their breath and breathing deeply during times of distress is invaluable as the following examples from people in my classes illustrate:

Case Example 3.11.

David was a 46-year-old man who enrolled in The Wellness Program after being diagnosed with high blood pressure. He worked for a computer software company. His direct supervisor had a hostile temperament and was a micromanager always quick to find fault with David's work. When his supervisor walked into his office, David's response was to panic. His shoulders would tense and he would hold his breath. After learning diaphragmatic breathing, he began focusing on his breath whenever he was in his supervisor's presence. He was stunned to realize just how calm he could remain. Much to David's surprise, as he grew less reactive to his supervisor's criticism and hostility, his supervisor paid him less attention.

Case Example 3.12.

Debbie was a 32-year-old woman diagnosed with chronic fatigue syndrome. While enrolled in The Wellness Program, her physician had given her a new medication. She had a bad reaction and described feeling as if all of her muscles were buzzing. Frightened, she phoned her physician, who told her to drink water and discontinue the medication. She was told to ride out the reaction and to call the physician back only if she worsened or did not improve by late that afternoon. She could feel herself starting to panic and knew this would only make things worse. She put on her favorite classical music, lay down, and focused on her breathing. She described the breathing practices as a lifeline. No matter what was happening, she could still breathe. This calmed her. The intensity of the buzzing sensation in her muscles decreased. She was still uncomfortable for several hours, but she was able to manage the situation by maintaining her focus on breathing in a deep and steady manner.

Case Example 3.13.

Marion was a 38-year-old nurse who suffered chronic constant pelvic and right hip pain following the traumatic birth of her first child. Her physician's continual advice following the birth was to rest. After 2 years of a very low level of activity with minimal improvement in her pain, she entered The Wellness Program wanting to gradually increase her fitness level and learn additional pain management strategies. Her desire was to have a second child. She completed The Wellness Program, enrolled in a community-based gentle yoga class, and received additional treatment by a physical therapist specializing in pelvic floor disorders. Two years after she finished the program and after the birth of her second child, I received the following e-mail from her:

> Alexa is 6 months old now and so beautiful. Her birth was awesome. I showed up at the hospital at 11:30 PM. fully dilated and effaced! My labor nurse asked how I could walk with a smile on my face and, when I saw an old friend, chat and laugh with ease. "Well," I answered, "I've been in a lot of pain the last few years … this isn't much worse."
>
> "Oh, what from?" she asked.
>
> "From the *last childbirth!*" I laughed.
>
> "Oh, gosh," she exclaimed. "Do you take something for it?"
>
> "No," I answered. "I just breathe."

Mindful breathing exercises are powerful. They can be taught as brief 5-minute practices or, in a more extended form, as a component of a mindfulness meditation practice.

Mindfulness Meditation

When people perform breathing practices on a daily basis for 15 to 60 minutes or longer over a period of years, the ability to rest the mind in the present moment is profoundly strengthened. A quality of awareness that is stable and nonreactive in the face of changing circumstances is cultivated. People grow increasingly able to maintain inner equanimity while experiencing pleasure or pain, joy or sorrow, mental calm or distress. They touch the full range of the human experience with increasing compassion, understanding, acceptance, and wisdom. They often have experiences of insight, inner peace, and well-being. Such a practice is called mindfulness meditation.

The word *meditation* means to "engage in contemplation and reflection."[5] There are many kinds of meditation, and every major religion has a practice that can be identified as a type of meditation. Mindfulness meditation is a systematic experiment in the conscious and thorough investigation of present moment life experience. It is a careful and deliberate examination of any phenomena arising in one's awareness, including thoughts, mental images, sense impressions, and emotions, with an unwavering quality of attention. Although it is a type of meditation found in some religious traditions, developing a skillful means to closely observe and experience life as it happens in the here and now does not require the study or adoption of any religious view. For some people, spiritual study enriches their experience of meditation; however, association with a religion is not required for people to benefit from training in mindfulness meditation.

Mindfulness meditation has special applications to health, wellness, and rehabilitation because of its emphasis on the breath, body awareness, the present moment, and its inherent affirmation of the capacity of people to embrace the full range of life's experiences. When we face something unpleasant, such as a sensation of pain or a feeling of grief, our reaction is often to avoid it. This reluctance to acknowledge something unwanted usually adds to our inner distress and turmoil. This distress can cloud our understanding and lead to poor decision making. Our desire to avoid unpleasant aspects of our experience can drive addictive behaviors. We may turn to drugs, alcohol, work, TV, shopping, or overeating to find temporary comfort and avoid facing the truth.

Mindfulness meditation trains the practitioner to do just the opposite. It asks the practitioner to look toward and into what is unpleasant and unwanted. This direct and whole-hearted examination of difficult experiences and circumstances is the first step in effectively and wisely responding to them. Mindfulness meditation provides direct insight into the nature of self and suffering. It offers a profound shift in the misguided focus that something outside can bring lasting peace and well-being and affirms that the roots of peace and well-being are ultimately found within us. Teaching mindfulness meditation in a group wellness program is substantially different from teaching brief breathing exercises. A teacher trained in mindfulness meditation coaches people in the depth and breadth of this transformative practice and guides people to experience mindfulness as a way of life.

When people hear the word meditation, the image of a monk sitting cross-legged and silent in a monastery often comes to mind. It is a mistake to limit meditation to this image. Meditation is practiced by people from many walks of life and is a growing component of health care services and medical school training nationwide.[6-8]

Scientific Research in Mindfulness Meditation

Research studies investigating the neurobiology of mindfulness meditation are few and further investigation is warranted, especially as interest in this approach increases. In a randomized clinical trial laboratory study conducted by Davidson et al, employees at a biotech company received an 8-week training course in mindfulness meditation, termed Mindfulness-Based Stress Reduction (MBSR).[9] Participation in the training program was found to be associated with increased left frontal cortical activation in the brain as measured by EEG. Research suggests that this increased left frontal cortical activity is associated with more effective processing of negative emotional states and therefore with reduced stress reactivity.[10] In addition, the employees receiving the intervention mounted a significantly higher antibody response to a viral challenge (influenza vaccine) following the MBSR program than did the wait-list controls. Immune enhancement correlated strongly with the brain activation patterns observed in the intervention group. Significant psychological changes were also observed in the meditators but not in the wait-list control group.

Lazar et al used functional magnetic resonance imagery to identify and characterize brain regions active during meditation.[11] Significant signal increases were observed in those areas associated with attention and autonomic nervous system regulation.

Sudsuang et al studied serum cortisol and total protein levels, blood pressure, heart rate, and lung volume in 52 meditators.[12] Following meditation, serum cortisol levels were significantly reduced, serum total protein was significantly increased, and systolic and diastolic pressure and heart rate were significantly reduced.

Tooley et al observed nighttime melatonin plasma levels following a period of meditation.[13] Experienced meditators showed significantly higher plasma melatonin levels following a period of meditation compared with levels on a control night.

As the general public increasingly pursues complementary medicine services, the practical application of mindfulness meditation to patient care is receiving increased attention among medical practitioners and researchers. Research remains preliminary, and additional large-scale studies with long-term follow-up are needed; however, initial studies show that mindfulness has a promising role in managing several chronic conditions, including heart disease, cancer, multiple sclerosis, fibromyalgia, and chronic pain.

In a study that did follow an intervention group for 4 years, Patel et al examined the health outcomes of providing instruction in breathing exercises, meditation, and relaxation to people with two or more risk factors for heart disease.[14] One hundred ninety-two men and women were randomly assigned to an intervention group or control group. Both groups received written health education information on reducing blood pressure. In addition, the intervention group met for 1 hour for 8 weeks and received instruction in breathing exercises, meditation, and relaxation. Significantly greater reductions in systolic and diastolic blood pressure were demonstrated in the intervention group at program completion and at 4 years following the intervention. In addition, at 4 years follow-up, the incidence of ischemic heart disease, fatal myocardial infarction, and electrocardiographic evidence of ischemia was significantly decreased in the treatment group compared to controls.

Kabat-Zinn et al examined the effect of an 8-week training in MBSR on the symptoms of 90 patients with chronic pain compared to a control group of 20 patients receiving regular care at a medical center pain clinic.[15] Following the intervention, significant reductions were observed in measures of pain, anxiety, depression, and pain-related medication use when compared to controls. Improvements were maintained in the intervention group at 15 months follow-up on all measures except present moment pain.

Drawing from the Kabat-Zinn model, other researchers have examined the role of MBSR in medical and nonmedical populations. Speca et al used a randomized, wait-list controlled design to examine the effects of participation in a meditation program on mood disturbance and symptoms of stress in 45 cancer outpatients.[16] The intervention was adapted from the MBSR model and consisted of three primary components: (1) theoretical material related to meditation and the mind-body relationship, (2) the experiential practice of mindfulness meditation in class and at home, and (3) group process focusing on adherence to the home program, the effective integration of mindfulness into daily life, and the supportive interactions among group members. The intervention group met once a week for 90 minutes for 7 weeks. On completion of the program, the treatment group had significantly lower scores on total mood disturbance and on subscales of depression, anxiety, anger, and confusion. They also had fewer physical symptoms of stress, including fewer cardiopulmonary and gastrointestinal symptoms, than the control group.

In a pilot study, Singh et al examined the role of mindfulness meditation and mindful movement on function, pain perception, and mood state in 20 patients with fibromyalgia.[17] The group met once a week for 2.5 hours for 8 consecutive weeks. Standard outcome measures showed significant reduction in pain, fatigue, and insomnia and improvement in function, mood state, and general health on completion of the 8-week intervention.

In another pilot study, Mills and Allen examined balance and multiple sclerosis symptoms in eight patients with multiple sclerosis after a six-session individual training program in mindfulness and mindful movement compared with a control group.[18] The treatment group showed significant improvement on a balance test and on self-reported symptoms. This improvement was sustained at 3 months following the intervention. The researchers conclude that mindfulness and mindful movement may be promising for people with multiple sclerosis; however, because of the small sample size, the findings need to be treated with caution and additional research is required.

Williams et al examined the role of MBSR in a randomized controlled study of community volunteers in a university setting with high levels of perceived stress.[19] Fifty-nine participants were assigned to the intervention group and 44 adults served as the control group. The intervention was adapted from the MBSR curriculum to meet the needs of a nonclinical population. Participants in the intervention group reported significant reductions in daily hassles, psychological distress, and number of medical symptoms from baseline. No significant change from baseline was reported in the control group receiving educational materials and referral to community resources only.

Because these studies are relatively few in number and have not been replicated, the efficacy of mindfulness meditation remains an area for further medical investigation; however, converging lines of evidence suggest that significant health benefits can be gained through this practice.

Clinical Practice

The growing interest in mindfulness meditation among health researchers, providers, and the public opens a door for clinicians to train in mindfulness meditation and initiate the integration of this practice into health promotion and wellness programs. The ability to effectively teach mindfulness meditation depends directly on a clinician's personal experience with the practice. Although any clinician can teach brief breathing exercises, teaching meditation is substantially different and requires years of training. Kabat-Zinn and Santorelli, pioneers in bringing mindfulness meditation into medicine, have established minimum qualifications for what they identify as a Level 1 MBSR provider that include a daily meditation practice, 3 years of consistent meditation practice, and two 5- to 10-day mindfulness meditation retreats.[20] Meditation training centers are listed at the end of this chapter.

In many instances, clinicians teaching wellness programs and participants enrolling in them may have no interest in meditation. This should not deter a clinician from learning and teaching basic diaphragmatic breathing exercises and introducing the concept of present moment awareness to a group. At first glance, the instruction may appear simplistic. The effects of mindful breathing and present moment awareness, however, should not be underestimated. For example, several years ago I taught my mother, who was in her early eighties at the time, diaphragmatic breathing and the concept of present moment awareness over the telephone. This minimal instruction lasted perhaps 5 to 10 minutes. My mother has never practiced formal meditation of any kind, yet she frequently reports taking deep breaths when she drives, cannot sleep, or is worried about something. She often tells me that she repeats to herself, "The moment. Life is about the moment."

Respiratory Muscle Anatomy and Function

A basic understanding of respiratory muscle anatomy and function is helpful when teaching breathing exercises. This information is a review for many clinicians, but some health care practitioners teaching wellness programs may find this material to be new.

Inspiratory Muscles[21]

The primary muscles of inspiration, which are active during quiet breathing in a healthy individual, are the diaphragm, the scalenes, and the parasternal intercostals muscles.

The *diaphragm* arises from the margins of the lower six ribs, from the posterior aspect of the xyphoid process, and from the anterolateral aspect of L1 to L3 vertebrae. Fibers from these origins radiate inward to insert into the central tendon. When the diaphragm contracts, muscle fibers shorten and its dome shape descends to compress abdominal contents. The resting tension of the abdominal muscles creates an increased pressure in the abdominal compartment during inspiration. The downward movement of the diaphragm, which is opposed by the abdominal contents, pulls the ribs upward and outward. The lower rib cage expands, causing intrathoracic pressure to decrease and inspiration to occur. This action of the diaphragm performs approximately 70% to 80% of the work of quiet breathing in a healthy individual.

The *scalene muscles* originate on the transverse processes of the lower five cervical vertebrae and insert into the upper surface of the first and second ribs. These muscles lift and expand the rib cage during inspiration.

The *parasternal muscles* attach to the sternum and run between the costal cartilages in a downward and outward direction. When they contract, the ribs lift and the anterior posterior diameter within the rib cage increases.

Expiratory muscles

In a healthy individual, expiration is a passive process achieved by the elastic recoil of the lungs. The abdominal muscles assist in expiration. Their contraction decreases the size of the rib cage. Their activity also increases intraabdominal pressure, pushing the abdominal contents upward. This action decreases lung volume and lengthens the diaphragm at the end phase of expiration.

Described succinctly, during inspiration in healthy individuals, the diaphragm descends and the ribs move upward and outward, increasing the size of the thoracic cavity. A negative pressure is created and air is drawn into the lungs. The inspiratory muscles then relax and expiration occurs passively.

Mindful Breathing Exercises

Several breathing exercises that can be included in a wellness program are described as follows. They are presented in a brief practice format. Personally practice

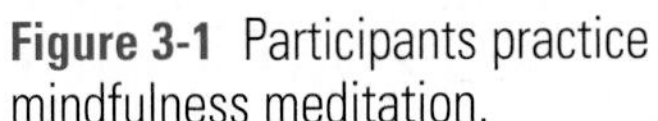

Figure 3-1 Participants practice mindfulness meditation.

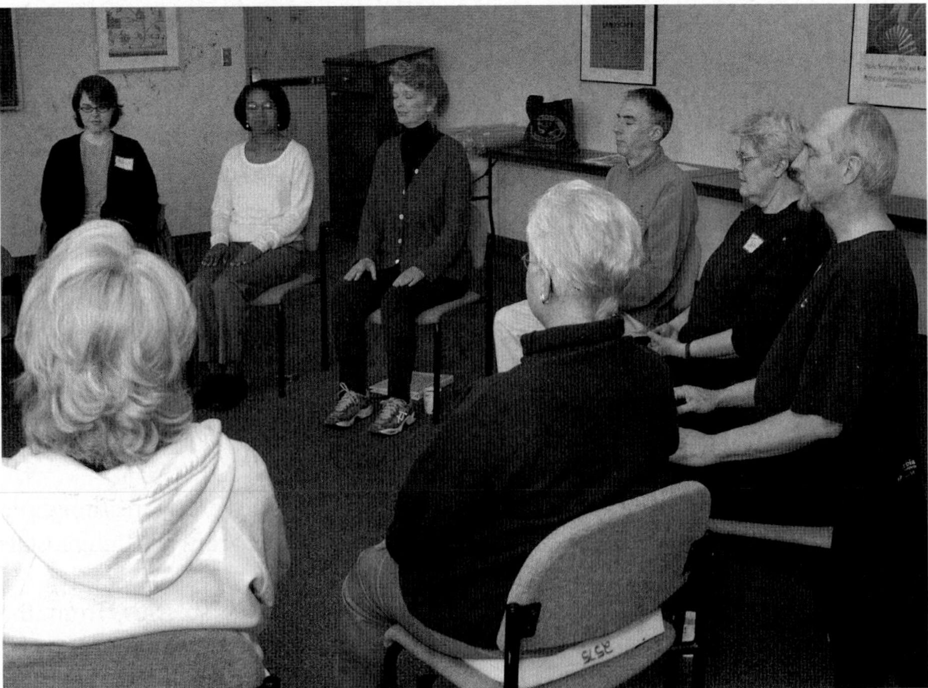

each exercise several times on your own before introducing it in a class. For the clinician who is trained in mindfulness meditation, these exercises can be extended for increasing time periods for the purpose of meditation training (Figure 3-1).

When presenting these exercises in a group, allow for a period of discussion, enabling participants to share their experiences and have questions answered. The amount of time for this discussion will vary with the number and complexity of questions.

Exercise 1: Mindfulness of Breathing

Sit comfortably. Avoid slouching. Sit so that your shoulders are aligned over your hips. Place both feet on the floor. Close your eyes. Consider the quality of awareness you might bring to something in nature. For example, think of how you might look at a mountain range or the ocean. This quality of awareness is open and nonjudging.

Now bring this same quality of awareness to your inner landscape and observe your breathing. As you inhale, simply feel what part of your body moves as you inhale. As you exhale, simply feel what part of your body moves as you exhale. Do not attempt to consciously manipulate or alter your breathing in any way. This is an opportunity to observe your breathing just as it is.

You can experience the movement of your breath in different places in your torso. You might notice your belly moving, your rib cage rising and falling, or your upper chest or even shoulders moving as you breathe. Each breath is unique. Simply experience the movement of your body however it is occurring, moment to moment.

(Pause to allow participants to practice.)

Now, place one hand on your upper chest, on top of your breastbone. Draw your stomach in slightly and breathe into your hand. Allow your breath to be of average size. You should feel your breast bone, upper chest, and rib cage rise and fall. Observe these sensations. This is called upper chest or shallow breathing.

(Pause to allow participants to practice.)

Observe how you feel.

Now, place your hand on your abdomen at the level of your navel. As you inhale, imagine breathing into your hand. You should experience your stomach pushing forward into your hand as you breathe in. You might also feel your lower ribs flare out to the side slightly. As you exhale, your stomach should gently fall. This is called diaphragmatic breathing, abdominal or belly breathing.

(Pause to allow participants to practice.)

Observe how you feel.

Now allow your breathing to return to whatever feels comfortable and natural for you. Again, simply observe your experience just as it is.

(Brief pause)

Now, slightly round your shoulders and assume a slouched posture. Notice how this affects your breathing.

(Pause to allow participants to practice.)

Now, return to sitting upright and slightly draw your shoulder blades together and down your spine. Lift your breastbone slightly upward. This movement should be small and done gently. Notice how this movement affects your breathing.

(Pause to allow participants to practice.)

Now, return to a comfortable posture and breathing pattern that feels natural for you. Once again, observe your in breath and out breath.

(Pause to allow participants to practice.)

And now, gradually return your awareness to the room and let your eyes open.

Exercise 2: Diaphragmatic Breathing

We are now going to explore the practice of diaphragmatic breathing more closely. When we are under stress, in pain, or sometimes when exercising, our breathing pattern becomes more shallow and rapid. This pattern of upper chest or shallow breathing results in a decrease in oxygen intake and reinforces the body's stress reaction. In contrast, diaphragmatic breathing is a powerful strategy to ensure that your lungs receive a healthy volume of oxygen with your inspiration. Diaphragmatic breathing also decreases the body's stress reaction and promotes calming your mind and body.

Sit comfortably. Avoid slouching. Sit so that your shoulders are aligned over your hips. Place both feet on the floor. Close your eyes. As you observe your experience, meet yourself with a quality of fundamental kindness and self-acceptance. Your body is doing the very best it can, and there is no need to judge yourself or your experience as good or bad, right or wrong.

As you inhale, simply feel what part of your body moves as you inhale. As you exhale, simply feel what part of your body moves as you exhale.

Now, let your awareness rest in your belly. As you breathe in, allow your breath to move deep into your lungs, your stomach to gently move outward, and your lower ribs to move out to the side slightly. As you breathe out, allow your stomach to gently fall. You do not have to take an exceptionally large breath. Your breath can be of average size. The key is to allow your breath to fill the bottom of your lungs. You know this is happening when your stomach rises slightly on the in breath and falls as you exhale.

If you have ever rested on a raft on the ocean, you may have had the experience of the raft gently rising and gently falling as each wave passes by. Observing diaphragmatic breathing is somewhat similar. Instead of experiencing the gentle rise and fall of the raft with each passing ocean wave, you are observing the rise and fall of your stomach and rib cage with each wave of the breath. As you breathe in, become aware of the sensations of breathing in, and as you breathe out become aware of the sensations of breathing out.

When observing the breath, it is common for the mind to wander. Suddenly we are thinking about something that happened yesterday or we are planning tomorrow. When this happens, simply observe that your mind has wandered and return your attention to your breath. Consider your mind to be like the sky and thoughts to be like small clouds floating by. Simply observe the thought as you might observe a cloud pass by in the sky and return your awareness to your breathing.

Practice for 5 minutes.

Exercise 3: Diaphragmatic Breathing with Verbal Cues

One practice that both calms the mind and body and helps build present moment concentration is to repeat a word or phrase to yourself in concert with your breath. The simplest of these is "breathing in" on the in breath and "breathing out" on the out breath. Or more briefly, "in"…"out."

You can use any word or phrase that has meaning for you. For example, you may know the experience of having a very long day and finally making it home. You open the door, step into your home, and experience a feeling of calm and ease automatically come over you. Drawing on this experience, you can use the words "arriving" on the in breath and "home" on the out breath. As you repeat these words, you can experiment with recreating some of that feeling of ease in your body. In this instance, you are not arriving to your external home, but rather to an internal one. Arriving home to yourself, to your center, to the foundation of who you are. Also you are arriving home to the present moment–to the here and now.

Other examples of phrases you might use in concert with your breath include repeating your own name on the in breath followed by the phrase "let go" on the out breath, or "present moment" on the in breath and "only moment" on the out breath. If you practice within a religious tradition, you can use a word or phrase from spiritual writings or the phrases "let go" on the in breath, "let God" on the out breath, or "in the Kingdom of God"…"I dwell."

Sit comfortably. Place both feet on the floor. Close your eyes. As you observe your experience, let go of any preconceived ideas you have about breathing or expectations of how you think you should breathe and what should happen. Experience your breath as if each breath was your first breath, each moment a new moment.

Choose any word or phrase that speaks to you, and repeat this phrase in concert with your breathing. When your mind wanders, simply observe that your mind has wandered and return your attention to your breath and the phrase.

Practice for 5 minutes.

Exercise 4: Diaphragmatic Breathing with Counting

Another practice that both calms the mind and body and helps build present moment concentration is to count each exhalation from 1 to 10. When you reach the tenth exhalation, then begin again at 1. With the first breath, on the exhalation, say to yourself "one," on the second "two," on the third "three," and so on until you reach the tenth exhalation. Then return to 1 and begin again.

If you find that your mind wanders, simply observe your thoughts as you might observe a small cloud floating by in the sky and return your attention to your breath and begin again with "one."

Practice for 5 minutes.

Exercise 5: Mindfulness of Breathing and the Body

Once you have the ability to maintain your awareness on your breath, you can expand your awareness beyond the breath to the whole body. Begin by letting your awareness rest with the rhythm of your breathing. Gradually expand your awareness beyond the breath to include sensations of your body. You might notice the sensations of your feet inside your shoes or the sensation of your thighs and buttocks against the chair. You might notice how you've chosen to hold your arms and hands in your lap. Or observe how you are holding your head over your spine. Is your head forward of your spine? Does it feel like you are leaning slightly to the left or right? Or does it feel centered? Just observe different sensations. Ultimately, allow the field of your awareness to take in your body as a whole, from the soles of your feet to the crown of your head.

If you find that your mind wanders, simply observe your thoughts as you might observe a small cloud floating by in the sky and return your attention to your breath and to your body as a whole.

Practice for 5 minutes.

Exercise 6: Mindfulness of Thoughts and Feelings

Just as you can observe the sensations of your body in the present moment, so too, you can observe your thoughts and feelings. Thoughts and feelings come and go, they flow and change. Mindfulness enables you to observe this changing landscape of your experience just as it is. You become an impartial observer, watching your thoughts and feelings without judging your experience or trying to change it in any way. It is much like observing different weather patterns pass by. Sometimes the cloud patterns are dark and turbulent, whereas other times they are fair-weather ones.

Sit comfortably. Place both feet on the floor. Close your eyes. Observe your breath. As you observe your experience, meet yourself with a quality of fundamental kindness, compassion, and self-acceptance. Remember, there is no need to judge yourself or your experience as good or bad, right or wrong. As you observe your experience, let go of any preconceived ideas you have about what you think should happen. Let your breath serve your mind as an anchor, always bringing your awareness home to the present moment.

Now observe your thoughts. Notice how each thought has its own life span. It appears, has its moment in your awareness, then disappears. Notice a thought, accept it, and let it go. Thoughts are just thoughts.

(Pause to allow participants to practice.)

Now observe your feelings. Each feeling has its own life span as well. Feelings come and go, flow and change. Feelings can be pleasant, unpleasant, or neutral. Sometimes we are not feeling anything, and if that is the case, simply observe the experience of not feeling anything. Again, your awareness remains stable as you observe feelings.

(Pause to allow participants to practice.)

Observe any relationship that might exist between your thoughts and your feelings.

(Pause to allow participants to practice.)

Observe any relationship that might exist between your thoughts and feelings and your body. Notice how different thoughts and feelings influence physical sensations.

(Pause to allow participants to practice.)

Practice for 5 to 10 minutes.

These exercises are a first step in offering people one strategy to respond to symptoms and to daily stress. They provide people with an introduction to observing automatic physical, mental, and emotional habit reactions throughout their day, in any situation. This awareness is the first step toward change. People can gain a beginning insight into how certain reactions contribute to symptom severity and overall distress and make it possible for them to choose alternative responses. People also glimpse the experience of living in the present moment—the only moment we have available for living.

These breathing exercises in their brief form can be integrated into any wellness program. They can be used as an opening exercise. People often arrive to class with their attention still at work or with an event that happened earlier in the day. They may be physically tense from driving or from rushing to arrive on time. Breathing exercises help people release mental stress and physical tension. Participants shift their attention from the other areas of their life to their present moment experience sitting in the classroom. Afterward, they are more present to the class experience and the learning process.

These exercises can also be practiced before and/or after a stretching and strengthening exercise program. They are a wonderful way to help people begin to pay attention to their body before exercising and promote healthy respiration. At the end of an aerobic exercise program, these exercises can be easily integrated into the closing of a cooldown sequence.

These breathing exercises can also be used to close a group session, inviting people to pay attention to what they are experiencing after the time period of being together. At the end of a breathing exercise, an instructor can include a positive affirmation or dedication as a simple way to close a class. One example of a dedication I use at the end of a breathing exercise at the close of a class is the following:

> This time we have taken together has generated something supportive and positive in our lives. You can dedicate the benefit of this time and these activities to your own well-being. May our efforts together truly serve you and be of benefit. In addition, it is important to recognize when we take time for ourselves in this manner, we never do this for ourselves alone, but we are always interconnected in a much larger family of humanity. You can dedicate the merit of our time together not only to your own well-being, but you can also imagine extending it out to benefit others. Perhaps there is someone in your life who is suffering. You can imagine any positive and nourishing qualities of our time together touching that person. Ultimately you can dedicate the merit of this time together to the benefit of all people.

I have found that people deeply appreciate this closing reminder of their connection with others and that somehow, even if not readily apparent, their efforts in the class might not only help themselves, but might also be helpful to others.

Dealing With Common Difficulties

Most people learn diaphragmatic breathing quickly and easily; however, some individuals have problems with these exercises. There are no cookbook answers to people's difficulties with breathing exercises. A clinician must always attend to the individual person and circumstances. Following are three problems that people occasionally experience. Keeping in mind each person and situation is unique, possibilities for responding are suggested.

1. *"I can't sit still."* Occasionally someone expresses anxiety about sitting still. For people who are always on the go, constantly doing one task after another, the idea of simply sitting still and observing the breath, even for 5 minutes, can evoke panic. It is helpful to meet these people with understanding and reassurance and ask them to continue with the exercises even though they find them difficult. For example, an instructor might respond as follows:

   > If you are a person who is always on the go, it is understandable that you might experience anxiety about these exercises. You are

being asked to do something that is foreign and unfamiliar. Often when we first step out of our comfort zone in any area of our lives, we can feel uncertain and anxious. Practicing breathing exercises is like learning anything new. At first it might feel uncomfortable and awkward, but with time and practice it becomes easier and more comfortable. So for now, I'm going to ask that you acknowledge your feelings of anxiety as an understandable response to doing something that is very new for you and to stick with the exercises. If you can, experiment with meeting these feelings with openness and curiosity. Observe what it is like for you to be at your learning edge and moving into new territory with compassion.

2. *"I get more anxious when I pay attention to my breathing."* For some people, observing their breathing evokes anxiety. They "try too hard" or worry about "doing it right." They may have an anxiety disorder or sitting quietly may allow them to notice their anxiety about an individual situation. These people benefit from acceptance, understanding, and reassurance. An instructor might respond as follows:

   Sometimes when we actually observe our breath for the first time, we can become flustered, wonder if we are breathing correctly, or become nervous about breathing. Sometimes we notice uncomfortable emotions. We are breathing constantly but usually are not consciously aware of these sensations. Your body has been breathing from the moment you were born. Your body knows how to breathe. However you have been breathing has been good enough. You might think of this process of observing your breath as similar to observing ocean waves come up to the shoreline and recede. Some waves come quite far up on the shore, whereas others come in only a small distance. Each wave is unique. So too each breath is unique. One breath may be shallow; one, deep; and one, somewhere in between. Accept each breath just as it is. Instead of observing your breath as it moves through your torso, you can experiment with observing the sensation of the breath moving in and out of the nostrils. This might be more comfortable for you.

   If you can, experiment with observing the anxiety with curiosity. This is an opportunity to experiment with relating to unpleasant feelings in new ways. Can you step back in a sense and notice what you are saying to yourself about your breathing? Perhaps just observe the story. If it becomes very difficult, you might shift your attention to a different physical sensation for a period of time. For example, you might observe the sensation of your thighs and buttocks resting against the chair and directly sense a quality of stability of your body in sitting. It is fine to rest your mind with the present moment sensations of your thighs and buttocks against the chair and when you feel comfortable, experiment with shifting your attention to your breath for one or two breaths then back to the sensation of your thighs and buttocks against the chair.

3. *"I can't deep breathe."* For people with a longstanding pattern of shallow breathing, diaphragmatic breathing can be difficult. It is helpful to have different ways of describing the process of deep breathing. Sometimes a

person requires additional individual assistance. An instructor might respond as follows:

> The body already carries the knowledge of deep breathing. If you have ever watched infants breathe, this is how newborn babies breathe; their bellies rise and fall. So we were all born using our diaphragm as a natural part of our breathing. We are just remembering something that is already there. You are working with your body just as an athlete does. You are listening to your body, learning about your body, and working with it to maximize its function. Don't worry. Avoid working too hard at this practice. Your body is extraordinary as it is, and your breathing has been doing a fine job. Accept each breath just as it is. If you feel you would like additional individual instruction, come talk with me at the break.

The Informal Practice of Breathing Exercises

In addition to the formal exercises described previously, awareness of breathing can be applied to activities of daily living. This important practical application enables people to bring the benefits of diaphragmatic breathing and present moment awareness into their often busy lives. Instruct participants to rest their awareness in the present moment and observe their breath from time to time during their day. Wherever they find themselves, whatever the time of day, ask that they take a moment to bring their attention into the here and now and observe their breath. Encourage participants to observe their breath during simple daily activities such as when sitting at a red light in traffic, standing in line at the grocery store, or waiting in a doctor's office. This sounds elementary, yet the benefits are powerful.

Most people learn quickly that they can often relax their body and calm their mind to some degree using this strategy. Breathing also enables them to observe their physical, mental, and emotional reactions to daily stress and make conscious choices that support their health. They also touch more deeply and live more fully the moments of their lives. The challenge is remembering to pay attention. To help people integrate mindful breathing into daily activities, I provide them with "Breathe" stickers, made at a local print shop. Participants are instructed to place them on the dashboard of their car, computer terminal, telephone, or anywhere else the stickers might catch their eye and remind them to pause and breathe with awareness. Participants love them.

Home Exercise Program

Breathing exercises can easily be included in a home program. Home practice can include the 5-minute practice of breathing exercises daily and the integration of awareness of the breath during daily activities. For a wellness program that includes meditation training, a daily meditation practice can be an integral component of a home program.

The Mindful Body Scan

Imagine seeing a blueprint for the perfect house; however, the home you live in is far from the ideal and can never be accommodated to match it. Imagine waking up every morning and noticing what is wrong and the ways in which your home never measures up. As you are reminded daily of the ideal, a voice of constant criticism takes hold. Your house is never enough, never right. If only you could have that perfect place, everything would be okay. Without it, you will never be happy. This is how many people experience their bodies. These attitudes are enough to create conflict and distress and drain away feelings of vitality and well-being.

People have a wide range of attitudes toward their bodies that influence their health choices. Many have destructive beliefs based on negative messages from childhood or media images of the body that contribute to feelings of self-judgment, shame, and low self-esteem. Add the feelings of anger, fear, and confusion that can accompany the diagnosis of a medical condition, and people are often left alienated from their bodies. Burdened with these negative feelings, it can be difficult to generate the energy and motivation to exercise and make additional healthy lifestyle choices. If you fundamentally like your house, you put time and energy into keeping it in good condition. If you do not like your house in some basic way, you are more likely to neglect it and allow parts to fall into disrepair. The body is no different.

Well-being requires a healing of this alienation. Our body is our first home. Learning to feel at home and at ease in the body is a necessary ingredient for well-being. To achieve this goal, people need to change how they experience the body. Rather than know the body only through a constant comparison to a fabricated ideal that emphasizes external appearance, people need to directly experience what is true and authentic about the body from the inside. They need to put preconceived concepts aside and learn to listen to and appreciate the body just as it is. The mindful body scan exercise provides a means to achieve this shift.

The mindful body scan is an exercise in *how* to listen to the body. It is also an exercise in present moment awareness. The qualities of mindfulness, which were described earlier in this chapter, offer an effective approach to paying attention to the body in a healthy and healing manner. People let go of self-defeating approaches and experience the body in a new way. Not only does this exercise help release people from distorted concepts and beliefs about the body, but it is also a powerful tool for building mind-body awareness. It also promotes muscle relaxation and, with practice, an inner experience of peace.

The mindful body scan should not be confused with relaxation exercises. There are important and fundamental differences between the two. Relaxation exercises assume a dualistic viewpoint. Tension is perceived as "bad" and something to decrease or eliminate. Relaxation is seen as "good" and something to attain. If you achieve relaxation, you are "successful." If you do not relax, you are "unsuccessful." When you perform relaxation exercises you are actively striving to change the present moment experience of muscle tension into one of relaxation. In contrast, practicing the mindful body scan, you are not trying to accomplish anything other than to observe your present moment experience just as it is. There is nothing to improve, change, or eliminate. Muscle relaxation and muscle tension are observed without labeling one as "good" and desirable and the other as "bad" and undesirable. The meditative mind is equally at ease with both tension and relaxation. Muscle relaxation and states of serenity are often reported and are natural outcomes of the mindful body scan, but they are *not* preset goals that a practitioner strives to attain.

Teaching The Mindful Body Scan

The mindful body scan is a form of meditation. As with any meditation practice, extensive personal experience is required before presenting it in a group setting.

Experience with mind-body therapies such as yoga or Feldenkrais enhances a practitioner's skill in teaching this practice. If you include this practice in your program and ask participants to perform the practice 6 days a week, you should do the practice 6 days a week along with them. Your personal experience of this practice and its transformative effects in your own life will directly affect the skill and effectiveness you bring to your teaching.

The exercise is verbally delivered in a manner that promotes the control and power of the participants. That is, active commands are minimized and the participle form of the verb is used. For example, instead of "Now, bring your awareness to your right foot," the instructor guides, "Now, *bringing* your awareness to your right foot." In the former, the power is in the instructor's hands as he or she tells participants what to do. In the latter, more power remains with the participants as they are guided, not commanded, to move the focus of their awareness. This may appear to be a small and subtle change in language, yet it is an important one that supports participant control.

Another phrase that promotes participant control is "I'll now *invite you* to bring your awareness to your right foot." Again, the instructor is not voicing a command, but rather an invitation.

Following is a script for the mindful body scan exercise. For clinicians with no previous experience of mindfulness meditation, it is presented as an introduction to the practice. Because it is difficult to experience the full benefit of the exercise while reading the text, you may ask a colleague to read it to you or make a cassette or CD recording of the text for later listening. In addition, professional recordings of this exercise are available. Sources for these are listed at the end of this chapter.

For the clinician who is experienced in mindfulness meditation, the following script introduces one approach to guiding the exercise. It is not meant as a formula to be parroted. The delivery of this material in a group is unique to both the presenter and the moment in which it is presented. Its power and effectiveness come from the combination of the depth of the clinician's personal experience and the present moment presentation. Depending on the time available and the pace, this exercise requires 30 to 40 minutes.

The script begins with a mindfulness of breathing exercise and then guides participants to bring mindful awareness to different body areas. It guides participants to imagine breathing into and out from these body regions. Upon completing a scan of the entire body, participants are invited to rest their awareness with their experience of the body and experience a sense of wholeness and completeness.

Guided Script for the Mindful Body Scan Exercise

Close your eyes. As you observe your experience, whatever it might be, experiment with meeting yourself with a quality of fundamental kindness and self-acceptance. Your body is doing the very best it can, and there is no need to judge yourself or your experience as good or bad, right or wrong.

During this exercise, at some point you might find your mind wandering. Maybe you find yourself planning tomorrow or thinking about something that happened yesterday. When this happens, simply observe that your mind has wandered and return your attention to your breathing and the instructions.

Observing your breathing. As you inhale, simply feeling what part of your body moves as you inhale. As you exhale, simply feeling what part of your body moves as you exhale. Focusing your awareness on your present moment experience.

And now, letting your awareness rest with your belly, as you breathe in, allowing your breath to move deeply into your lungs and your stomach to gently rise. As you breathe out, allowing your stomach to gently fall.

Perhaps you have had the experience of resting on a raft on the ocean and felt the raft gently rising and falling as each wave passes by. Observing diaphragmatic breathing is somewhat similar. Instead of experiencing the gentle rise and fall of the raft with each passing ocean wave, you are observing the rise and fall of your stomach and rib cage with each wave of the breath. It is a calming and peaceful rhythm. Breathing in, breathing out.

As you observe your experience, experiment with letting go of any preconceived ideas you have about your body or expectations of how you think your body should feel or look. These are only concepts. They are just notions or ideas that may have little bearing on what is true and authentic about this human body. Letting them drop away. Observing your direct experience, just as it is.

Breathing in, aware of the in breath. Breathing out, aware of the out breath.

Now, shifting the focus of attention to the right foot. Becoming aware of whatever the feelings are in this area of the body. Just feeling the right foot as it is. You may feel warmth, coolness, or moisture. If you do not feel anything when you observe this region, then just notice this experience of not feeling anything.

And now moving your awareness to your right ankle. Becoming aware of whatever the feelings are in this area of the body. Feeling the ankle just as it is. And now moving your awareness to your right lower leg. Observing sensations in this area of the body.

And now moving your awareness to your right knee. Observing sensations in this area of the body. Just feeling the knee as it is. And now moving your awareness to your right thigh. Observing sensations in this area of the body. Listening as if for the first time to the sensations arising from your right thigh. And observing your right hip.

Observing your entire right leg and foot. Bringing acceptance to your experience just as it is. And, as you breathe, you can imagine breathing into your right leg and foot and out from your right leg and foot. Your breath is like a gentle, healing, comforting river washing through your body. And now on the out breath, letting go of the right leg and foot and moving your awareness to your left foot.

Now, shifting the focus of attention to the left foot. Becoming aware of whatever the feelings are in this area of the body. Just feeling the left foot as it is.

You may feel warmth, coolness, or moisture. If you do not feel anything when you observe this region, then just notice this experience of not feeling anything. And now moving your awareness to your left ankle. Becoming aware of whatever the feelings are in this area of the body. Feeling the ankle just as it is.

And now moving your awareness to your left lower leg. Observing sensations in this area of the body. And now moving your awareness to your left knee. Observing sensations in this area of the body. Just feeling the knee as it is. And now moving your awareness to your left thigh. Observing sensations in this area of the body. Listening as if for the first time to the sensations arising from your left thigh. And observing your left hip.

Observing your entire left leg and foot. Meeting your experience with friendliness and compassion. Accepting your experience just as it is. And, as you breathe, you can imagine breathing into your left leg and foot and out from your left leg and foot. Your breath is like a gentle, healing, comforting river washing through your body.

And now on the out breath, letting go of the left leg and foot and moving your awareness to your lower torso. Observing your pelvis and genitals. Noticing the sensations arising from your buttocks. Observing your abdomen and the inner organs of your lower torso.

And, as you breathe, you can imagine breathing into your lower torso and out from your lower torso. Your breath is like a gentle, healing, comforting river washing through your body.

And now guiding your awareness to your back. Becoming aware of your entire back. Listening and observing, moment to moment, to the feelings and sensations arising in this part of your body. Now bringing present moment awareness to your lower back. And now observing the middle part of your back. And observing your upper back. Listening again to your entire back. Observing your back with nonjudging awareness. Listening with a beginner's mind, as if you were listening to your back for the first time.

And, as you breathe, you can imagine breathing into your back and out from your back. Your breath is like a gentle, healing, comforting river washing through your body.

And now, bringing this present moment awareness to your chest and rib cage. Listening and observing any sensations that arise here. Listening to this home of your heart, here in your chest. And, as you breathe, you can imagine breathing into your chest and rib cage and out from your chest and rib cage.

Now, shifting the focus of attention to the right arm and hand. Observing your hand on the right side. Becoming aware of whatever the sensations are in this area of the body. You may feel warmth, tingling, or coolness. Observing your hand, moment to moment.

And now moving your awareness to your right wrist. Becoming aware of whatever sensations are arising in this area of the body. Observing the wrist just as it is. And now moving your awareness to your right forearm. Observing sensations in this area of the body.

And now moving your awareness to your right elbow. Observing sensations in this area of the body. And now moving your awareness to your right upper arm. Observing sensations in this area of the body. Listening as if for the first time to the sensations arising from your right upper arm.

Observing your entire right arm and hand. Bringing acceptance to your experience just as it is. And, as you breathe, you can imagine breathing into your right arm and hand and out from your right arm and hand. Your breath is like a gentle, healing, comforting river washing through your body. And now on the out breath, letting go of the right hand and arm and moving your awareness to your left side, to your left hand and arm. Noticing how your left hand and arm feel compared to your right.

Now, shifting the focus of attention to the left hand. Becoming aware of whatever the feelings are in this area of the body. Just observing the left hand as it is. And now moving your awareness to your left wrist. Becoming aware of whatever the feelings are in this area of the body. Feeling the wrist just as it is.

And now moving your awareness to your left forearm. Observing sensations in this area of the body. And now moving your awareness to your left upper arm. Observing sensations in this area of the body. Listening as if for the first time to the sensations arising from your left upper arm.

Observing your entire arm and hand. Bringing acceptance to your experience just as it is. And, as you breathe, you can imagine breathing into your left arm and hand and out from your left hand and arm. Your breath is like a gentle, healing, comforting river washing through your body.

And now, bringing this present moment awareness to your shoulders. Noticing the sensation here. Does your right shoulder feel the same as your left or are there differences? Observing sensations, moment to moment.

And observing your neck. And, as you breathe, you can imagine breathing into your shoulders and neck and out from your neck and shoulders. Your breath is like a gentle, healing, comforting river washing through your body.

And now, observing your face. Noticing your jaw, the area around your mouth, your tongue. Bringing present moment awareness to your cheeks, your eyes. Noticing your forehead. Observing your ears and temples. Listening to the back of your head and the crown of your head. Now taking in the whole of your face and head. Listening in the here and now to sensations as they arise in this part of your body. And, as you breathe, you can imagine breathing into your face and head and out from your head and face.

And now, letting your awareness rest again with your breath. Aware of the in breath and aware of the out breath.

Now, observing the whole of your body from the soles of your feet to the crown of your head. Experiencing your body as a whole. Allowing your mind to rest in the present moment with your experience just as it is. Meeting your experience with an open heart and an open mind, with kindness and compassion. Letting yourself experience wholeness and completeness. Letting things just be, just as they are in each moment.

Allow for 2 to 5 minutes of silence.

You might ask yourself, "Who is doing the observing?"

Once again, observing your breathing. Now, gradually begin to bring your awareness back to the room and, when you are ready, allow your eyes to open. You may wish to wiggle your toes or stretch your legs gently. If you are lying on your back, please roll to one side. Rest on your side for a moment before pushing up to sitting.

People can experience a wide range of reactions to this exercise. Some are positive, whereas others can be very negative. It is essential that the instructor have personal experience in meditation and the mindful body scan in order to effectively respond to these reactions. Frequently people report feeling calm and relaxed. Many describe becoming aware of places in the body where they carry tension that, before the exercise, they did not notice. Others report that deep breathing was easier by the end of the exercise.

If several participants share positive experiences of the exercise, it is very important for the instructor to ask, "Who had problems with this exercise?" Often people who are having difficulty are reluctant to speak up when others are describing new insights and good feelings. They can feel isolated and confused, telling themselves, "Everyone else is getting this but me." It is important to draw them out and reassure them that the difficulties they are having are common and can be addressed.

Mindfully Responding to Pain

Rather than feeling calm and relaxed, people sometimes become more aware of physical pain, tension, or emotional distress. They feel worse, not better. If you were teaching relaxation exercises, this might be viewed as a problem, something to change or eliminate. In contrast, an instructor trained in mindfulness meditation meets this reaction that appears unwanted or unpleasant with acceptance and curiosity. It is not to be avoided or eliminated, but rather observed with the qualities of mindful awareness.

Some people with chronic pain initially experience an increase in pain with this practice. If they have coped with pain by constantly distracting themselves from it, the mindful body scan can initially heighten their awareness of pain. Clinicians must respond with understanding and confidence in the capacity of these people to experiment with responding to their pain in new ways. An example of a mindful response to pain is the following:

Think of a large garden. If a plant is in poor condition, you take time to examine it, notice the soil, the stalk and leaves, how much sunlight and water it receives. By paying attention, you can more effectively respond to caring for that plant. So too, by mindfully observing pain and your reaction to pain, you can gain insight and understanding of pain and your reactions to it. You can develop effective ways of responding to pain that can never occur if you are constantly distracted from the pain. I want to emphasize that this requires time and practice.

Observing your breathing. Letting your breath serve your mind as a foundation for your attention. Now allowing your awareness to observe the pain. If the pain is severe, this might occur for just a brief moment. Noticing physical qualities. Perhaps it feels hot or burning, maybe it is cold or tingling, maybe there's a sensation of vibration or oscillation. These sensations may alter and fluctuate. Observing just the pure physical sensation you label "pain." If it gets too difficult, return your awareness to your breath. Allowing your awareness to remain with your breath until you are ready to observe the pain again.

Now becoming aware of the thoughts you have about the pain. Perhaps you tell yourself, "I hate this pain" or "This pain has ruined my life." Recognize that these are thoughts *about* pain. They are not the pain itself, but rather a story you tell yourself about the pain. Bringing awareness to the story. As thoughts arise, observe them, accept them. Observing the story and recognizing the difference between the direct physical sensation of pain and thoughts about the pain. Returning to your breath whenever you need to.

Now becoming aware of the feelings you have about the pain. Maybe you feel angry or frightened or confused. Recognize these as the feelings you have in *reaction* to the pain. Again there is a difference between the direct sensation of pain and how you feel in reaction to the pain. The physical sensation of pain is one thing. Your emotional reaction to the pain is something else.

Observing all of this with kindness, compassion, and self-acceptance. Do not judge yourself or your experience. Do not try to change your experience in any way. With very stable attention, observe the pain and your reaction to it. Assuming the position of an impartial witness, watching sensations, thoughts, and feelings.

The outcome of bringing mindful awareness to the experience of pain can be quite powerful, as the following example demonstrates:

Case Example 3.14.

Julie was a 74-year-old woman with severe arthritis. Her main complaint was that her pain woke her up at night. She remained awake, tense, anxious, and unable to return to sleep. At first, she was reluctant to bring mindful awareness to her pain. She worried that her pain would increase. With practice, her attitude changed. She commented, "When I looked into the pain, I saw there was the sensation of pain and my fear of the pain. The fear was making my situation even more difficult. I said to myself, 'I've been dealing with this pain for 10 years, what is there to be frightened of? Focus on the now.'

"This gave me a kind of confidence. The fear left me and I wasn't so tense. I focused on breathing with the pain. Now I use this technique every night. Sometimes I fall back asleep. Other times it is still very uncomfortable, but I am not so tense and anxious about it. Some part of me is very calm even though I am in pain. The part of me that is relaxed and calm is stronger than the pain."

As Julie's example demonstrates, mindfulness of pain can be an effective strategy to strengthen a person's insight and confidence. A central tenet of this whole approach is that the clinician continually meets people with compassion and acceptance just as they are, and when they are experiencing something unpleasant or difficult, helps them find in themselves the courage and capacity to examine it with mindful awareness. This approach inherently affirms that which is good, positive, capable, and healthy already within the individual. This process is not easy. A teacher must have personal experience with mindfulness in order to have this level of confidence in others.

One Thanksgiving morning while listening to a public radio special broadcast, I was struck by a powerful metaphor for the mindful examination of difficult circumstances unknowingly shared by one of the speakers. Charles Laughton, the British actor, was discussing his friendship with the sculptor, Thomas Moore. He described asking Moore to reveal his inspiration for the circular form found in many of his sculptures. Moore replied, "I was cutting so deeply into the heart of the stone, I found the sky on the other side." This image mirrors the application of mindfulness to the experience of pain and other unpleasant, unwanted experiences. At first glance, they may appear cold, hard, dark, and impenetrable; however, by continuing to look deeply into that which we find unpleasant and unwanted, a profound shift in experience and insight can occur. We can, in a sense, discover the sky on the other side.

Home Exercise Program

If a clinician is choosing this approach, the regular practice of the body scan exercise is an important component of a home exercise plan. An instructor may choose to professionally record a cassette tape or CD that can be used daily by class participants. Body scan tapes and CDs are also commercially available. To promote adherence, participants can be provided with a daily log in which they record their experience of the exercise.

Summary

Mindfulness means present moment awareness or paying attention. Awareness is important to maintain health, prevent injury, maximize rehabilitation potential, minimize the distress of unpleasant medical treatments, cope with chronic pain and illness, and enhance quality of life. The qualities of mindful awareness include present moment attention, fundamental kindness, nonjudging, nonstriving, accepting, not knowing, and letting go. Mindful breathing exercises are a powerful strategy that can be easily integrated into a wellness program. They emphasize diaphragmatic breathing, concentration, and present moment observation of physical sensations, thoughts, and feelings. They ensure optimal respiratory function, facilitate relaxation, build body awareness, and promote self-control. They can be effectively integrated into daily activities to control the body's stress reaction and manage symptoms.

The mindful body scan exercise teaches people how to listen to the body in a positive and health-promoting manner. It is guided in a manner that encourages participant control. It includes mindful breathing, scanning the body with mindful awareness, and a closing period of rest during which a feeling of wholeness and completeness is introduced. In addition, these exercises can be further developed into a practice of mindfulness meditation. The growing interest in the medical applications of mindfulness meditation among health researchers, clinicians, and the public offers new opportunities for health care practitioners to train in meditation and integrate this practice into healthcare services.

References

1. Faucett J. Depression in painful chronic disorders: The role of pain and conflict about pain. *J Pain Symptom Manage* 1994;9(8):524.
2. Kabat-Zinn J. *Full Catastrophe Living: Using the Wisdom of Your Body and Mind to Face Stress, Pain and Illness.* New York: Delacorte Press, 1990.
3. Gunaratana H: *Mindfulness in Plain English.* Boston: Wisdom Publications, 1994.
4. McCracken LM. Learning to live with pain: acceptance of pain predicts adjustment in persons with chronic pain. *Pain* 1998;74:21-27.
5. *Webster's New Collegiate Dictionary.* Springfield, Mass: G & C Merriam Co., 1974, p. 714.
6. Wetzel MS, Eisenberg DM et al. Courses involving complementary and alternative medicine at US medical schools. *JAMA* 1998 Sep 2;280(9): 784-787.
7. Eisenberg DM, Davis RB et al. Trends in alternative medicine use in the United States, 1990-1997: Results of a follow-up national survey. *JAMA* 1998;280(18):1569-1575.
8. Gordon NP, Sobel DS, Tarazona EZ. Use of and interest in alternative therapies among adult primary care clinicians and adult members in a large health maintenance organization. *West J Med* 1998 Sep;169(3): 153-161.
9. Davidson RJ, Kabat-Zinn J, Schumacher J et al. Alterations in brain and immune function produced by mindfulness meditation. *Psychosomatic Medicine,* 2003 (in press).
10. Davidson R, Abercrombie H, Nitschke JB, Putnam K. Regional brain function and disorders of emotion. *Curr Opin Neurobiol* 1999;9(2): 228-234.
11. Lazar S, Bush G et al. Functional brain mapping of the relaxation response and meditation. *Neuroreport* 2000 May 15;11(7): 1581-1585.

12. Sudsuang R, Chentanez V, Veluvan K. Effect of Buddhist meditation on serum cortisol and total protein level, blood pressure, pulse rate, lung volume and reaction time. *Physiol Behav* 1991 Sep;50(3):543-548.
13. Tooley GA, Armstrong SM et al. Acute increases in nighttime plasma melatonin levels following a period of meditation. *Biol Psychol* 2000 May;53(1):69-78.
14. Patel C, Marmot MG et al. Trial of relaxation in reducing coronary risk: four year follow up. *Br Med J* 1985 Apr 13;290(6475):1103-1106.
15. Kabat-Zinn J, Lipworth L, Burney R. The clinical use of mindfulness meditation in the self-regulation of chronic pain. *J Behav Med* 1985;8(2):163-190.
16. Speca M, Carlson LE et al. A randomized, wait-list controlled clinical trial: the effect of a mindfulness-based stress reduction program on mood and symptoms of stress in cancer outpatients. *Psychosomatic Medicine* 2000 Sept-Oct;62(5):613-622.
17. Singh BB, Berman BM et al. A pilot study of cognitive behavioral therapy in fibromyalgia. *Altern Ther Health Med* 1998 Mar;4(2):67-70.
18. Mills N, Allen J. Mindfulness of movement as a coping strategy in multiple sclerosis: a pilot study. *Gen Hosp Psych* 2000;22:425-431.
19. Williams KA, Kolar MM et al. Evaluation of a wellness-based mindfulness stress reduction intervention: a controlled trial. *Am J Health Promot* 2001;15(6):422-432.
20. Santorelli SF. Mindfulness-Based Stress Reduction: Qualifications and Recommended Guidelines for Providers. In Kabat-Zinn J, Santorelli SF (eds); *Mindfulness-Based Stress Reduction Professional Training: Resource Manual.* Worcester, Mass, Center for Mindfulness in Medicine, Health Care and Society, 1999.
21. Reid WD, Dechman G. Considerations when testing and training the respiratory muscles. *Phys Ther* 1995 Nov;75(11):971-974.

Annotated Bibliography

Farhi D. *The Breathing Book: Good Health and Vitality Through Essential Breath Work.* New York: Henry Holt, 1996. Yoga instructor Donna Farhi presents a thorough, simple, and practical guide to breathing techniques. This accessible and comprehensive manual provides basic information on respiratory anatomy and mechanics and offers exercises to increase awareness of breathing and promote a healthy breathing pattern. This text is especially useful to the clinician who is new to breathing exercises and instruction.

Gunaratana H. *Mindfulness in Plain English.* Boston: Wisdom Publications, 1994. The Venerable Henepola Gunaratana, ordained as a Buddhist monk at the age of 12, holds a Ph.D. in philosophy. In this text, he offers an accessible, straightforward introduction to mindfulness meditation in very simple language. He provides a clear exploration of what meditation is and isn't, describes the practice of meditation, and makes suggestions for responding to the common problems people experience. Using examples that the reader can easily relate to daily life, he offers a convincing description of the powerful and practical applications of mindfulness meditation to living in the modern world.

Kabat-Zinn J. *Full Catastrophe Living: Using the Wisdom of Your Body and Mind to Face Stress, Pain and Illness.* New York: Delacorte Press, 1990. This book describes in detail a nationally recognized mindfulness-based stress reduction group program founded and taught at the University of Massachusetts Medical Center and School since 1979. Kabat-Zinn offers a thorough examination of mindfulness and its practical application to the circumstances of people living with chronic medical conditions. The many experiences of participants in the program described in this text offer a rich perspective and valuable insight into the direct application of mindfulness to the care of people with chronic medical conditions.

Kabat-Zinn J. *Wherever You Go, There You Are: Mindfulness Meditation in Everyday Life.* New York: Hyperion, 1994. With great clarity, humor, and wisdom, Kabat-Zinn introduces mindfulness as an activity that can be easily integrated into everyday life. He offers practical information on meditation practices and provides relevant anecdotes to demonstrate how mindfulness can be applied to common daily activities. A delightful and insightful book, this is a wonderful introduction to mindfulness.

Langer EJ. *Mindfulness.* Cambridge, Mass: Perseus Books, 1989. Ellen Langer, Ph.D., a Professor of Psychology at Harvard, draws on her extensive research experience to explore mindfulness from the perspective of Western science. She begins by examining how mind*less*ness in daily life undermines our potential and well-being and creates problems and suffering. She leads the reader from an investigation of mindlessness to an examination of the role of mindfulness in living and learning. Clinicians with an interest in geriatrics will find her research with seniors of special interest.

Nhat Hanh T. *Peace Is Every Step: the Path of Mindfulness in Everyday Life.* New York: Bantam Books, 1991. Thich Nhat Hanh is a Zen master and teacher who was nominated for the Nobel Peace Prize in 1967 by Martin Luther King, Jr. for his tireless efforts for peace during the Vietnam War. Through meditations, personal anecdotes, and stories from his life as a peace activist, he shows how mindfulness can be brought to small acts of daily living and to difficult circumstances to promote healing, well-being, and peace. He reminds the reader that peace is as close as each step taken. Beautifully written, this book is an accessible and inspiring introduction to mindfulness.

Resources

For Guided Meditation CDs

www.carolynmcmanus.com: Meditation and relaxation CDs by the author

For Mindfulness in Medicine

The Center for Mindfulness in Medicine, Health Care and Society
University of Massachusetts Medical School
Shaw Building, 55 Lake Ave. North
Worcester, MA 01655
(508) 856-2256
www.umassmed.edu/cfm/

For Mindfulness Meditation Instruction

Many groups and organizations provide training in mindfulness meditation. Following are five well-established and well-respected organizations. Contemplative Outreach Ltd., offers meditation instruction within a Christian religious tradition. The other four groups offer meditation instruction within a Buddhist tradition.

Contemplative Outreach Ltd.
P.O. Box 737
Butler, NJ 07405
(937) 838-3384
www.centeringprayer.com

Insight Meditation Society
1230 Pleasant St.
Barre, MA 01005
(978) 355-4378
www.dharma.org

Green Mountain Dharma Center
P.O. Box 182
Hartland-Four-Corners, VT 05409
(802) 436-1103
www.plumvillage.org

Spirit Rock Meditation Center
P.O. Box 169
Woodacre, CA 94937
(415) 488-0164
www.spiritrock.org

Deer Park Monastery
2499 Melru Lane
Escondido, CA 92026
(760) 291-1003
www.plumvillage.org

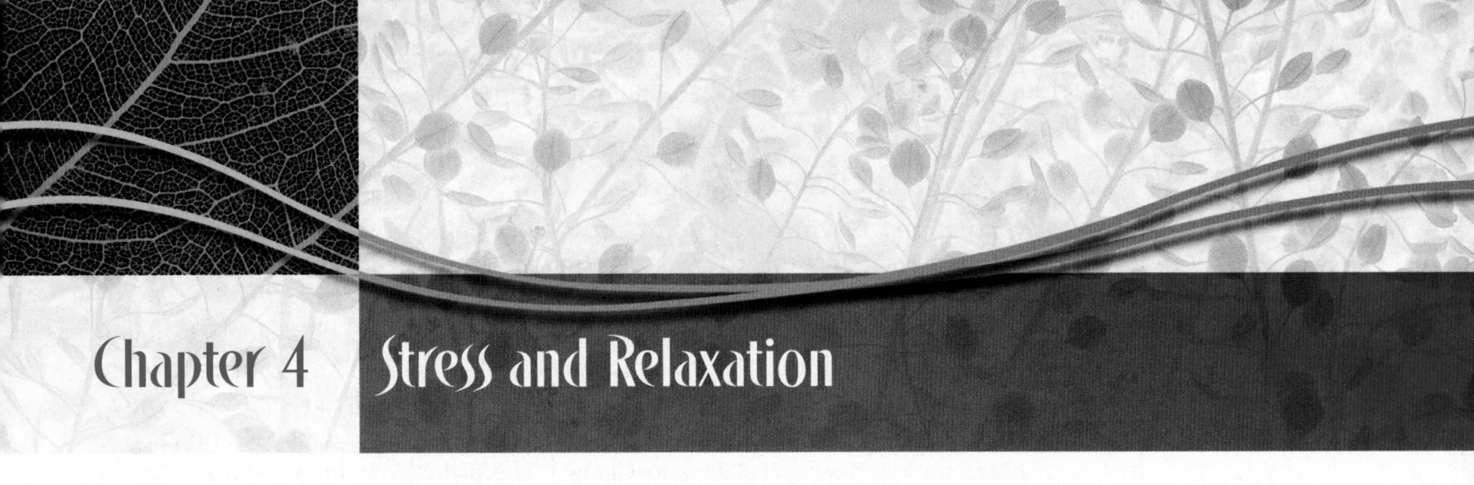

Chapter 4 Stress and Relaxation

Medical evidence suggests that stress and stress management interventions influence the course of several medical conditions. This chapter offers an overview of the stress reaction and identifies the roles that stress and stress management interventions play in cardiovascular disease, diabetes, immune system function, wound healing, and musculoskeletal pain. Relaxation and guided imagery exercises are described. Suggestions for dealing with the difficulties people sometimes experience with these exercises are discussed. A specific class structure for teaching these topics in a group program is presented.

Overview of the Stress Reaction

You are already running late when you notice your next patient is new and scheduled for only 30 minutes instead of the standard 45 minutes. You complain to the secretary and hope the person has a simple problem. You step into the room and as introductions are exchanged, you realize the person does not speak English and is joined by a translator. They begin a complex story of car accidents, surgeries, and previous treatment.

This scene would likely lead to a stress reaction in a busy health care professional. Although mentally you attempt to set priorities, physically your body readies for a fist-fight or sprint to the exit. Your neck, shoulder, and back muscles tense. Your breath becomes shallow. Your heart rate increases and blood pressure rises. Digestion slows as blood is drawn away from the stomach and intestines and is directed to major muscle groups. You prepare to fight or run for survival just as your Stone Age ancestors once did.

Although the challenges and adversities we face today are far different from those of our cave-dwelling predecessors, our biology is unchanged. We remain physiologically equipped to deal with stress that is short-lived and resolved by running or fighting. The long-term and complex stress of modern life can cause the chronic activation of the body's alarm mechanism, increasing the risk for diseases and exacerbating existing medical conditions.

Stress is a household word commonly used to describe the pressures and demands we face in daily life. It is used to describe an internal experience, as in the expression, "I feel stressed." It is also used to describe an external circumstance, as in the comment, "My job is stressful." Stress is best understood as the interaction of both internal and external factors. It is the result of a situation *and* a person's individual reaction to the situation.

Not all stress is negative. Life constantly presents changes and challenges that promote learning, growth, and optimal functioning. People successfully respond and adapt to many of life's changes and challenges; however, when people lose their capacity to successfully respond and adapt, a condition of chronic negative stress results.

The body's physical reaction to stress was first described and labeled "fight or flight" by Walter Cannon in the 1920s.[1] In the 1930s Hans Selye formalized this concept and borrowed the term stress from engineering to describe animals' adaptive responses to extreme conditions.[2] Selye also identified a relationship between chronic stress and disease states.

Under conditions of homeostasis, the body maintains a physiological equilibrium primarily through a dynamic balance of actions of the sympathetic and parasympathetic nervous systems. A perceived threat results in increased sympathetic nervous system (SNS) activity. The following overview of SNS function is based on a review by Petzke and Clauw.[3] The principle components driving the stress reaction are the neural and adrenomedullary elements of the SNS and the hypothalamic-pituitary-adrenal (HPA) axis. The neural component of the SNS consists of nerve networks innervating the cardiovascular system, reticuloendothelial organs, and salivary and sweat glands. The primary neurotransmitter released by this system is norepinephrine. The adrenomedullary component of the SNS response consists of the adrenal medulla and its neurotransmitter, epinephrine. Together, norepinephrine and epinephrine increase heart rate, respiratory rate, and shunt blood flow to major muscles. They promote the release of glucose from the liver and relax visceral muscles, decreasing digestive tract activity. Epinephrine and norepinephrine act within seconds of the onset of a stress reaction.

The HPA axis regulates release of glucocorticoids, including cortisol, from the adrenal cortex. This response begins with the discharge of corticotropin-releasing hormone by the hypothalamus, which triggers corticotropin release from the pituitary. Corticotropin in turn acts on the adrenal cortex to stimulate the release of glucocorticoids. Glucocorticoids increase blood sugar release from the liver, inhibit insulin production, inhibit vitamin D activity necessary for calcium uptake by bone, decrease digestive tract activity, and inhibit immune system function. Glucocorticoids act within minutes or hours of the onset of a stress reaction. In addition, the pituitary secretes vasopression, an antidiuretic hormone, and the pancreas releases glucagon that acts to increase blood sugar levels.

Disruption and damage to the body's equilibrium and health occur when this reaction, which is designed for short-term activation, becomes a long-term physiological condition.

Stress and Disease

Considerable medical evidence identifies stress as an influencing factor in the course of several medical conditions, including cardiovascular disease, diabetes, immune system function, wound healing, and musculoskeletal pain. A detailed discussion of this evidence is beyond the scope of this text. The role stress may play in these conditions is briefly examined in the following sections. Studies exploring the application of relaxation exercises and stress management in treatment are noted. The intent is to provide a brief introduction to the role of stress and stress management in these conditions. For a more thorough examination of this topic, see the annotated bibliography at the end of this chapter.

Cardiovascular Disease

Convincing medical evidence exists for the significant role of stress in the pathogenesis and progression of cardiovascular disease.[4,5] The stress-induced release of catecholamines and corticosteroids results in increases in heart rate, cardiac output, blood pressure, platelet aggregation, and blood viscosity.[6] In those patients already diagnosed with coronary artery disease, these combined changes may promote the progression of atherosclerosis and increase the risk of myocardial ischemia, coronary thrombosis, and myocardial infarction.[7]

Sensitive imaging techniques in laboratory studies demonstrate an association between acute mental or negative emotional stress and the incidence of myocardial ischemia.[8-10] Anger may play an especially potent role in provoking ischemia.[11,12] One proposed mechanism for these occurrences is stress-induced arterial vasospasm.[8,9] Excessive SNS activation may also precipitate a decrease in the electrical stability of the heart during acute stress and increase the occurrence of cardiac dysrhythmias.[10] A relationship has been identified between myocardial ischemia induced by mental stress and subsequent clinical events, including cardiac death, myocardial infarction, coronary artery bypass surgery, and angioplasty.[14,15]

In most studies examining stress management and heart disease, relaxation exercises are a component of a multiple strategy program. In one study, however, Grossman et al examined the effectiveness of breathing exercises alone on reducing blood pressure.[16] Thirty-three patients with uncontrolled blood pressure were randomly assigned to an intervention or control group. The two groups were matched by initial blood pressure, age, gender, body mass index, and medication. The intervention group practiced 10 minutes of musically guided breathing exercises daily for 8 weeks. Both in-clinic and at-home blood pressure measurements were significantly lower in the intervention group. The at-home data showed an average decline in blood pressure of −5.0/−2.7 mm Hg in the intervention group, whereas the changes in the control group were −1.2/+0.9. Although additional research is warranted, this preliminary evidence suggests that the daily practice of simple breathing exercises may benefit some people with elevated blood pressure.

Present evidence supports a role for comprehensive stress management programs in the treatment of patients with heart disease. In a meta-analysis of 23 controlled trials evaluating stress management programs that included relaxation exercises along with patient education, cognitive restructuring, and/or problem solving, reductions in blood pressure, heart rate, serum cholesterol levels, and psychological distress were identified.[17] In one study, Blumenthal et al compared outcomes of exercise, stress management, and usual treatment in cardiac patients with myocardial ischemia.[18] One hundred seven patients with coronary artery disease and documented stress or exercise-induced ischemia were randomly assigned to a 4-month stress management or exercise group. The stress management intervention included progressive relaxation, patient education, and cognitive restructuring. Patients living a distance from the facility comprised the control care group. Nine percent of the stress management group, 21% of the exercise group, and 30% of the control group experienced combined fatal and nonfatal infarctions or angina requiring coronary revascularization during a follow-up period of 5 years. These data suggest that relaxation exercises, when combined with a multistrategy stress management program, benefit cardiac patients with evidence of myocardial ischemia.

Diabetes

Insulin resistance increases in response to the release of stress hormones. In people with diabetes, changes in glucose levels resulting from increases in stress hormones vary considerably from person to person.[19-22] For some, an increase in glucose levels takes place. For others, a decrease occurs.

Glycemic control in individuals with diabetes depends on the complex relationship of meal planning, exercise, and medication compliance. Stress can indirectly affect metabolic control by triggering maladaptive coping responses, including poor diet and lack of exercise.

Research examining the role of relaxation exercises in diabetes treatment is minimal.[23-26] The few studies examining the role of relaxation exercises as an isolated intervention in Type 2 diabetes have demonstrated no consistent effects on glycemic control.[24,25] Using a design that combined progressive relaxation exercises with other stress management strategies, Surwit et al found a small improvement in metabolic control in people with Type 2 diabetes.[26]

Regular exercise and proper diet are key self-management interventions in the treatment of diabetes. High stress levels are associated with decreased adherence to exercise and healthy eating habits. As a treatment intervention, stress management may help people with diabetes to decrease stress levels and minimize the use of poor coping responses that undermine adherence to regular exercise and proper diet.

Immune System Function

The body's mechanisms for fighting disease and infection are highly intricate and complex, involving cells originating in bone marrow, thymus, and lymph nodes. For a description of the immune system and its actions, the reader is referred to an excellent review article by Cohen and Herbert and texts listed in the annotated bibliography at the end of this chapter.[27]

In a meta-analysis of the medical literature on stress and human immunity, Herbert and Cohen conclude that substantial evidence exists for a relationship between stress and decreases in functional immune measures, including decreases in peripheral responses to mitogens and in natural killer cell activity.[28] They also identify an association between stress and decreases in numbers and percentages of circulating white blood cells and immunoglobulin levels. They conclude that specific health consequences of these changes in immune measures have not been established.

In a meta-analysis and critique of relaxation exercises and additional psychological interventions on immune response, Miller and Cohen conclude that only modest evidence exists for the hypothesis that these interventions have a positive impact on immune measures.[29] Relaxation exercises alone showed little capacity to promote immune changes, while disclosure and stress management programs demonstrated only scattered success. Findings indicated that hypnosis with immune system suggestion had some success in modulating immune system response. In addition, conditioning interventions yielded immune system changes. Conditioning interventions involve administering a neutral stimulus followed by an immune-modulating agent. This pairing is repeated for several days, after which the neutral stimulus is presented alone. The expected outcome is for the subject to respond to the neutral stimulus as if the immune-modulating agent had been administered. Preliminary findings suggest that conditioning interventions can increase natural killer cell cytotoxicity.

In addition, the authors of this analysis concluded that no evidence supports the claim that relaxation exercises alone or other psychological interventions promote improved immune measures in medical populations; however, Miller and Cohen suggest that although the literature on the whole remains unsupportive, under certain conditions, specific interventions may have some capacity to bring about consistent immune changes. In one provocative study, Antoni et al examined the effects of a multistrategy stress management intervention on anxious mood, perceived stress, 24-hour urinary catecholamine levels, and changes in T lymphocyte subpopulation cell counts in symptomatic HIV-positive men.[30]

Seventy-three men were randomly assigned to a 10-week group intervention or a wait-list control group. The weekly classes included 45 minutes of relaxation exercises and 90 minutes of additional stress management strategies. At posttreatment and 6- and 12-month follow-up, the intervention group demonstrated significant reductions in anxiety, mood disturbance, perceived stress, and had less norepinephrine output compared with controls. Greater decreases in norepinephrine output and greater frequency of practicing relaxation exercises at home during the intervention were associated with higher T lymphocyte subpopulation cell counts at follow-up. These results, although preliminary, suggest that interventions that teach people to relax, develop effective coping strategies, and experience greater mastery may decrease anxious mood and offer immune system benefits in a medical population.

Although relaxation exercises have not been shown to influence immune measures in cancer patients, they have been shown to significantly reduce nausea and vomiting during chemotherapy treatment.[31] It has been suggested that psychological in addition to pharmacological reactions may account for these side effects to chemotherapy treatment.[32] As many as 60% of patients receiving antiemetics for treating nausea and vomiting continue to experience nausea.[33] Nausea and vomiting can cause electrolyte imbalance, dehydration, and nutritional deficiencies and can contribute to decreases in function and quality of life. Relaxation exercises may serve as a simple self-management resource for people to decrease these treatment side effects during chemotherapy.

Wound Healing

Several research studies have shown that stress slows wound healing.[34-36] One proposed mechanism for this impaired healing process is a stress-induced decrease in levels of pro-inflammatory cytokines, central to the early stages of wound repair, at the wound site.[36-38] These studies and analyses have been conducted by the same principle investigators and need to be replicated by others to confirm the validity and reliability of results.

Rarely have studies been conducted that explore the effects of relaxation exercises on wound healing. In one study examining the effects of relaxation and guided imagery on healing following cholecystectomy, however, those patients who listened to a relaxation and guided imagery audiotape demonstrated less anxiety, lower cortisol levels postsurgery, and less surgical wound erythema than the control group.[39] Although further research is warranted, this finding suggests that surgical patients may benefit from practicing relaxation exercises before and after surgery. Relaxation exercise instruction offered in a group class format may help some people facing surgery to optimize healing and minimize distress.

Musculoskeletal Pain

The etiology and prognosis for musculoskeletal disorders is multifactorial and includes the complex interaction of physical and psychological factors. Among these factors, stress is consistently identified as playing a role in the onset and prognosis of musculoskeletal pain.[40-47] Psychological stress may double later risk for low-back pain.[48] The specific physiological mechanism by which stress impacts musculoskeletal pain is not well understood. Sustained SNS activity causing abnormal muscle function is one proposed pathway.[47] Researchers suggest that chronic activation of the SNS may induce the constant activation of motor units and block normal patterns of rest and recovery, leading to pain. In addition, acute stress may cause excessive activation of motor units with activity and increase the risk of injury.[49] In fibromyalgia, research has suggested that dysregulation of the HPA axis may be a factor in symptom development.[50]

In studies examining musculoskeletal pain treatment, relaxation exercises are often a component of a comprehensive stress or self-management program.[51-53] These exercises may be most effective when taught in combination with other treatment strategies.[54] In one study, Halroyd et al examined the efficacy of three sessions of relaxation exercise instruction and cognitive therapy in the treatment of chronic tension headaches.[53] Two hundred three adults were randomly assigned to receive stress management training, a tricyclic antidepressant, or a combination of stress management and medication. Stress management training and antidepressant medication were each effective at significantly reducing headache pain. When combined, they produced the greatest reductions in headache pain.

Self-Managing the Stress Reaction

Mindfulness meditation, described in Chapter 3, is a powerful strategy to observe and develop skills to self-manage the stress reaction. It enables people to pay attention in a nonreactive manner to their physical, cognitive, and emotional responses to stress. With practice, it promotes the discovery of an inner stability in the midst of changing physical sensations, thoughts, and emotions. This awareness often produces a shift in understanding or new insight and makes it possible for a person to respond to stress in new ways.

In addition, relaxation exercises promote a decrease of the fight-or-flight response and are a common component of chronic illness self-management programs. Providing instruction in relaxation to groups does not require the years of practice that is recommended to teach mindfulness meditation. Education in many health care disciplines includes instruction in relaxation exercises, and most clinicians feel confident in teaching these strategies without additional training. Any teacher of relaxation should have personal experience with the techniques and their practical application to symptom management and daily life.

Relaxation exercises include diaphragmatic breathing, progressive relaxation, autogenic training, relaxation body scan, and guided imagery.

Teaching Relaxation Exercises

People should be as comfortable as possible for these exercises. Avoid letting the room temperature grow cool. What is too hot for one person is often too cool for the next, so remind people to dress in layers. These exercises can be done sitting or supine. If mats are available, people may want to lie down for progressive relaxation, autogenic training, relaxation body scan, and guided imagery exercises (Figure 4-1). If supine is a particularly difficult position for a participant, side lying or sitting in a chair are options. If mats are not available, these exercises can also be done with group members sitting. Performing the exercises while sitting is also a good reminder that relaxation can be done in any posture. Lying down is not a prerequisite for relaxation.

Diaphragmatic Breathing

For a detailed description of diaphragmatic breathing exercises, see Chapter 3. Breathing exercises one through three described in Chapter 3 can easily be adapted to relaxation instruction. Exercises one and two build body awareness and the skill

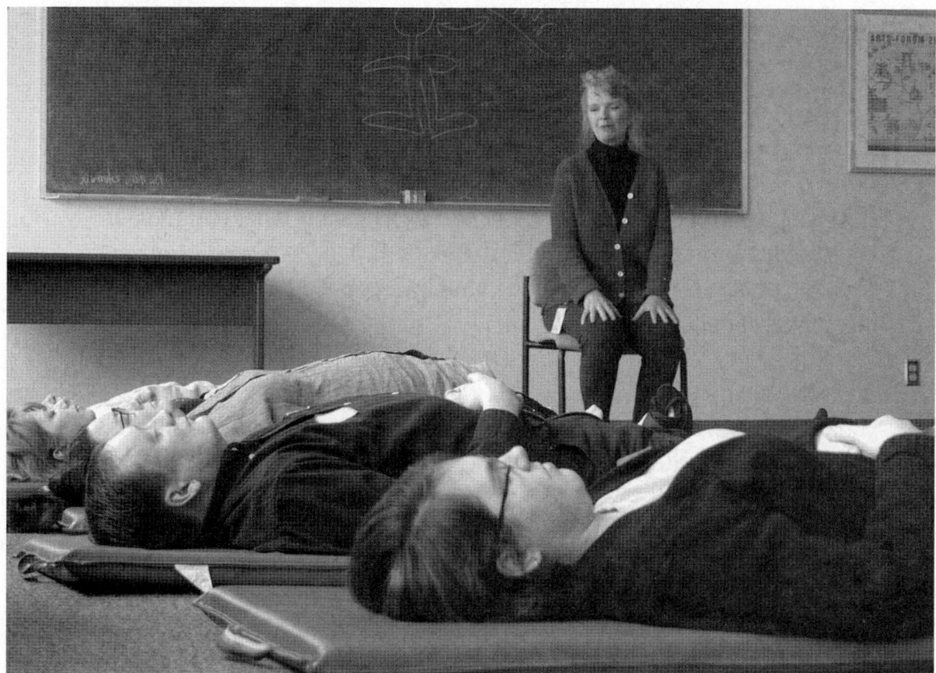

Figure 4-1 Participants practice relaxation exercises.

of diaphragmatic breathing. Exercise three invites people to choose a word or phrase to repeat to themselves in concert with their breath. People can choose calming single or multiple word phrases, such as "peace," "I grow calm," or their own name followed by the phrase "let go." The goal of repeating calming verbal cues is to cultivate a sensation of physical relaxation.

Progressive Relaxation

Edmund Jacobsen, a Chicago physician, developed a series of exercises in the 1920s designed to teach muscle awareness and relaxation.[55] These exercises progress through the body and involve contracting and relaxing different muscle groups. They are especially helpful to people who have little or no body awareness and who may not be aware of the chronic patterns of tension they carry. Because of the active nature of the exercises, they can also be helpful to people who have difficulty sitting still or concentrating.

Guided Script for Progressive Relaxation

In this exercise you will be guided to tense and then relax different muscle groups throughout your body. This exercise builds body awareness and gently guides you into a state of relaxation. It is important to tense muscles only as is comfortable for you. It is okay to be gentle as you tense your muscles. Avoid overdoing it and tensing muscles in an aggressive manner that might cause you pain or discomfort.

Close your eyes. As you observe your experience, whatever it might be, experiment with meeting yourself with a quality of fundamental kindness and self-acceptance.

During this exercise, at some point you might find your mind wandering. Maybe you find yourself planning tomorrow or thinking about something that happened yesterday. When this happens, simply observe that your mind has wandered and return your attention to your breathing and the instructions.

Observing your breathing. As you inhale, simply feeling what part of your body moves as you inhale. As you exhale, simply feeling what part of your body moves as you exhale. Focusing your awareness on your present moment experience.

And now, letting your awareness rest with your belly, as you breathe in, allow your breath to move deep into your lungs and your stomach to gently rise. As you breathe out, allow your stomach to gently fall.

Imagine resting on a raft on the ocean and experience the raft gently rising and falling as each wave passes by. Observing diaphragmatic breathing is somewhat similar. Instead of experiencing the gentle rise and fall of the raft with each passing ocean wave, you are observing the rise and fall of your stomach and rib cage with each wave of the breath. It is a calming and peaceful rhythm. Breathing in, breathing out.

As you observe your experience, let go of any preconceived ideas you have about your body or expectations of how you think your body should feel or look. These are only concepts. Letting them drop away. Observing your body, just as it is.

Breathing in, aware of the in breath. Breathing out, aware of the out breath.

Now, shifting the focus of attention to your right hand. Become aware of whatever the feelings are in this area of the body. Now, gently make a fist with your right hand. Hold the tension. Breathe deeply. Observe sensations of tension in your hand. And relax. Observe sensations of relaxation. And again, make a fist, hold the tension, breathe, and relax. Once more, make a fist, breathe, observe the sensation of tension, and relax. And observe the sensation of relaxation in your hand.

Now, make a fist with your right hand and gently bring it up to your shoulder, tensing the muscles in your upper arm. Hold the tension, notice how this feels in your upper arm, breathe, and relax. Letting your arm return to rest at your side. Once again, make a fist and bring it up toward your shoulder, hold the tension, breathe deeply, and relax. And again, bring your fist toward your shoulder, hold, breathe, and relax. Notice the feelings of relaxation in your hand, forearm, and upper arm.

And now bring your awareness to your left hand and arm. Observe how your left hand and arm feel compared with your right. Now, make a fist with your left hand and gently bring it up to your shoulder, tensing the muscles in your upper arm. Hold the tension, notice how this feels in your upper arm, breathe, and relax. Letting your arm return to rest at your side. Once again, make a fist and bring it up toward your shoulder, hold the tension, breathe deeply, and relax. And again, bring your fist toward your shoulder, hold, breathe, and relax, letting your left arm return to rest at your side. Notice the feelings of relaxation in your left hand, forearm, and upper arm.

And now, bring your awareness to your shoulders and neck. Notice how your neck and shoulders feel. And gradually tense your shoulders by bringing your shoulders toward your ears and holding them there. Continuing to breathe deeply, observe sensations of tension throughout your shoulders and neck. And relax and release, letting all of the tension go. Once more, gradually tense your shoulders by bringing your shoulders toward your ears and hold. Breathe deeply, observing sensations of tension. And relax, letting all of the tension go. And again, bring your shoulders toward your ears and hold. Continuing to breathe deeply, observe sensations of tension throughout your shoulders and neck. And relax and release, letting all of the tension go. Allowing your shoulders to rest soft and relaxed, and observe any sensations of relaxation.

Next bringing your awareness into your face. Observing how your face feels. Now gently close your eyes tightly and wrinkle your forehead, hold the tension. Breathe. Observe sensations of tension throughout your face. Then relax, letting all of that tension go. Observe sensations of relaxation. And again, close your eyes tightly and wrinkle your forehead, hold the tension. Breathe. Observe sensations of tension throughout your face. Then relax, letting all of that tension go. Once more, close your eyes tightly and wrinkle your forehead, and hold. Breathe. Then relax, letting all of that tension go. Observe sensations of relaxation throughout your face.

Now guide your awareness into your back. Gently tense your back by drawing your shoulder blades together and slightly arching your back. Hold. Continue to breathe deeply. Notice sensations of tension in your back. And relax. Observe the release of tension and the experience of muscle relaxation along your spine. And again, gently tense your back by drawing your shoulder blades together and slightly arching your back. Hold. Continue to breathe deeply. Notice sensations of tension in your back. And relax. Once more, gently tense your back by drawing your shoulder blades together and slightly arching your back. Hold. Continue to breathe deeply. Notice sensations of tension in your back. And relax. Observe the release of tension and the experience of muscle relaxation along your back.

Now, observe your buttocks and hips. Tighten your buttocks muscles. Hold the tension. Continue to breathe deeply. And relax. And again, tighten your buttocks muscles. Hold the tension. Continue to breathe deeply. And relax. Once more, tighten your buttocks muscles. Hold. Breathe deeply. And relax. And observe any sensations of relaxation throughout your hips and buttocks.

Next, observe your thigh muscles. Gently tighten your thigh muscles by pushing your knees downward and drawing your thigh muscles to your thigh bones. Hold the tension. Breathe. And relax, letting all of that tension go. And again, gently tighten your thigh muscles by pushing your knees downward and drawing your thigh muscles to your thigh bones. Hold the tension. Breathe. And relax, letting all of that tension go. Once more, gently tighten your thigh muscles, and hold. Breathe. And relax, letting all of that tension go. And observe how your thighs feel.

Now, guide your awareness to your lower legs and feet. Tense your lower legs by bending your ankles, drawing your forefeet and toes toward your face. And hold. Breathe. Notice sensations of tension throughout your lower legs and feet. And relax. And again, tense your lower legs by bending your ankles, drawing your forefeet and toes toward your face. And hold. Breathe. And relax. Once more, tense your lower legs. Hold. Breathe. Notice sensations of tension throughout your lower legs and feet. And relax. Allow your lower legs to rest, soften, and relax. Notice any sensations of relaxation here in your lower legs and feet.

And now, allow your awareness to rest again with your breath. Aware of the in breath and aware of the out breath.

Observe your entire body from the soles of your feet to the crown of your head. Allow your mind to rest in the present moment. Allow your entire body to rest and relax.

Allow for 2 to 5 minutes of silence.

Once again, observing your breathing. Now, gradually begin to bring your awareness back to the room and, when you are ready, allow your eyes to open. You may wish to wiggle your toes or stretch your legs gently. If you are lying on your back, please roll to one side. Rest on your side for a moment before pushing up to sitting.

Autogenic Training

Autogenic training is a systematic program that requires the repetition of key verbal phrases that induce a relaxation response. It is a popular relaxation technique in Europe that evolved from studies in hypnosis by psychiatrist Johannes Schultz.[56] Schultz recognized that individuals could experience states of relaxation similar to hypnosis by thinking of the heaviness and warmth of their limbs. He developed a series of phrases that incorporate these sensations and others that, when repeated, result in relaxation.

Initial autogenic sessions are brief, lasting 1 to 2 minutes, and are repeated five to eight times per day. As individuals become more skilled, the session length increases to 30 minutes and is repeated once or twice per day. During brief sessions, individuals focus on one or two groups of phrases. During longer sessions, several groups of phrases are repeated. During training sessions, individuals are encouraged to avoid trying too hard. They are asked to develop passive concentration, remaining alert yet relaxed, observing their experience but not analyzing it or attempting to force a particular sensation to happen.

Following is a script for a 30-minute autogenic training session. Individual groups of phrases can be selected from this longer sequence for brief session practice.

Guided Script for Autogenic Training

Close your eyes. As you observe your experience, whatever it might be, let your attention be focused, yet relaxed. Avoid trying too hard or analyzing your experience. Accept whatever you experience without judgment. This exercise involves repeating key phrases to yourself that promote relaxation.

During this exercise, at some point you might find your mind wandering. When this happens, simply observe that your mind has wandered and return your attention to the instructions.

Choose a position that is comfortable for you. You may be sitting or lying down. You can allow your eyes to gently close or to remain softly open.

Now, guiding your awareness to your right arm, repeat to yourself the phrase, "My right arm is heavy." Focus on the sensation of heaviness in your arm as you repeat to yourself, "My right arm is heavy." Experiencing the feeling of heaviness in your arm, repeat to yourself, "My right arm is heavy."

Now, moving your awareness to your left arm, repeat to yourself the phrase, "My left arm is heavy." Focus on the sensation of heaviness in your arm as you repeat to yourself, "My left arm is heavy." Experiencing the feeling of heaviness in your arm, repeat to yourself, "My left arm is heavy."

Now, guiding your awareness to your right leg, repeat to yourself the phrase, "My right leg is heavy." Observing the sensation of heaviness in your leg as you repeat to yourself, "My right leg is heavy." Experiencing the feeling of heaviness in your leg, repeat to yourself, "My right leg is heavy."

Now, moving your awareness to your left leg, repeat to yourself the phrase, "My left leg is heavy." Focus on the sensation of heaviness in your leg as you repeat to yourself, "My left leg is heavy." Experiencing the feeling of heaviness in your leg, repeat to yourself, "My left leg is heavy."

And now, repeating to yourself, "My arms and legs are heavy. My arms and legs are heavy. My arms and legs are heavy."

Now, cultivating a feeling of warmth in your limbs, guide your awareness back to your right arm and repeat to yourself the phrase, "My right arm is warm." Focus on the sensation of warmth in your arm as you repeat to yourself, "My right arm is warm." Experiencing the feeling of warmth in your arm, repeat to yourself, "My right arm is warm."

Now, moving your awareness to your left arm, repeat to yourself the phrase, "My left arm is warm." Focus on the sensation of warmth in your arm as you repeat to yourself, "My left arm is warm." Experiencing the feeling of warmth in your arm, repeat to yourself, "My left arm is warm."

Now, guiding your awareness to your right leg, repeat to yourself the phrase, "My right leg is warm." Observing the sensation of warmth in your leg as you repeat to yourself, "My right leg is warm." Experiencing the feeling of warmth in your leg, repeat to yourself, "My right leg is warm."

Now, moving your awareness to your left leg, repeat to yourself the phrase, "My left leg is warm." Focus on the sensation of warmth in your leg as you repeat to yourself, "My left leg is warm." Experiencing the feeling of warmth in your leg, repeat to yourself, "My left leg is warm."

And now, aware of your limbs, repeat to yourself, "My arms and legs are heavy and warm. My arms and legs are heavy and warm. My arms and legs are heavy and warm."

And now, bringing your awareness to your chest and repeat to yourself, "My heartbeat is calm and regular. My heartbeat is calm and regular. My heartbeat is calm and regular." Some people have difficulty focusing on their chest and heartbeat. If this is true for you, substitute the phrase, "I feel calm."

And now, bring your awareness to your breath, repeat to yourself the phrase, "My breath is calm and at ease." Allowing your breath to move gently deep in your lungs. Allowing your stomach to gently rise on the in breath and gently fall on the out breath. Repeat to yourself the phrase, "My breath is calm and at ease. My breath is calm and at ease." Breathing at a rate that feels comfortable and natural for you.

And now, bring your awareness to your abdomen, repeat to yourself the phrase, "My abdomen is calm and warm. My abdomen is calm and warm. My abdomen is calm and warm." Experience a feeling of calm, ease, warmth, and relaxation in your abdomen.

And now, bring your awareness to your forehead, repeat to yourself the phrase, "My forehead is calm and cool. My forehead is calm and cool. My forehead is calm and cool." Experience a feeling of calm, ease, coolness, and relaxation in your forehead.

And now, bring your awareness to your entire body and the whole of your experience. And now, take this time to repeat a phrase that is personally meaningful to you. It can be a phrase you have already repeated during this exercise or you can create a new phrase that focuses on a feeling or quality you would like to strengthen in yourself. Taking this time to repeat your personal phrase.

And now observe your entire body.

Keeping with you a feeling of calm as you now begin to move your awareness from your inner experience back to the room. You may wish to wiggle your toes or move your ankles gently back and forth.

Keeping with you any nourishing elements of this experience as you open your eyes if they have been closed and move from the position you have been in. Knowing that the ways in which you have been nourished by this practice will remain with you as you participate in the activities of daily life.

The Relaxation Body Scan

The relaxation body scan requires guiding your awareness through your body systemically, relaxing each body area. It is a simple and commonly used relaxation technique.

Guided Script for the Relaxation Body Scan

This exercise is called the relaxation body scan practice. You will be guided through your body systematically and encouraged to relax and release tension in each body area. This is a time just for you, to nourish yourself and allow your body to deeply rest and relax.

Let the quality of attention you bring to yourself during this exercise be basically kind and friendly. You might find that some parts of your body relax easily while others remain tense or guarded. Should you find an area of your body that remains tense, remember this is a common experience and nothing to worry about. Meet this area of your body with understanding, compassion, and acceptance. There is no need to push or force your body in any way. Your body already carries the knowledge of relaxation and will release tension in a manner that is just right for you. Trust the process. Remember it can take time to release longstanding patterns of tension.

During this exercise, as you move your awareness through your body, if, for any reason, it is difficult for you to let your attention rest with a particular body part, know that this is not a problem and guide your awareness back to your breathing. Allow your awareness to rest with your breathing until you are ready to continue.

Choose a position that is comfortable for you. You may be sitting or lying down. You can allow your eyes to gently close or to remain softly open.

Now, guiding your awareness to your breathing, observing your breathing. Aware of the in breath. Aware of the out breath.

Notice the sensations in your torso as you breathe. As you breathe in, observing what part of your body moves with the in breath. As you breathe out, observing what part of your body moves as you breathe out.

This calm rhythm is not unlike the calm rhythm of ocean waves meeting the shoreline. And just as each wave is different, so too each breath is unique.

Should you find your breath is shallow and only filling your upper chest, ever so gently, explore the possibility of allowing your breath to move a little more deeply into your lungs, so that your stomach rises slightly with the in breath and falls with the out breath.

Remember there is no need to push or force your body in any way. You are working with your body's own natural rhythms and wisdom.

As you breathe in, observing your stomach gently rise. As you breathe out, observing your stomach gently fall. This deep breathing pattern helps the body to naturally release unneeded tensions.

Breathing in. Breathing out.

As you breathe, noticing the surface on which you are resting. Letting your body receive the full support of this surface. Allowing yourself to feel the complete support of this surface.

Should your mind begin to wander at any time, that's not a problem. You can imagine your mind is open and boundless like the sky, and a thought is like a mere cloud drifting by. Note that your mind has wandered as you might observe a cloud drift by in the sky, and then gently and firmly guide your attention back to your breath and the sensations of the in breath and sensations of the out breath.

Thoughts come and go, flow and change. They are no big deal. Simply note them when they arise and come back to your breath.

Sometimes it is helpful to repeat a word or phrase in concert with your breath. This can help steady the mind and develop concentration and focus. Maintaining your attention on the sensations of the breath, repeating to yourself, "in" on the in breath, "out" on the out breath. In, out.

Or, you can repeat your name on the in breath followed by the phrase "let go" on the out breath. You can choose any word or phrase that speaks to you. It is important, however, to continue to be aware of the physical sensations of the breath as you repeat the word or phrase. Breathing in, aware of breathing in, breathing out, aware of breathing out.

Now becoming aware of how your body feels, from the soles of your feet to the crown of your head.

From this place of observing your entire body, now guiding your awareness into your right foot. Observing the feelings and sensations in your right foot. As feels comfortable for you, allow your right foot to soften and relax.

Now guiding your awareness to your lower leg on the right side. And gently allow your lower leg to soften and release.

Moving your awareness to your right thigh. Observing this area of your body from your knee to your hip. And allow your right thigh to soften and relax.

Now guiding your awareness into your left foot. Observing the feelings and sensations in your left foot. As feels comfortable for you, allow your left foot to soften and relax.

Now guiding your awareness to your lower leg on the left side. And gently allow your lower leg to soften and release.

Moving your awareness to your left thigh. Observing this area of your body from your knee to your hip. And allow your left thigh to soften and relax.

And now, guiding your awareness to your lower torso. Observing your buttocks, hips, and pelvis, allowing this area of your body to soften and relax. And noticing your abdomen. Allowing your abdomen to soften, relax, and release.

Next, moving your awareness to your back and the muscles along your spine. Observing your lower back and allowing your lower back to relax. Noticing your midback, and allowing your midback to soften and release. And listening to your upper back. Allowing your upper back to release and relax. Imagine any tensions along your spine that are ready to be released, just melting away so that your back deeply rests, calm and at ease. It may feel as if your back were sinking into the surface on which you are resting.

Now guiding your awareness to your right hand. Observing feelings and sensations. And allowing your hand to soften and relax. Observing your forearm. And allowing your forearm to soften and release. Guiding your awareness to your upper arm and allowing your upper arm to relax.

Now guiding your awareness to your left hand. Observing feelings and sensations. And allowing your hand to soften and relax. Observing your forearm. And allowing your forearm to soften and release. Guiding your awareness to your upper arm on the left side and allowing your upper arm to relax.

Now guiding your awareness to your shoulders. Observing your shoulders. Allowing your shoulders to soften and relax, release and let go.

And guiding your awareness into your neck. Observing your neck. Allowing your neck to soften and release.

And noticing your face, allowing the muscles of your face to soften and relax. Relaxing your jaw and the muscles around your mouth. Relaxing your cheeks and the muscles just under your eyes. Imagining your forehead softening and releasing. And your temples, relaxing and letting go of tension. You can imagine relaxing the back of your head and the crown of your head.

And now, returning your awareness to your breath. Aware of the in breath. Aware of the out breath. Breathing at a rate that feels natural and comfortable for you.

And now listening to your entire body from the soles of your feet to the crown of your head. Taking in your experience just as it is.

If there is an area of your body that is in discomfort, you can imagine breathing into that area and out from that area. Your breath, like a gentle, calming, healing river washing through this area of your body.

Just listening to your entire body, resting calm and at ease. Resting now in a state of relaxation and well-being, balance and harmony, calm and peace.

Once again observing your breathing. Aware of the in breath and aware of the out breath. Keeping with you a feeling of calm as you now begin to move your awareness from your inner experience back to the room. You may wish to wiggle your toes or move your ankles gently back and forth.

Keeping with you any nourishing elements of this experience as you open your eyes if they have been closed and move from the position you have been in. Knowing that the ways in which you have been nourished by this practice will remain with you as you participate in the activities of daily life.

Guided Imagery

Guided imagery exercises can be taught to promote relaxation and engage the mind-body relationship in a healing process. Images can be general, such as "Imagine yourself in a calm and peaceful place." Or they can be specific, such as "Imagine your strong, healthy immune system cells cleansing your body of weak, feeble cancer cells." The images introduced in guided imagery exercises must be appropriate to the participants. For example, the instruction "Imagine being in the state of health you desire" is fine for a recreational athlete with a good prognosis following an injury but can evoke feelings of sadness in someone with a chronic medical problem grieving the loss of an active lifestyle. "Imagine being in a state of well-being, harmony, and peace" guides the listener to experience dimensions of wellness that can occur independent of physical function. Following are scripts for a general guided imagery exercise and a guided imagery for cancer treatment.

General Guided Imagery Script

Begin this exercise by guiding the group through a brief relaxation body scan, then continue with the guided imagery:

And now imagining yourself in a calm, tranquil, and peaceful place. Imagining yourself somewhere serene, a place where you feel at ease. A place embodying beauty, harmony, and peace. Bringing the image of this place clear in your mind.

Engaging your senses. Taking in what you see. The colors of this place.

Taking in the sounds of this place. Observing textures, smells. Noticing the temperature. Bringing this place alive in your imagination. Feeling the ground under your feet. And the experience of your body. Noticing how your body feels.

Experiencing yourself in harmony with these surroundings. Interwoven, interconnected in this wondrous web of life.

Noticing how you feel in this place. Allowing yourself to feel at ease. Cultivating an inner experience of wholeness, peacefulness, well-being, and joy.

Taking this time to rest here. To be nourished by the beauty and serenity of this place. To dwell in an experience of wholeness, peacefulness, well-being, and joy. Alive, nourished, and renewed with this experience of wholeness, peacefulness, well-being, and joy.

Imagine generating any quality or feeling you would like to strengthen in yourself. Imagining this feeling coming alive and increasing within you.

Now imagine drawing the positive and nourishing feelings you experience in this image into your body as you rest here and now. Imagine the positive and nourishing feelings you experience in this image as residing in each cell of your body, here and now, so that each cell becomes radiant with these feelings and qualities. Bringing the feelings from the image into your body.

Each cell illuminated with these feelings and qualities. Every cell remembering what it is to be in balance, in harmony. Every cell awakened to the experience of peacefulness, well-being, and joy. Every cell alive with whatever qualities you would like to strengthen in yourself.

Now increasing these qualities, this radiance in your body as if you were turning up the volume on your favorite piece of music. Each cell alive with your inner resources for well-being, balance, harmony, joy, peacefulness, and any other nourishing qualities.

Knowing that these qualities and inner resources are always here within you.

Knowing that this calm, serene place and these qualities are always here within you. And now, returning your awareness to your breath.

And now just listening to the whole of your body. Dwelling in an inner place of renewal.

Once again observing your breathing. Aware of the in breath and aware of the out breath. Keeping with you any nourishing feelings as you now begin to move your awareness from your inner experience back to the room. You may wish to wiggle your toes or move your ankles gently back and forth. Taking your time.

Keeping with you any nourishing elements of this experience as you open your eyes and move from your resting position. Knowing that the ways in which you have been nourished by this practice will remain with you as you participate in the activities of daily life.

Guided Imagery for Cancer Treatment

Begin this exercise by guiding the group through a brief relaxation body scan, then continue with the guided imagery:

And now just listening to the whole of your body.

Remembering that the same intelligence that brings us spring is also alive in every cell of your body. Acknowledging the profound and powerful creative intelligence you carry within you at the cellular level. This same intelligence that brings us sunlight and the night sky, the oceans and the mountains, flowers and a grain of sand is also alive within you. Experiencing your connection with all of life and this profound and powerful creative intelligence alive within the cells of your body. Recognizing your own body's capabilities and tremendous inner resources for healing.

Important immune system cells begin their journey deep inside your thigh bones. Bringing your attention to your thigh bones. Your immune system cells are born here, deep in the marrow of these bones. Imagining billions of cells being born here. Many kinds of cells whose life mission is to support and protect you. Know that you have many kinds of cells that work tirelessly, supporting your health and well-being, protecting you from disease and infection.

Among these cells are those responsible for eliminating cancer cells. Imagining that your body is abundant with these cells. Knowing that your body is abundant with these cells whose mission is to cleanse your body of cancer cells. Imagining these immune cells as strong, powerful, and resourceful. Imagine these robust, intelligent immune system cells in any fashion that comes easy to you. Experience these cells as mobile, vibrant, intelligent, and capable. They are ever alert, ready to cleanse from your body any disease or even potential for disease. A mere touch by one of these powerful immune cells paralyzes a cancer cell and causes the cancer cell to completely dissolve. Imagining these immune system cells as powerful, strong, and capable. Vibrant, intelligent, resourceful.

Now imagining any cancer cells as weak, feeble, and confused. Imagining these debilitated cells in any fashion that is easy for you. Imagining any diseased cells as deficient and feeble, frail and weak. Imagining any diseased cells as sedentary and sluggish, confused, and easily overcome by your immune system.

Now imagining your strong, healthy, vibrant immune system cleansing your body of any disease or potential for disease. Imagining your immune system as powerful and capable, eliminating any diseased cells or even potential for disease.

And imagining your treatment team assisting and supporting you in this process. Recognizing in each community that there are those who are gifted, trained, and experienced in healing. Recognizing the many strengths of your treatment team, imagining the members of your team as capable and powerful healers, supporting your own inner capacities for healing and renewal. Imagining them surrounding you and experiencing yourself as strengthened by their presence and their gifts and powers. Experiencing yourself supported and strengthened by this powerful team of healers.

And imagining your treatment as a helpful and powerful ally. Imagining that your own cells know your treatment is a co-worker in your healing process. Imagining your treatment cooperating with your own cells to eliminate any disease. Imagining your treatment as strong, intelligent, and effective at targeting only diseased cells and avoiding healthy ones. Imagining your treatment targeting only diseased cells. Imagining your treatment effectively cleansing from your body any cancer cells while your own healthy cells become even stronger.

Imagining your own strong, capable, and healthy immune system continuing to eliminate any cancer. Imagining the healing powers of your health care team and your treatment cooperating in this process, ridding your body of these deficient cells. Imagining your healthy cells becoming stronger.

And now bringing to mind your family, friends, and all members of your support system and community. Letting yourself receive the love, healing wishes, and healing energy from these people. Experiencing yourself nourished, strengthened, and empowered by this love, by these healing wishes and prayers, and by this healing energy of family, friends, and all members of your support system and community. Imagining this energy strengthening you, further fueling your capacities to cleanse your body of any disease. Imagining your body free of disease and potential for disease.

And now, imagining yourself in a state of well-being. Experiencing wholeness, well-being, dwelling in a state of harmony and balance.

Now, gradually bring your awareness back to your breath. Aware of the feeling of the in breath. Aware of the feeling of the out breath. Knowing that the suggestions, images, and powers of this practice will continue to support and strengthen you even after the exercise is over.

Keeping with you any nourishing feelings as you now begin to move your awareness from your inner experience back to the room. You may wish to wiggle your toes or move your ankles gently back and forth. Taking your time. Keeping with you any nourishing elements of this experience as you open your eyes and move from your resting position.

Addressing Difficulties People Experience

Most people respond positively to these exercises; however, some individuals have negative reactions. Following are four problems people occasionally experience and suggestions for responding to them. Keep in mind that there is no single correct response to a problem. A clinician must be sensitive to the individual and the circumstance.

1. *"I cannot feel my feet."* When some people first do relaxation exercises, they do not feel anything in parts of their body. This inability to perceive sensation in a body part can be disturbing. Reassurance and instructions on how to respond are helpful. A possible response is as follows:

   It is common when first paying attention to your body to have a vivid experience of sensations in one part of your body and to feel very little or nothing in another part. This happens frequently and is neither good nor bad. There is no need to be troubled by not feeling anything. Just observe it and continue with the relaxation exercise. With time and practice you can begin to experience sensations in these areas where you originally feel nothing.

2. *"I'm too restless."* When some people are introduced to autogenics, relaxation body scan, or guided imagery, they experience a strong desire to move or a general restlessness. They can further react with feeling frustrated or criticize themselves for having difficulty just being still. This does not occur as often with progressive relaxation because of the active muscle contraction and movement required during the exercise. Reassurance and instructions on how to handle these feelings are helpful. An instructor might respond as follows:

   When asked to stop and pay attention to the body in this manner, some people experience a strong impulse to move. Others feel a general restlessness or describe a jumpy or jittery feeling in their legs. This is common. Remember, many of us are constantly moving and our minds are constantly racing, so this exercise is a radical shift from this usual habit. It is important to avoid becoming critical of yourself and labeling the experience of restlessness or desire to move as bad or wrong. Simply observe it. Meet it with understanding. Keep your focus on your breathing as best you can. If it becomes unbearable for you, change your position.

3. *"I fall asleep."* When some people close their eyes and begin to quiet internal conversation, they fall asleep. It is helpful for these people to do relaxation exercises sitting rather than lying down. They can also keep their eyes softly open. Bright lighting in a room is helpful. They can also avoid doing the exercise right before bed when they are likely to be tired.

   For people with insomnia, these exercises can help improve sleep patterns. Many people will do the exercise before bed because it helps them fall asleep and achieve a more deep and restful sleep. This is a very helpful benefit of the exercise. Ultimately, relaxation exercises are about building awareness and learning to relax, not falling asleep. If participants use the exercises to fall asleep, they may also want to do it at some other time during the day and maintain alertness.

4. *"I'm in too much pain."* For people who are experiencing pain, the first practice of relaxation exercises decreases pain intensity for many people. For some people, however, pain intensity increases. For those who have coped with pain through constant distraction, relaxation exercises can increase their awareness of pain. It is important to remind participants that learning to relax and effectively manage pain takes time, practice, and patience. It requires a willingness to experiment and courage to try new things. It is not always easy. Following are four additional strategies for responding to people who complain of increased pain:

   a. *Remind participants that pain is a physical sensation.* It is not who they are. The pain is not their identity. The sensation of pain arises in a context of a much larger experience of being human. This is one dimension, not the whole picture.

   b. *Explain the pain-tension cycle.* When we experience pain, we often tense our muscles in reaction to the pain. This constant muscle tension only increases pain. We get caught in a cycle of pain triggering more muscle tension, then more tension leads to more pain. Relaxation exercises can be an initial step toward breaking that cycle. Sometimes, however, when we first pay attention to what is actually happening, we feel more pain. I am going to ask you to continue doing the exercises as best you can because with continued practice, a shift often occurs.

With practice, you learn to control your response and can relax rather than tense your muscles. This prevents the escalation of pain that occurs from increasing muscle tension.

Also, your relationship *to* the pain can change. You can find new confidence in coping with pain and controlling your reaction to pain. This requires time and practice. Do the best you can. When it is very difficult, let your awareness return to your breath. If it becomes unbearable, you can always stop the exercise. Avoid criticizing yourself if this happens. This criticism only makes things worse. Meet yourself with understanding and take small steps. You might choose to spend 5 minutes performing the breathing exercises three or four times a day if the full-body exercises are too difficult. This is a wonderful place to begin.

c. *The application of mental imagery is helpful in responding to pain.* An instructor might employ one or a combination of the following images:
   1) *Imagine for a moment, your body is like a garden.* Relaxation is like taking a walk through this garden, bringing water and plant food to the plants. Your symptom—in this case, pain—is a like plant in the garden that is not doing well. First, you are taking time to survey your whole garden. A good gardener knows to pay attention not only to a plant in need, but to the whole garden as well. This enables the gardener to prevent the rest of the garden from falling into neglect and provides perspective on the troubled plant. The relaxation exercises enable you to take this approach with the body. You deliberately focus on different areas in the body one by one. By letting your awareness rest in different areas of your body, your attention touches those places that are functioning well. You have the big picture. You experiment with taking care of and relaxing those areas of the body that are not in pain. This is key to your overall health and can provide a new perspective on what is problematic.
   2) *Imagine your mind is vast like the sky.* In whatever way is comfortable for you, connect with a quality of great spaciousness, of being boundless and open like the sky. Now imagine the pain is like a cloud or a weather pattern in this vast sky of your mind. The physical sensation is still there, but you are creating a quality of great openness and spaciousness around the pain.
   3) *Imagine that you carry an ocean of compassion in your heart.* Imagine you carry within your heart a quality of compassion that is boundless, immeasurable, and infinite. Now imagine the pain is like a small piece of driftwood floating on this great ocean of compassion. The physical sensation is still there. You are not trying to change it or get rid of it, but to create a sense of openness and spaciousness around the pain and surround it with this ocean of compassion.
   4) *Another strategy for responding to pain is to breathe into the pain.* You can imagine your breath is like a healing wind, a healing river, or like a flowing stream of light. As you breathe in, imagine the breath flowing into the pain. As you breathe out, imagine the breath flowing through and out from the pain. Imagine the healing energy of the breath flowing through the pain.

Home Exercise Program

If a clinician chooses to include this approach in a wellness program, the regular practice of relaxation exercises is an important component of a home exercise plan. An instructor can professionally record a cassette tape or CD that can be used daily by class participants. Relaxation and guided imagery tapes and CDs are also commercially available. To promote adherence, participants can be provided with a daily log in which they record their experience of the exercise.

Introducing the Stress Response to a Group

Important health consequences are not the only reasons for including stress reduction techniques in a wellness program. Everyone has personal experience with the topic. People are often eager to share their concerns and ready to learn all they can to manage stress more effectively. One class structure for teaching this topic is offered as follows. Clinicians can build from this initial framework based on their training and experience and the needs of an individual group.

1. Ask group members to define stress. Write the list of responses on a blackboard or flip chart.
2. When the group members have exhausted their responses, point out that stress is not easily defined and has different meanings to different people. Introduce the following equation:

   Stress = The Situation + Our Reaction

   Point out how the group members' responses, although varied, fit into this simple equation.
3. Provide additional descriptions and examples that further clarify this model. Explain how stress can be broken down into two components. The first is the situation itself. The second is our reaction *to* the situation. Acknowledge that people can have very different reactions to the same situation. For example, a man and his son are sitting in a car at a railroad crossing watching a train go by. The man is frustrated and tense, thinking to himself, "Oh no. How long is this going to go on? I hate getting stuck at this crossing." On the other hand, the little boy is delighted. He is thinking to himself, "Oh boy, this is wonderful! I love trains!" Same situation. Two very different reactions.
4. Provide examples, appropriate to your group, that demonstrate how some situations can be changed to decrease stress. If your group consists of working people, the following scenario may be appropriate: An employer assigns you a complex work task to be completed in a brief time frame. The stressful situation is the work assignment with a fast-approaching deadline. To change the situation, you can attempt to extend the deadline or enlist the help of co-workers.

   If your group is made up of retirees, a different example is needed: You invited a friend for lunch, but you feel tired, your symptoms have flared up, and you are not up to all the preparation. You decide to give your friend a call and suggest meeting at a local restaurant.
5. Introduce examples of situations that cannot be changed. These include experiencing chronic pain or illness, a decision by company owners to downsize the office, or getting stuck in traffic on the way to an important engagement. When we cannot change the situation to reduce our stress, we can look inward and take charge of our response.

6. Identify the three components of our response to stress. One is a physical reaction, the second is a cognitive reaction, and the third is an emotional reaction. These three components are interconnected and influence one another. This session examines the body's response to stress.
7. Invite participants to describe what they physically experience when they are stressed. To avoid responses related to thoughts, emotions, and behaviors, emphasize that you are asking what they directly experience in their bodies. Write the list of responses on a blackboard or flip chart. When the group members have exhausted their responses, introduce the fight-or-flight reaction and its health effects, referring to the list of responses as appropriate. Following a question-and-answer period, introduce relaxation exercises.

Summary

Stress has adverse consequences when people fail to successfully respond and adapt to it. Although the types of stress we face are far different from our Stone Age ancestors, our biological response is unchanged. Through a cascade of neuroendocrine processes, the SNS directs the body to prepare to fight or run. The chronic activation of this alarm mechanism may have a role in the course of several medical conditions, including cardiovascular disease, diabetes, immune function, wound healing, and musculoskeletal disorders. Both the potential health consequences of chronic stress and the eagerness among many people to learn effective coping tools make stress management an important component of any wellness program. Mindfulness meditation, described in Chapter 3, promotes the self-regulation of the stress reaction. Relaxation exercises are also effective strategies to decrease the fight-or-flight reaction and are easily incorporated into a wellness program. These exercises include diaphragmatic breathing, progressive relaxation, autogenic training, relaxation body scan, and guided imagery.

References

1. Cannon WB. *The Wisdom of the Body*. New York: W.W. Norton, 1939.
2. Selye H. *The Stress of Life*. New York: McGraw Hill, 1956.
3. Petzke F, Clauw DJ. Sympathetic nervous system function in fibromyalgia. *Curr Rheumatol Reports* 2000;2:116-123.
4. Rozanski A, Blumenthal JA, Kaplan J. Impact of psychological factors on the pathogenesis of CVD and implications for therapy. *Circulation* 1999;99:2192-2217.
5. Pickering TG. Mental stress as a causal factor in the development of hypertension and cardiovascular disease. *Curr Hypertension Rep* 2001;3(3):249-254.
6. Krantz DS, Sheps DS, Carney RM et al. Effects of mental stress in patients with coronary artery disease: evidence and clinical implications. *JAMA* 2000;283(14):1800-1802.
7. Krantz DS, Kop WJ, Santiago HT, Gottiener JS. Mental stress as a trigger for myocardial ischemia and infarction. *Cardiol Clin* 1996;14:271-287.
8. Schoder H, Silverman DH, Campisi R et al. Effect of mental stress on myocardial blood flow and vasomotion in patients with coronary artery disease. *J Nucl Med* 2000;41(1):11-16.

9. James PR, Taggart P, McNally ST et al. Acute psychological stress and the propensity to ventricular arrhythmias: evidence for a linking mechanism. *Eur Heart J* 2000;21(12):1023-1028.
10. Kop WJ, Krantz DS, Howell RH et al. Effects of mental stress on coronary epicardial vasomotion and flow velocity in coronary artery disease: relationship with hemodynamic stress responses. *J Am Coll Cardiol* 2001;37(5):1359-1366.
11. Mittleman MD, Maclure M, Sherwood JB et al. Triggering of acute myocardial infarction onset by episodes of anger. *Circulation* 1995;92:1720-1725.
12. Moller J, Hallqvist J, Diderich F et al. Do episodes of anger trigger myocardial infarction? A case cross-over analysis in the Stockholm Heart Epidemiology Program (SHEEP). *Psychosom Med* 1999;61(6):842-849.
13. Muller JE, Tofler GH, Stone PH. Circadian variation and triggers of onset of acute cardiovascular disease. *Circulation* 1989;79:733-734.
14. Jiang W, Babyak M, Krantz DS et al. Mental stress-induced myocardial ischemia and cardiac events. *JAMA* 1996;275:1651-1656.
15. Krantz DS, Santiago HT, Kop WI et al. Prognostic value of mental stress testing in coronary artery disease. *Am J Cardiol* 1999;84:1292-1297.
16. Grossman E, Grossman A, Schein MH et al. Breathing control lowers blood pressure. *J Hum Hypertens* 2001;15(4):236-239.
17. Linden W, Stossel C, Maurice J. Psychological interventions for patients with coronary artery disease: a meta-analysis. *Arch Internal Med* 1996;156:745-752.
18. Bleumenthal JA, Jiang W, Babykok MA et al. Stress management and exercise training in cardiac patients with myocardial ischemia: effects on prognosis and evaluation of mechanisms. *Arch Int Med* 1997;157: 2213-2223.
19. Kramer JR, Johannes L, Manos G et al. Stress and metabolic control in diabetes mellitus: methodological issues and an illustrative analysis. *Ann Behav Med* 2000;22(1):17-28.
20. Surwit RS, Schneider MS, Feinglos MN. Stress and diabetes mellitus. *Diabetes Care* 1992;15(10):1413-1422.
21. Surwit RS, Schneider MS. The role of stress in the etiology and treatment of diabetes mellitus. *Psychosom Med* 1993;55(4):380-393.
22. Goetsch VL, Weibe DJ, Velyum LG et al. Stress and blood glucose in type 2 diabetes mellitus. *Behav Res Ther* 1990;28(6):531-537.
23. McGrady A, Bailey BK, Good MP. Controlled study of biofeedback-assisted relaxation in type 1 diabetes. *Diabetes Care* 1991;14(5):360-365.
24. Aikens JE, Kiolbasa TA, Sobel R. Psychological predictors of glycemic change with relaxation training in non-insulin dependent diabetes mellitus. *Psychother Psychosom* 1997;66:302-306.
25. Lane JD, McCaskill CC, Ross SL. Relaxation training for NIDDM. Predicting who may benefit. *Diabetes Care* 1993;16(8):1087-1094.
26. Surwit RS, vanTilburg M, Zucker N et al. Stress management improves long-term glycemic control in type 2 diabetes. *Diabetes Care* 2002;25(1):30-34.
27. Cohen S, Herbert TB. Health psychology: psychological factors and physical disease from the perspective of psychoneuroimmunology. *Ann Rev Psych* 1996;47:113-142.

28. Herbert TB, Cohen S. Stress and immunity: a meta-analytic review. *Psychosom Med* 1993;55:364-379.
29. Miller G, Cohen S. Psychological interventions and the immune system: a meta-analytic review and critique. *Health Psychology* 2001;20(1):47-63.
30. Antoni MH, Cruess DG, Cruess S et al. Cognitive-behavioral stress management intervention effects on anxiety, 24-hr urinary norepinephrine output, and T-cytotoxic/suppressor cells over time among symptomatic HIV-infected gay men. *J Counsel Clin Psychol* 2000;68(1):31-45.
31. Molassiotis A, Yung HP, Yam BM et al. The effectiveness of progressive muscle relaxation training in managing chemotherapy-induced nausea and vomiting in Chinese breast cancer patients: a randomized controlled trial. *Support Care Cancer* 2002;10:237-246.
32. Burish TG, Tope DM. Psychological techniques for controlling the adverse side effects of cancer chemotherapy: findings from a decade of research. *J Pain Symptom Manage* 1992;7:287-301.
33. King CR. Non-pharmacologic management of chemotherapy-induced nausea and vomiting. *Oncol Nurs Forum* 1997;24(Suppl 7):41-48.
34. Kiecolt-Glaser JK, Marucha PT, Malarkey WB et al. Slowing of wound healing by psychological stress. *Lancet* 1995 Nov;346(8984):1194-1196.
35. Marucha PT, Kiecolt-Glaser JK, Favegehi M. Mucosal wound healing is impaired by examination stress. *Psychom Med* 1998 May-Jun;6(3):362-365.
36. Glaser R, Kiecolt-Glaser JK, Marucha PT et al. Stress-related changes in proinflammatory cytokine production in wounds. *Arch Gen Psychiatry* 1999 May;56(5):450-456.
37. Kiecolt-Glaser JK, Page CG, Marucha PT et al. Psychological influences on surgical recovery. Perspectives from psychoneuroimmunology. *Am Psychol* 1998;52(11):1209-1218.
38. Rozlog LA, Kiecolt-Glaser JK, Marucha PT et al. Stress and immunity: implications for viral disease and wound healing. *J Periodontol* 1999;70(7):786-792.
39. Holden-Lund C. Effects of relaxation with guided imagery on surgical stress and wound healing. *Res Nurs Health* 1988;11(4):235-244.
40. Linton SJ. The risk for back pain: a systemic review. *J Occ Rehab* 2001 Mar;11(1):53-66.
41. Lampe A, Sollner W, Krismer M et al. The impact of stressful life events on exacerbation of chronic low back pain. *J Psychom Res* 1998 May;44(5):555-563.
42. Thorbornsson CB, Alfredsson L, Fredriksson K et al. Physical and psychological factors related to low back pain during a 24 year period. A nested case-control analysis. *Spine* 2000 Feb 1;25(3):369-374.
43. Lundberg U, Dohns IE, Melin B. Psychophysiological stress responses, muscle tension, and neck and shoulder pain among supermarket cashiers. *J Occup Health Psychol* 1999 Jul;4(3):245-255.
44. Nahit ES, Pritchard CM, Cherry NM et al. The influence of work related psychosocial factors and psychological distress on regional musculoskeletal pain: a study of newly employed workers. *J Rheumatol* 2001 Jun;28(6):1378-1384.
45. Van Susante J, Van de Schaaf D, Pavlov P. Psychological distress deteriorates the subjective outcome of lumbosacral fusion. A prospective study. *Acta Orthop Belg* 1998 Dec;64(4):371-377.

46. Schade V, Senmer N, Main CJ et al. The impact of clinical, morphological, psychosocial and work-related factors on the outcome of lumbar disectomey. *Pain* 1999;80(1-2):239-249.

47. Lundberg U. Stress responses in low-status jobs and their relationship to health risks: musculoskeletal disorders. *Ann NY Acad Sci* 1999;896: 162-167.

48. Power C, Frank J, Hertzman C et al. Predictors of low back pain onset in a prospective British Study. *Am J Pub Health* 2001;91(10):1671-1678.

49. Marras WS, Davis KG, Heaney CA. The influence of psychosocial stress, gender and personality on mechanical loading of the lumbar spine. *Spine* 2000;25(23):3045-3054.

50. Petzke F, Clauw DJ. Sympathetic nervous system function in fibromyalgia. *Curr Rheumatol Rep* 2000;2:116-123.

51. Moore J, Lorig K. A randomized trial of a lay person led self-management group intervention for back pain patients in primary care. *Spine* 1998;23(23):2608-2615.

52. Marhold C, Linton SJ, Melin L. A cognitive-behavioral return-to-work program: effects on pain patients with a history of long-term vs. short-term sick leave. *Pain* 2001 Mar;9(1-2):155-163.

53. Halroyd KA, O'Donnell FJ, Stensland M et al. Management of chronic tension-type headache with tricyclic antidepressant medication, stress management therapy, and their combination: a randomized controlled trial. *JAMA* 2001 May 2;285(17):2208-2215.

54. Keel PJ, Bodoky C, Gerhard U et al. Comparison of integrated group therapy and group relaxation training for fibromyalgia. *Clin J Pain* 1998 Sep;14(3):232-238.

55. Jacobson E. *Progressive Relaxation*. Chicago: University of Chicago Press, 1974.

56. Sadigh M. *Autogenic training: a mind-body approach to the treatment of fibromyalgia and chronic pain.* Binghamton, NY: Haworth Press, 2001.

Annotated Bibliography

Payne RA. *Relaxation Techniques: a Practical Handbook for the Health Care Professional* 2nd ed. New York, Churchill Livingston, 2000. Rosemary Payne, MCSP, is a clinical therapist and specialist in relaxation instruction. This text offers the health care professional a thorough introduction to a wide range of relaxation techniques applicable for an individual or group format. Detailed descriptions of breathing exercises, progressive relaxation, autogenic training, and several visualization exercises for relaxation and well-being are included. Practical guidelines for providing relaxation instruction and specific relaxation scripts are presented. The background theory, advantages, and disadvantages of each method are reviewed. This is an excellent resource for clinicians who want to learn or broaden their skills in relaxation training.

Rabin BS. *Stress, Immune Function and Health: the Connection*. New York, Wiley, John & Sons, 1999. Bruce S. Rabin is a Professor of Pathology and Psychiatry at the University of Pittsburgh and a leading researcher in the field of stress and immune system function. In this detailed and authoritative text, Rabin provides an overview of the immune system and the nervous system–immune system connection. Drawing extensively from scientific studies, he examines how stress hormones alter the immune system and may influence immune-related diseases. In addition, he identifies health behaviors that buffer the adverse effects of stress.

Sapolsky RM. *Why Zebras Don't Get Ulcers: an Updated Guide to Stress, Stress-related Diseases and Coping*. New York, NY: Henry Holt & Co., 1998. Robert Sapolsky, Professor of Biological Sciences and Neuroscience at Stanford University, offers an examination of the stress response and the role chronic stress may play in a range of physical and mental afflictions, including heart disease, metabolic and digestive disorders, cognitive impairment, and depression. Combining pertinent research, clinical applications, and humor, he provides a readable and entertaining exploration of the topic of stress and disease.

Sternberg E. *The Balance Within: the Science Connecting Health and Emotions*. New York, W.H. Freeman and Co., 2000. Esther Sternberg, M.D., is the Director of the Molecular, Cellular, and Behavioral Integrative Neuroscience Program and Chief of the Section on Neuroendocrine Immunology and Behavior at the National Institutes of Health. In this book, Sternberg offers a fascinating journey into the research discoveries that are the scientific foundation of mind-body medicine. Drawing from historic vignettes and recent experiments, she describes how science researchers uncovered the links between the mind and body. She offers a detailed examination of the connections between the nervous system and immune system and identifies the influences of stress on immune function. This book provides the clinician with a thorough background in the history of mind-body medicine research and the current scientific evidence for promoting a whole person approach to patient care from a leading researcher in the field.

Resources

For Guided Relaxation CDs

www.carolynmcmanus.com: Relaxation and meditation CDs by the author

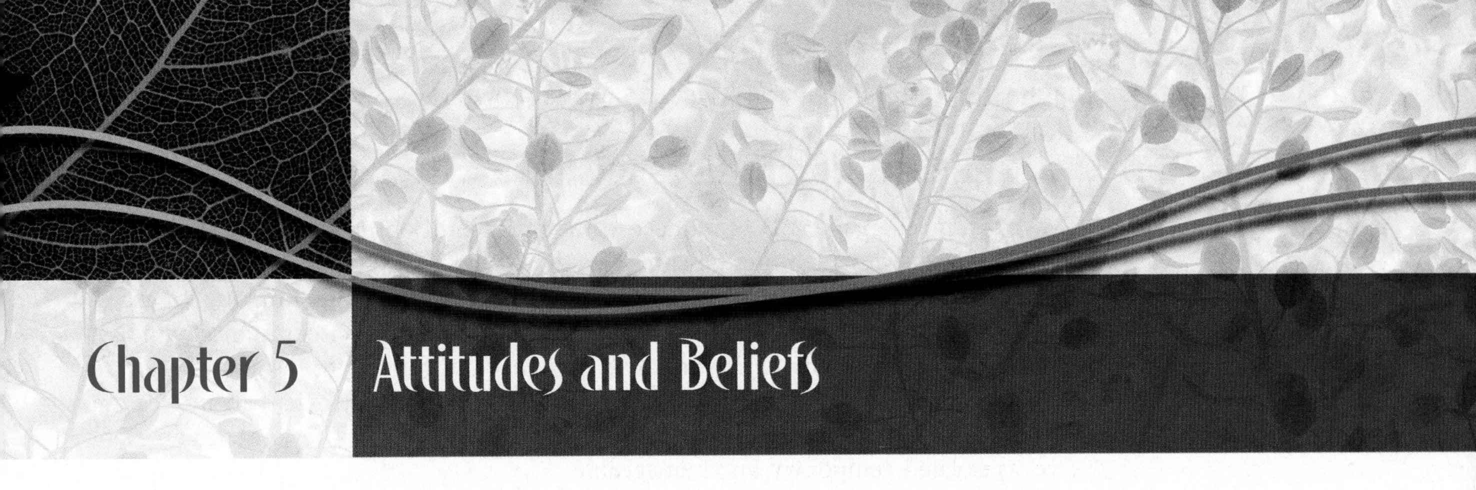

Chapter 5 Attitudes and Beliefs

People's attitudes and beliefs about health and illness play an important role in their ability to adapt to the challenges of living with a chronic medical condition. This chapter examines research from the fields of psychology, rehabilitation, and pain management that demonstrates a direct link between attitude and beliefs and physical and psychosocial function. Cognitive restructuring, a model from psychology commonly applied to changing maladaptive thinking habits, is described. The applications of mindfulness to cognitive restructuring are discussed.

The Role of Attitudes and Beliefs in Health

There are certain people and patient care experiences a clinician remembers. Often they surprise us, teach us something, or inspire us to think in new ways. Kathy was one of those people. A middle-aged woman who limited herself to the use of a wheelchair following multiple knee surgeries, she was referred to physical therapy for reconditioning and gait training. As part of her rehabilitation program, I taught her relaxation exercises for pain management. During one treatment session, I included a brief guided imagery, inviting her to imagine walking along a beach. I described the gait cycle in detail using such phrases as "experience the sensations of your legs moving through space and your feet touching the sand, feel the movement of your hips and spine with each step." When I was finished, I asked her to describe her experience. She spoke of the beauty of the beach, a feeling of peace, and the physical sensations of relaxation in her body; however, she never took a step. She could not imagine walking. This response came as an unexpected surprise to both of us and stimulated a discussion of her pessimistic outlook and inability to believe she could someday walk. She left our session determined to give this subject further thought, to explore a more positive attitude, and to experiment with the image of walking.

There is no way to determine how Kathy's initial inability or subsequent choice to imagine walking affected her rehabilitation progress. It was one of many experiences I had with patients early in my career as a physical therapist that led me to wonder how a person's attitude about his or her health and medical condition impacted rehabilitation, function, and quality of life. I began to ask new questions: Were people limited not only by their medical condition but also by how they *thought* about their condition? Was it possible for people with negative attitudes to change their outlook through education, coaching, and encouragement? Was there a constructive and healthy way to think about pain and illness?

Researchers from the fields of psychology, rehabilitation, and pain management have explored these questions, examining optimism versus pessimism, the role of attitude in chronic pain, and perceived locus of control.

Optimists Versus Pessimists

Martin Seligman, M.D., a pioneer in the research of optimistic versus pessimistic response styles, identifies pessimists as those who adopt a fatalistic outlook when faced with unpleasant events.[1] They are prone to catastrophic thinking, to excessively blaming themselves, to believing an unpleasant circumstance will last forever, and to generalizing negative thoughts and feelings from one situation to other aspects of their lives. Optimists, on the other hand, view an unpleasant circumstance in perspective and do not fall into self-blame. They see such an event as isolated, temporary, and manageable.

Individuals with pessimistic explanatory styles have poorer physical health, are prone to depression, and are more frequent users of health care services than optimists.[1] In addition, a pessimistic explanatory style is associated with increased mortality.[2] Researchers suggest that if pessimistic thinking puts people at increased risk for illness and premature death, it may be worthwhile to help people develop an optimistic outlook and reduce negative thinking.[2-4]

Beliefs, Catastrophic Thinking, Coping, and Chronic Pain

Numerous studies have examined how beliefs, catastrophic thinking, and coping relate to physical disability and psychosocial function in people with chronic pain conditions.[5-10] Although beliefs, thinking patterns, and coping ability are interdependent processes, researchers have examined them separately to identify how each may influence adjustment to chronic pain.

A *belief* is a trusted concept or assumption about reality. It creates the filter through which a person interprets, understands, and explains the world. Beliefs that solicitous responses by others to pain complaints are appropriate, that pain indicates damage, and that one is disabled by pain are associated with increased physical disability.[5-8]

Catastrophic thinking is a cognitive process of exclusive focus on negative thoughts and self-statements that emphasize the adversity of a situation, misinterpret an event as overwhelmingly negative, or project a disastrous outcome.[5] Negative thoughts and self-statements such as "I am useless" and "I am going to become an invalid" are associated with increased physical disability and depression.[5,8-10]

Catastrophic thinking has also been identified as a potential precursor for pain-related fear and subsequent avoidance behaviors.[11-13] A statement such as "If I sit at the computer, my back will hurt and I will end up in bed" creates fear of an activity in *anticipation* of pain. A person avoids activity because of an *imagined* experience of pain rather than because of actual pain. Continued avoidance of activity because of fear of pain results in deconditioning and decreased function and may be more disabling than pain itself.[12,14,15] In addition, people who are assessed with high fear of pain demonstrate attention bias toward pain-related somatic information compared with those who are identified with low fear of pain.[16] This finding suggests that people with a high fear of pain are vulnerable to increased pain experiences because of a biased attention process.

Coping is a process of changing thoughts and behaviors to adjust to and manage demands assessed by an individual as excessive. Self-limiting coping strategies, including muscle guarding, restricting activity, and asking for assistance, are associated with increased physical disability in patients with chronic pain.[17]

Several research studies suggest that interventions designed to change maladaptive beliefs, promote constructive self-talk, and provide effective coping strategies improve physical and psychosocial function.[18-23] In a review and meta-analysis of 25 randomized controlled trials of cognitive behavioral interventions for chronic pain in adults, Morley et al concluded that, when compared with control conditions, cognitive behavioral interventions were associated with significant improvements in pain experience, positive cognitive coping and appraisal, pain behavior, activity level, and social role function.[20]

Locus of Control

Locus of control (LOC) identifies the perceived sources of power that control a person's circumstances.[24] The two major categories of LOC are internal and external. People with an internal LOC believe they are responsible for and can directly influence their health status. Those with an external LOC believe their health status depends on outside forces. These outside forces include luck, chance, fate, or powerful others, such as health care providers or family members.

Diminished internal control and a belief that one's health is unpredictable is associated with depression. In addition, people with chronic pain who believe their health is contingent on outside forces report greater depression and anxiety, feel more helpless to deal with their pain, and employ more maladaptive coping strategies when compared with those patients with an internal LOC.[24,25]

On completion of a multidisciplinary treatment program for chronic pain, patients have shown an increase in perceptions of internal LOC and decreased external LOC.[24,26] In one study, 73 people with chronic pain underwent a 4-week outpatient treatment program that included cognitive therapy, relaxation exercises, coping skills training, and exercise utilizing both individual and group formats.[24] Following treatment, participants experienced a significant increase in their perceived control over their pain and a decrease in their perceptions that their pain was the result of fate, chance, or powerful others. This study suggests that pain beliefs can be changed. Additional research is needed to determine if these changes are sustained over time.

Promoting Healthy Thoughts, Attitudes, and Beliefs

A group wellness program provides an ideal opportunity to encourage practical and healthy attitudes and beliefs about living with chronic medical problems. Changing maladaptive thoughts, attitudes, and beliefs requires conscious effort. Cognitive restructuring is a model from the field of psychology that articulates a method for changing unhealthy thinking habits. Cognitive restructuring is a therapeutic process that offers step-by-step guidance to change negative and unconstructive thinking habits by first observing a thought and then evaluating and challenging its validity. The final step in this process is to replace a maladaptive thought with a more reasonable, realistic one.[27,28] By decreasing negative thoughts and replacing them with more rational responses, greater well-being is achieved. Cognitive restructuring does not deny or minimize the genuine suffering people experience, but rather provides the guidance necessary to address difficult situations with greater cognitive insight and skill.

Although many health care providers do not have formal psychology training in cognitive restructuring, it is introduced here as a potential subject for wellness programs because its core principle is straightforward and its healing potential in chronic illness populations is so great. Many people with chronic medical conditions lack the desire or financial resources to receive psychological services; however, they can benefit immensely from the main tenet of cognitive restructuring. Many health care professionals do not have extensive training in psychology, yet they are on the frontlines of patient care, constantly providing emotional and psychological support, coaching, and encouragement daily. The underlying principle of cognitive restructuring can provide an additional tool for helping people. Clinicians must always recognize and respect the limitations of their training in psychology and refer people for appropriate psychological services when necessary. Each clinician must recognize his or her own comfort level with the basic theme of cognitive restructuring. Those who are not at ease with the material or who seek an extensive exploration of the subject by an expert may want to invite a psychologist as a guest speaker to present to a group.

For the clinician without training in cognitive restructuring, its main principle can be presented to a group in a simplified manner by introducing the concept that we all are constantly telling ourselves stories. We have an experience and then we tell ourselves a story *about* that experience. For example, in the raisin exercise described in Chapter 3, a person has a direct experience of the raisin, observing the tactile sensation of the raisin against the skin, its color and texture, its taste, and so on. In addition, the person tells a story about the raisin: "I like raisins. The last time I ate raisins I was hiking in the Grand Canyon. That was such a great trip." The raisin is *not* the story. If the story we tell ourselves is somehow inaccurate and unskillful, it distorts our experience in a negative way. The mind, caught in maladaptive thinking patterns, is like a distorted mirror in a circus fun house. Just like the mirror grossly alters an image, the mind, clouded with distorted thinking, grossly alters our perception of reality. We can make the mistake of assuming that our biased story is accurate and selectively filter out evidence that challenges our viewpoint. Unfortunately, we make choices and adopt behaviors based on these maladaptive views that often compound our distress. These distorted concepts limit our possibilities and potential. On occasion, they can put our health at risk, as the following example demonstrates:

Case Example 5.1.

Olivia, a participant in my program, preferred to receive care from alternative health care practitioners and had a strong aversion to mainstream medical providers, particularly doctors. Diagnosed with a complex immune disorder, she was asked to see a rheumatologist by her naturopath. She didn't want to. She believed her approach to her body was so different from the mainstream medical model that she would only experience emotional distress and conflict if she had to deal with doctors. She feared they would never listen to her concerns and their only answer to her problems would be drugs that she did not want to take. She viewed all conventional doctors as authoritarian, insensitive, and as having an agenda incompatible with her own.

Olivia had a maladaptive story about doctors, including this rheumatologist whom she had never met, that was unrealistically negative and potentially jeopardizing to her health.

Psychiatrist David Burns, a pioneer and leader in the field of cognitive therapy, identifies the following common patterns of distorted thinking.[27] Introducing these categories in a wellness program heightens awareness of the different kinds of maladaptive stories we commonly get caught in.

1. *All or nothing thinking.* A person assesses a situation in black-and-white terms. It is either all good or all bad. "Since this back injury, my life is destroyed. If only someone could fix my back, everything would be perfect."
2. *Overgeneralization.* A person views one negative situation as evidence of a never-ending pattern. "I tried exercising once and it didn't help my pain, so I don't see any point in trying again. No exercise will help me. It would only be a waste of my time."
3. *Mental filter.* A person identifies and dwells only on the negative element in a situation. "Now that I have knee pain, my jogging days are over. My body is really falling apart now."
4. *Disqualifying the positive.* A person diminishes or rejects something good. "The people in this program are friendly and helpful, but I know they don't like me. They are just being kind because they feel sorry for me."
5. *Jumping to conclusions through mind reading or fortune telling.* Mind reading occurs when someone imagines others are reacting to him or her in a negative way. "I know my family hates me and resents me because I am sick." Fortune telling occurs when a person predicts a negative outcome without evidence to support his or her view. "I feel some tension in my shoulders and I just know it will turn into a bad headache and I'll have to spend the day in bed."
6. *Magnification or minimization.* A person amplifies the negative and/or diminishes the positive. "Since starting this walking program, I've doubled my distance, but I haven't lost a single pound. My clothes fit a little better, but what good is walking if it doesn't pay off by losing weight?"
7. *Should statements.* Should statements reflect idealized expectations and unrealistic demands a person places on him- or herself or others. "I should put in the overtime on this project, even though I don't feel well."
8. *Labeling.* A person narrows and limits his or her understanding by attaching a label to him- or herself or others. "I didn't do my exercises this week. I am a total failure."
9. *Emotional reasoning.* A person mistakenly concludes that feelings are evidence of reality. "I feel afraid to do the exercises. The exercises are harmful."
10. *Personalization and blame.* A person assumes excessive responsibility in a situation or inappropriately relinquishes responsibility. "It's all my fault I have cancer. If only I were a better person, I wouldn't be sick." "It's all the doctors' fault that I am sick. None of them know how to help me."

Think of the mind as a garden. Ruminating over negative stories is similar to watering the weeds. We can water the weeds or water the flowers. The choice is always ours.

We often make a difficult situation worse by our thinking. Sometimes changing how we think changes an experience in a powerful way. Replacing a horror story with a healing story can influence a person's symptoms and function, as the following experiences of people in my class demonstrate:

Case Example 5.2.

Lucy was a 62-year-old woman diagnosed with osteoarthritis. Her main complaint was right low back and hip pain that was severe when she stood up from a chair. After walking a few yards, the pain would diminish. Halfway through The Wellness Program, she reported the following

> experience: "I noticed how I would anticipate the pain when I was sitting. I began to think, "Oh no, here it comes. It's going to be bad. I hate this pain. I'm going to end up an invalid someday, just like my mother." I could feel myself tense. Based on what I've learned here, I decided to try something different. I now say to myself, "Look, there is more right with your body than wrong. Your left hip is great. So are your knees and ankles. When you get up, the pain won't last long. You can handle it." I also take a breath and try to relax a bit instead of tense before standing. I feel so much better emotionally, but the real surprise is the pain is much less intense and it is now easier to get up from a chair."

Sometimes changing deeply held beliefs requires determination and creativity. Olivia, described in Case Example 5.1, recognized she had a story about doctors that was adversely affecting her treatment options and possibly putting her health at risk. Changing her mind about physicians, however, would not be easy. In one class, she told the following experience: "I knew I had to do something to change my negative attitude, so I brought a book on mindfulness meditation to read while I waited for the doctor. I thought this would put my mind in a more open and calm state rather than a hostile one. When the doctor walked in, he asked me what I was reading. I said, "A book about meditation."

He responded, "Oh, I could really use that. It would probably help me a lot, but I don't have time." In that moment, I realized he suffered, too, and I immediately felt compassion for him. Me? Feel compassion for a doctor? It changed everything. I was still uneasy, but my defensiveness and hostility went way down. He turned out to be kind and helpful."

I had a dream that provides a striking image of the insubstantial nature of negative and distorted thought patterns. During a tumultuous time in my life, I dreamed that my negative interpretation of events was written as a story across the sky in sky-writing. The words themselves began to break apart, with the individual letters separating and tumbling to the earth. They landed in a wheelbarrow and a man rolled the wheelbarrow away. This dream provided straightforward insight into the flimsy basis of my negative perspective and the unequivocal guidance to drop it!

Wellness and well-being, in the face of life's joys and sorrows, is a complex process involving the dynamic interaction of physical, mental, emotional, spiritual, social, and environmental factors. In many situations, cognitive restructuring is a useful and successful strategy for transforming distress. In other circumstances, the process is not such a simple one. The genuine sorrows and difficulties people experience must be acknowledged and embraced. Cognitive restructuring serves as one of many valuable tools in an expanding toolbox for transforming suffering.

Mindfulness and Cognitive Restructuring

Mindfulness meditation, described in detail in Chapter 3, is an exercise in the deliberate and nonreactive observation of thoughts, emotions, and physical sensations. As such, it provides an additional framework for the steps of cognitive restructuring. A person learns to observe thoughts and develop insight into the interdependent relationships of thoughts, emotions, and physical sensations.

When mindful, a person acknowledges thoughts as just thoughts. They are not infallible expressions of reality or necessarily evidence of the truth. Thoughts are not one's identity. They are just thoughts. In addition, thoughts are not labeled as good or bad. All thoughts are treated equally. This approach minimizes the likelihood of falling into self-recrimination for thinking negatively. Mindfulness takes the dominating power away from thoughts and, in doing so, creates new possibilities for self-knowledge, self-control, and opportunities for choice.

With a nonjudging attitude, a person can explore how a thought triggers physical sensations and emotions. This exploration alone can be powerful and promote greater insight, understanding, and wisdom. Once a person mindfully observes a thought, the additional cognitive restructuring steps of inquiry and evaluation can begin. Is this story helping or hurting? Is it a story I want to give my attention and energy to? Is there an alternative approach to thinking about this situation? What would a healing story be in this situation? After this reflective process, a conscious choice can be made, as demonstrated by the following example:

Case Example 5.3.

David enrolled in The Wellness Program looking for ways to help manage his high blood pressure. He talked about watching his mind one Saturday: "I observed how I was thinking about work, going over and over the details of a project I'm on, criticizing myself for a mistake I made. Then I noticed how tense I was getting. My jaw was clenching and my shoulders started to rise up. 'Wow, look at this,' I said to myself. 'It's my day off and I'm probably pushing my blood pressure up just thinking about this!' I decided to come back to the present moment. It was a beautiful day. Why not come back to the moment? I took a breath. I felt my body sitting in a chair on my deck. With my mind on my breath, I could step back and just observe the story. I began to calm down and find a better perspective. I saw all that negative thinking as just a story that I could change. I said to myself, 'Yeah, I made a mistake. Big deal. I can correct the problem. I do more right around there than wrong. Everyone makes mistakes. No one would die from this! In a hundred years, no one will even remember it.' I told myself to focus on the present moment. I noticed the blue sky and mountains in the distance. I know it sounds like a little thing, but I was amazed by the difference I could feel in my whole being. I relaxed."

Mindfulness also helps people manage and decrease pain-related fear. If a person feels fear, it is observed and accepted. The physical sensations and thoughts that accompany fear are observed. No effort is made to avoid or eliminate the fear. It is acknowledged as an emotion, not evidence of any reality or a concrete reason to avoid activity. A mindful examination of fear reveals that it is sometimes linked with unpleasant thoughts about the future. Mindfulness, with its emphasis on the present moment, provides a useful framework for responding to this future focus. Thoughts about the future are observed and understood as concepts and ideas and not proof of truth. This mindful exploration itself is a powerful experience for people. In addition, it sometimes leads to new insight and a shift in attention from disturbing stories about the future back to the present moment. A person is no longer limited by self-generated ideas about a negative future, but instead, is attentive to the present moment experience where new possibilities can arise. The present moment is often manageable, and fear frequently decreases in the process of this shift. Other times people examining fear experience a wavelike quality to its intensity. They observe feelings of fear increase and, as they maintain a steady, present moment focus, observe it decrease. Levels of fear may come and go, and they now have a skillful means of relating to the fear.

A decrease in fear of pain is one outcome I hear described over and over again from participants in The Wellness Program who have chronic pain. The following is one patient example:

Case Example 5.4.

Marsha was a 43-year-old woman who came to the program to help her manage pain from fibromyalgia and an unsuccessful back surgery. At the end of the program, she described the change that took place: "When I started the program, I was always running from the pain. It was a monster constantly chasing me and I could never stop running. I was never at ease or relaxed mentally or physically. Mindfulness helped me examine my pain and fear and stop running. The pain is the same, but the fear is gone. It is such a relief to no longer have that feeling of always running and have the confidence that I can deal with the pain."

The profound power of coaching someone to observe thought processes and recognize choices in combination with mindfulness meditation and yoga is reflected in the following letter (Figure 5-1) from a participant in The Wellness Program received by instructor Peggy Mass, PT.

Figure 5-1 Letter from a Wellness Program participant to her instructor.

Hi Peg,
I have thought of you and our class so often these past weeks and have been meaning to write you. I really wanted you to know how much your class has changed my life. Prior to the class I really was quite a negative person, always dwelling on what was wrong with my life and not being thankful for all the blessings I have been given. I really don't know how to thank you for making such a difference in my life. I am so much happier today than I can remember in a long time. It is like you turned a light switch on in my brain. The yoga and meditation has also been very helpful to me, especially during this stressful time in our county since September 11th. I notice a difference in how I feel when I don't do it for a few days, especially with the pain. I have to say that you have had the most positive impact on my life of anyone or anything else I have ever tried. I truly cannot thank you enough. I hope your life is filled with many blessings.

Thank you!!

Wendy

Summary

A person's thoughts about his or her medical condition impact function and quality of life. Research into optimism versus pessimism, locus of control and beliefs, catastrophic thinking, and coping identifies a direct relationship between these cognitive processes and physical and psychosocial function. Cognitive restructuring alone, or in combination with mindfulness meditation, provides reliable guidelines to transform maladaptive thoughts into health-promoting ones. Well-being is enhanced by replacing an irrational or excessively negative outlook with a realistic or positive one.

References

1. Peterson C, Seligman ME, Vaillant GE. Pessimistic explanatory style is a risk factor for physical illness: a thirty-five year longitudinal study. *J Pers Soc Psychol* 1988;55(1):23-27.
2. Maruta T, Colligan R, Malinchoc M et al. Optimists vs. pessimists: survival rate among medical patients over a thirty year period. *May Clin Proc* 2000;75:140-143.
3. Seligman ME. Optimism, pessimism and mortality. *May Clin Proc* 2000;75:133-134.
4. Optimism may affect health as much as diet, exercise. *Patient Focus Care Satisf* 1999;7(7):78-80.
5. Turner J, Jensen M, Romano J. Do beliefs, coping, and catastrophizing independently predict functioning inpatients with chronic pain? *Pain* 2000;85:115-125.
6. Jensen M, Romano J, Turner J et al. Pain beliefs predict patient functioning: further support for a cognitive-behavioral model of chronic pain. *Pain* 1999;81:95-104.
7. Jensen M, Turner J, Romano J et al. Relationship of pain-specific beliefs to chronic pain adjustment. *Pain* 1994;57:301-309.
8. Stroud M, Thorn B, Jensen M et al. The relationship between pain beliefs, negative thoughts and psychosocial functioning in chronic pain patients. *Pain* 2000;84:347-352.
9. Hassett A, Cone J, Patella S et al. The role of catastrophizing in the pain and depression of women with fibromyalgia syndrome. *Arthritis Rheum* 2000;43(11):2493-2500.
10. Turner J, Davorkin S, Mancl L. The roles of beliefs, catastrophizing and coping in the functioning of patients with temporomandibular disorders. *Pain* 2001;92:41-51.
11. Cromberg G, Eccleston C, Baeyens F. When somatic information threatens, catastrophic thinking enhances attentional interference. *Pain* 1998;75: 187-198.
12. Vlaeyen J, Linton S. Fear-avoidance and its consequences in chronic musculoskeletal pain: a state of the art. *Pain* 2000;85:317-332.
13. Severeijns R, Vlaeyen J, van der Hout M et al. Pain catastrophizing predicts pain intensity, disability and psychological distress independent of the level of physical impairment. *Clin J Pain* 2000;17(2):165-172.

14. Cromberg G, Vlaeyen J, Heuts P et al. Pain-related fear is more disabling than pain itself: evidence on the role of pain-related fear in chronic back pain disability. *Pain* 1999;80:329-339.

15. Vlaeyen J, Kole-Snijders A, Baeren R et al. Fear of movement/(re)injury in chronic low back pain and its relation to behavioral performance. *Pain* 1995;62:363-372.

16. Keogh E, Ellery D, Hunt C, Hannet I. Selective attentional bias for pain-related stimuli amongst pain fearful individuals. *Pain* 2001;91(1-2): 91-100.

17. Haythornthwaite J, Menefee L, Heinberg L, Clark M. Pain coping strategies predict perceived control over pain. *Pain* 1998;77:33-39.

18. Brown D, Wang Y, Ebbeling C et al. Chronic psychological effects of exercise and exercise and cognitive strategies. *Med Sci Sports Exerc* 1995;27(5):765-775.

19. Speckens A, van Hemert, Spinhoven P et al. Cognitive behavioral therapy for medically unexplained physical symptoms: a randomized control trial. *BMJ* 1995;311:1328-1332.

20. Morley S, Eccleston C, Williams A. Systematic review and meta-analysis of randomized controlled trials of cognitive behavior therapy and behavior therapy for chronic pain in adults, excluding headache. *Pain* 1999;80:1-13.

21. van Tulder M, Ostelo R, Vlaeyen J et al. Behavioral treatment for chronic low back pain. *Spine* 2000;26(3):270-281.

22. Jensen MP, Turner JA, Romano JM. Changes in beliefs, catastrophizing, and coping are associated with improvements in multidisciplinary treatment. *J Consult Clin Psychol* 2000;69(4):655-662.

23. Marhold C, Linton SJ, Melin L. A cognitive-behavioral return-to-work program: effects on pain patients with a history of long-term vs. short-term sick leave. *Pain* 2001;91(1-2):155-163.

24. Coughlin A, Badura A, Fleischer T, Guck T. Multidisciplinary treatment of chronic pain patients: its efficacy in changing locus of control. *Arch Phys Med Rehabil* 2000;81:739-740.

25. Gustafsson M, Gaaston-Johansson F. Pain intensity and health locus of control: a comparison of patients with fibromyalgia syndrome and rheumatoid arthritis. *Patient Educ Counsel* 1996;29:179-188.

26. Lipchik G, Miles K, Covington E. The effects of multidisciplinary pain management treatment and locus of control and pain beliefs in chronic non-terminal pain. *Clin J Pain* 1993;9(1):49-57.

27. Burns D. *Feeling Good: the New Mood Therapy*. New York: Penguin Books, 1980, pp. 28-47.

28. Wells-Federman C, Stuart-Shor E, Webster A. Cognitive therapy: applications for health promotion, disease prevention, and disease management. *Nursing Clin N Am* 2001;36(1):93-113.

Annotated Bibliography

Burns D. *Feeling Good: the New Mood Therapy.* New York: William Morrow and Co., 1999. Drawing from his extensive experience, psychiatrist David Burns describes how people can change negative moods and self-defeating behaviors through the steps of cognitive restructuring. Burns uses many examples of client experiences to demonstrate this systematic program for changing maladaptive thinking habits and the behaviors they trigger. This book, which was written for the general public, is a useful, detailed introduction to cognitive restructuring principles and practice.

Foster R, Hicks G. *How We Choose to be Happy*. New York: Berkley Publishing Group, 1999. Rick Foster and Greg Hicks, successful business consultants, define happiness as: "A profound, enduring feeling of contentment, capability and centeredness." They traveled around the country, interviewing happy men and women, single and married, wide ranging in ages and from diverse backgrounds, in varied situations to learn what made happy people tick. This book shares the results of their research. People's constructive attitudes and thinking about their circumstances is one recurring theme. Foster and Hicks present the nine principles these people had in common and, drawing from the lives of those interviewed, reveal how it is possible to choose happiness even under difficult circumstances.

Greenberger D, Padesky C. *Mind Over Mood*. New York: Guilford Publications, 1995. Dennis Greenberger, Ph.D., and Christine Padesky, Ph.D., are clinical psychologists. This practical manual guides the reader to examine automatic thoughts and their role in mood. It offers suggestions for developing alternative or balanced thinking habits and provides worksheets for experimenting with new thoughts and behaviors. Designed in a self-help workbook format for the general public, this book provides the nonpsychologist with a comprehensive and accessible introduction to cognitive restructuring.

Segal ZV, Williams MG, Teasdale JD. *Mindfulness-Based Cognitive Therapy for Depression: a New Approach to Preventing Relapse.* New York: Guilford Publications, 2001. Zindal Segal, Ph.D., Professor of Psychiatry and Psychology at the University of Toronto; Mark Williams, Ph.D., Professor of Psychology at the University of Wales; and John Teasdale, Ph.D., from the Medical Research Council's Cognition and Brain Sciences Unit in Cambridge, England, combine their expertise to describe designing and leading an eight-session mindfulness-based group program to prevent the relapse of depression. They identify the theoretical basis for mindfulness in the treatment of depression and describe a group format and offer illustrative transcripts of group sessions. They provide guidelines for awareness exercises and specific cognitive interventions. The authors discuss their own introduction to the practice of mindfulness meditation and how their personal experience with the practice became the foundation for their teaching. This easy-to-read, thorough examination of a mindfulness-based group format for treating depression is an important contribution to the health field and highly recommended reading.

Chapter 6 Nutrition

Kathleen Putnam

Health care providers have an important responsibility and key role in providing people with nutritional information and helping them achieve and maintain a healthy weight. This chapter identifies basic nutrition information and guidelines for promoting healthy weight management. Achieving a desired weight through sustainable lifestyle changes is discussed. Eating for physical versus psychological reasons is explored, and a scale to help people distinguish levels of physiological hunger is presented. A framework for introducing healthy eating to a group is offered.

Nutrition Information

Good nutrition is essential to sustain life, promote health, and prevent many diseases. Helping people develop optimal eating habits is both a science and an art. A working knowledge of the role of foods in health and disease and sensitivity to the anxieties people have about food, body image, and body weight are necessary. A group format offers an ideal opportunity to provide people with nutrition guidelines and support to make healthy food choices.

Although basic nutritional concepts are clearly defined, eating habits are highly personal and change with time as tastes and physiological requirements change. Food choices are influenced by multiple factors, including childhood experiences, ethnicity and tradition, stress, habit, availability, economics, values, body image, emotional comfort, social interactions, and convenience.[1] Consequently, helping people identify an optimal and achievable diet requires flexibility and creativity.

A diagnosis of a chronic medical condition can be a pivotal opportunity to introduce and promote healthy eating habits. People are often surprised and empowered by the profound impact dietary changes have on health, energy level, and medical symptoms. For example, a person with diabetes can improve blood sugar levels and decrease the role of diabetic complications by altering the quantity or types of foods eaten. A person living with cardiovascular disease can often decrease blood pressure and cholesterol levels with changes in diet combined with increases in activity levels. The direct health results of dietary changes can promote self-confidence, self-efficacy, and self-esteem.

If the wellness group consists of participants with a variety of medical conditions, fundamental guidelines for healthy eating can be presented. If all participants share the same health concerns, nutritional information specific to a single medical condition can be addressed. Inviting a dietitian to speak to a group to address specific interests and needs can be incorporated into the program. Specific nutrition information for individual medical conditions is beyond the scope of this text. References that address nutritional information for select medical conditions are listed at the end of the chapter.

Nutritional Concepts

Good nutrition is much of what your mother always told you: Eat your vegetables! The basic concepts of nutrition include whole foods, variety, balance, moderation, adequacy, and nutrient density. These concepts are important whether a person needs to lose weight or is a performing athlete. They apply to everyone but need to be tailored to meet individual nutritional needs.

Research has repeatedly shown that a variety of whole foods promote healthy bodies and prevent disease.[2] A whole food is the food at its most natural state with minimal altering.[3] For example, an apple is more whole than applesauce. Most of the time whole foods, not just individual supplements containing nutrients or food compounds, promote health. Whole foods protect the body against common diseases such as diabetes, heart disease, and cancer.[1]

Variety

Eating a variety of foods promotes adequate nutritional intake, helps deliver an optimal balance of energy, and keeps food and meals interesting. Many people think changing breakfast cereal or lunch every so often adds adequate variety into their diet. This is a start; however, introducing food variety can be achieved in many ways and include much more creativity. Variety can be achieved by eating locally, seasonally, and ethnically.

Eating locally means eating those foods grown close to home rather than those shipped from long distances. Whole foods rotate in the markets as they come into and out of season. Eating with the seasons naturally encourages variety. Eating with the seasons requires a willingness to eat what is in season, wait for favorites to come into season, and try unfamiliar foods. Another benefit of eating in season is that it ensures a person chooses the most flavorful, nutrient-packed, and economical food. Eating ethnically or eating the local food when traveling helps introduce a variety of foods into our diet.

Practical ways to encourage variety in the diet include the following:

- Eat foods from three food groups at each meal.
- Eat a variety within each food group (e.g., a variety of fruits).
- Eat seasonal foods.
- Eat ethnically at least twice a week.
- Try a new restaurant twice a month.
- Try a new vegetable, fruit, whole grain, or bean weekly.
- Try a new recipe once a month.
- Take a cooking class.
- Visit an ethnic grocery store (e.g., Italian or Indian).

Moderation

Moderation is particularly important in our culture in which the idea "more is better" prevails. Eating in excess of nutritional needs is reflected in the current state of our population in which 50% of the population is overweight.[1] Eating too much food, one food, or one ingredient is not healthy. Moderation levels are not universal but vary with individual needs and physiological responses to foods and nutrients. For example, some hypertensive individuals experience a decrease in blood pressure when modifying sodium intake, whereas others do not.[1] Although general nutrition concepts are important for everyone, specific individual needs must be kept in mind when making nutrition recommendations. Sweeping generalizations regarding restrictive recommendations should be avoided. An example of an inappropriate generalization would be "all people with hypertension should avoid sodium."

Moderation is key to maintaining a healthy weight range. When weight loss is the goal, moderation of total caloric intake combined with increased energy expenditure as permanent lifestyle changes are optimal behaviors for the permanent weight loss.

When modifying intake of any nutrient, food, or food component, completely omitting foods or a favorite food is not recommended. Most foods can be fit into a meal plan. Including those favorite foods is often necessary for successful lifestyle modification. Those who have lost weight and been successful with maintaining weight loss over 5 years found that occasionally including favorite high-calorie foods into a meal plan was key to the permanent lifestyle change and weight loss, along with regular exercise and plenty of plant foods.

Another key point when discussing a restriction is to discover suitable substitutes and emphasize what can be eaten in large quantities, such as fruit and vegetables. Invoking feelings of deprivation or shame around food desires can be detrimental. A food plan must be livable so people can see themselves being successful with the recommended changes. Most of the public gets their nutrition information from the media, friends, and books, and some of it may include inappropriate self-imposed restrictions. This may lead to food taboos or off-limit foods unnecessarily.

Adequacy

Adequacy means getting enough of the essential nutrients to prevent nutrient depletion and avoid an eventual overt deficiency.[1] The quality of the diet is very important in nutritional adequacy. A high-quality diet is one with minimal processed foods and consisting mostly of a high volume of whole foods. The more food is altered from its natural form, the more nutrients are lost. As food is chopped, rinsed, dried, milled, ground, extracted, and exposed to light, heat, and air, the more nutrients are lost. The more people choose to eat whole, fresh, or frozen food, the more likely their diet is to be adequate.

Nutritional deficiencies are more common as a result of eating an abundance of processed food. The most common nutritional deficiency is iron deficiency leading to anemia. Those at highest risk for this deficiency are women of childbearing age.[1] Another common nutritional deficiency is the lack of adequate calcium in the diet, which is associated with osteoporosis and colon cancer.

Balance

The concept of balance is essential for health and weight control. The term *balance* refers to the percentage of protein, carbohydrates, and fat calories in a diet as well as the ratio of plant to animal food sources. The balance between plant and animal foods has health implications as well. Improving the balance in favor of plant sources of food is desirable to prevent and manage numerous illnesses.

The optimal balance between proteins, fats, and carbohydrates has recently been a subject of hot debate among researchers. The recommended amounts by the U.S. Department of Agriculture are 55% to 60% of calories from carbohydrates, 10% to 20% from protein, and less than 30% from fat.[1] Adhering to the recommended balance between high-fat, low-fat, and high-fiber foods is a good approach to maintaining this nutritional concept on a daily basis.

Balancing textures in meals and dishes both maintains interest and enjoyment and creates the variety needed in the diet. Balance of colors within a meal can also help ensure healthy levels of nutrients in the meal or dish. Differing tastes, including salty, sweet, sour, and bitter, also creates balance and maintains interest in foods.

Balancing caloric intake with physical activity is essential to weight control. Half the American population is struggling with maintaining a healthy body weight.[1] Both incorporating regular physical activity and a well-balanced diet are often necessary to achieve a healthy weight. The amount of food and exercise required to reach a healthy weight varies from one person to the next.

Nutrient Density

Foods considered nutrient dense are those low in calories yet high in nutrients. An example of nutrient-dense foods are dark green leafy vegetables. Loaded with vitamins, minerals, and phytochemicals, these vegetables deliver many nutrients without many calories. For example, one cup of cooked kale contains 36 calories, 3 g fiber, 23 mg magnesium, 94 mg calcium, 296 mg potassium, and 53 mg vitamin C.[1] Whereas, one-half cup of butter contains 820 calories, 0 g fiber, and minimal magnesium, calcium, potassium, and vitamin C![1]

Foods lose nutrient density as high-calorie additives are included and heavily processed in the preparation from the whole food. For example, a potato prepared as French fries has lost its nutrient density and has become calorie dense. Unfortunately, many of our food-processing techniques compromise the nutrient density of foods.

Nutrients

Nutrients essential to a healthy diet are carbohydrates, protein, fat, omega 3 fatty acids, vitamins and minerals, water, and phytochemicals.

Carbohydrates

Carbohydrates are the preferred energy source of the body. When exerting our bodies, carbohydrates are the first type of fuel used by our muscles. In addition, carbohydrates are the preferred source of energy for the brain. High-quality carbohydrates are healthier than refined versions. High-quality carbohydrates, such as brown rice and whole-wheat products, are nutrient rich and promote adequate nutrition, whereas refined carbohydrates, such as white bread, are often depleted of nutrients. Ironically, heavily processed foods often have nutrients added to them to appear as nutritious as their whole-food counterpart. Although these processed foods remain nutrient inferior to whole foods, the customer is often deceived. For example, refined white flour has folate, niacin, riboflavin, thiamin, and iron added back in after refining; however, much more than just the B vitamins and iron are lost in the processing. Nutrients lost include fiber, zinc, magnesium, and B_6.[1] Choosing whole grains such as whole wheat, oats, and brown rice instead of the refined versions is central to a healthy diet and disease prevention.

Nutrients have been added to the refined flour as a result of diseases linked to nutrient-deficient diets; however, refined flour remains nutrient inferior to whole grains. For instance, people eating whole grains on a regular basis have a lower risk of developing Type 2 diabetes than those who do not. The effects of suboptimal levels of nutrients in the body continue to be researched and explored. Ways to ensure high-quality carbohydrate intake include the following:

- Eat whole grains as much as possible.
- Try an unfamiliar whole grain, such as quinoa or buckwheat.
- Eat vegetables at least three to four times daily.
- Eat whole fresh or frozen fruit as much as possible two to four times daily.
- Eat beans in soups, salads, dips, and spreads daily.

Protein

Protein, also known as the nutrient of life, is essential to growth, maintenance, and repair of the body. Not a preferred energy source for the body, the recommended percentage of calories of protein to the other energy nutrients is the lowest at 10% to 20% of total calories. High-quality proteins, containing moderate to low amounts of cholesterol and saturated fat, are essential to health.

The body does not require all amino acids to be present in the food we eat at once. Our bodies are able to combine amino acids from one meal with the next to produce the body proteins necessary for health. If all essential amino acids are eaten within a 24-hour period, the body's protein needs will be met. It was once thought that plant protein sources, other than soy, had to be combined in one meal to receive all of the essential amino acids needed by the body. We now know that is not true. Therefore, any legume is a good source of protein as long as grains, dairy, or meat/fish are also eaten in the same day. Eating a source of protein at each meal is recommended to achieve balance, moderation, adequacy, blood sugar, and calorie control.

High-quality protein sources include the following:

- Soy products (considered a complete protein)
- Legumes or dried beans
- Most nuts and seeds
- Lean meats such as chicken or turkey breast, fish, beef, or pork tenderloin
- Egg whites
- Nonfat or 1% dairy products

Fat

Although fat gets lots of negative press, it plays many important roles in the body's health. The absorption of fat-soluble vitamins provides insulation, organ protection, and the building blocks for hormones. Just as the quality of carbohydrate and protein is important for health, so is the quality of fat. The most desirable fats for our health are the monounsaturated fats, whereas the least desirable fats are hydrogenated and saturated fats.

Hydrogenated oils are unsaturated oils processed by adding hydrogen to make them solid at room temperature and more shelf stable. Saturated fats are "naturally" high in hydrogen and, just like hydrogenated fats, are solid at room temperature. Saturated fats are found in high-fat dairy and beef products, coconut, palm kernel, and cocoa. Hydrogenated fats include margarines and shortenings. Hydrogenated fat is manufactured to mimic or replace saturated fat and acts similar to saturated fat in our food products and in the body by raising cholesterol levels. An additional concern when using hydrogenated fats is the transfatty acids produced in the process of hydrogenation. Transfatty acids are found predominantly in margarines and shortenings and products containing them. Avoiding margarines, shortenings, and foods containing hydrogenated or "partially hydrogenated" oils limits transfatty acids in the diet. Transfatty acids are minimal in whole foods but are a product of hydrogenation and contribute to elevated blood cholesterol levels.[1]

Polyunsaturated fatty acids are chemically the most volatile oils, with multiple double bonds in the chemical structure, and have a higher rancidity potential. Consumption of these oils should be minimized because they potentially increase the risk for heart disease and some cancers. Polyunsaturated fatty acids include most vegetable oils, such as soybean, cottonseed, sunflower, safflower, and corn oil.

The optimal fatty acids are the monounsaturated fats. Monounsaturated fats contain only one double bond in the chemical structure. Monounsaturated fats aid in lowering the risk of developing high blood cholesterol levels and thus decrease the risk for cardiovascular disease. These fats include the fat predominantly found in olives, nuts, and avocados, as well as olive, canola, and peanut oils.

Practical ways to improve the quality of fat intake include the following:

- Use olive, canola, and peanut oils at home in cooking and food preparation.
- Use nut butters, olive oil, or olive tapenade on bread and toast instead of margarine or butter.
- Use guacamole instead of sour cream.
- Use avocado instead of cheese on sandwiches.

Omega 3 Fatty Acids

Omega 3 fatty acids are one type of fat linked with disease prevention. These fats have both anti-inflammatory and anti-clotting properties. They have been shown to lower triglyceride levels, protect against some cancers, and are associated with a significant reduction of sudden cardiac death in men. Omega 3 fatty acids, however, are very low in the average diet and are becoming less and less available in the food supply. The best sources of omega 3 fatty acids are fatty fish such as salmon, mackerel, tuna, sardines, and flaxseed oil or ground flaxseed, walnuts, and butternuts. To a much lesser extent, omega 3 fatty acids are found in olive and canola oil and dark green leafy vegetables.[1]

Vitamins and Minerals

Vitamins and minerals are referred to as micronutrients. Our bodies need these nutrients in small amounts compared to carbohydrates, fats, proteins, and water. Each vitamin and mineral has a specific function in the body, and all are essential to achieve and maximize wellness. Vitamins and minerals work together to produce their desired function. For example, the development of red blood cells requires vitamins B_6, B_{12}, folate, iron, and copper. If one of these nutrients is missing, the production of red blood cells is impaired. In the media, one nutrient is often focused on as being the "super nutrient" or the "age-defying nutrient" when in fact all nutrients are necessary for health and wellness.

Historically, how much of each nutrient we require was determined based on levels at which a nutrient deficiency was seen. As nutrition science has advanced, nutrient levels are determined not only by prevention of deficiency but also by promotion of health and the potential for protecting against disease. Optimal nutrient levels vary with age, gender, medical condition, and medications taken.

Supplements

Although not a substitute for a health-promoting balanced diet, nutritional supplements may help prevent deficiencies and protect against some diseases. Several over-the-counter multiple vitamin daily supplements are adequate. A range of 100% to 300% of the recommended dietary allowance is the appropriate range for any individual vitamin or mineral level in a supplement. Many supplements are toxic and can cause problems if taken in high doses without medical supervision. A balance among individual nutrients is important as well. This is especially true among the minerals. Taking too much of one mineral may induce a deficiency of another. For example, too much calcium alone may impair iron and magnesium absorption and eventually cause a deficiency.

Water

Water is the *most* essential of all the nutrients. Our bodies may go days, even weeks, without food but not without water. Almost all processes carried out in the body require water. Water is needed for regulating the body's temperature, transporting nutrients, and cushioning joints and body tissues. On average, an adult requires about 8 to 10 cups of water daily, with additional fluids required with physical exertion and hot weather.

Practical ways to ensure adequate water intake include the following:

- Carry a water bottle with you and drink from it throughout the day.
- Drink a full glass of water when taking medications.
- Drink a full glass of water before each meal.
- Drink a glass of water after urination.
- Take water breaks instead of coffee or soda breaks.
- Drink juice or carbonated water for a break.
- Drink additional water before, during, and after exercise.
- Eat plenty of fruits and vegetables throughout the day (lettuce is 95% water, watermelon is 92%, and broccoli is 91%).

Phytochemicals

Phyto is a Greek term meaning "plant." Phytochemicals come only from plant sources.[1] Phytochemicals are newly discovered plant compounds beneficial to health. Phytochemicals are beneficial in addition to the fiber, water, vitamins, and minerals also found in fruits, vegetables, and whole grains. Phytochemicals have been shown to protect the body against heart disease and various cancers.[1]

Eating to be Well

Healthy eating is a permanent lifestyle, not a short-lived experiment with a special diet. The problem with most diets is that we often go "on" them and then go "off" them, returning to old eating habits. Any benefit is lost over the long term. Ninety-five percent of diets fail because new eating habits are temporary and are not embraced as a lifestyle. Eating to be well can include recognizing our connection with food sources, combining foods, and nurturing ourselves in ways other than eating.

Connection

As the food industry has changed throughout the years, most of us have lost our connection with our food source. The art of growing and raising one's own food is rare. Honoring our food sources can improve our appreciation of our food and help us feel more connected and more mindful of our food.

Practical suggestions to connecting more with our food sources include the following:

- Shop at a farmer's market.
- Visit a local farm, orchard, or ranch.
- Grow your own vegetables.
- Start an herb garden.
- Participate in "pick your own" farms and orchards.
- Join a sustainable farm program.
- Participate in urban communal gardening.

Food Combinations

Eating a variety of foods throughout the day containing carbohydrates, proteins, and fats aids in achieving balance and may help satisfy hunger more than eating predominantly carbohydrates. Carbohydrates are the quickest digested of all the energy nutrients. By combining protein and fats with snacks and meals, managing balance, variety, and energy is easier to obtain.

Meal and snack ideas to incorporate a variety of nutrients include the following:

- Natural peanut butter and whole-grain bread
- Low-fat/nonfat milk and cereal
- Low-fat/nonfat yogurt and fruit
- Fruit and low-fat/nonfat cottage cheese
- Hummus or any bean dip and pita with vegetables
- Sandwich with whole-grain bread, lean meat, and vegetables
- Bean or lentil soup and a whole-grain roll

Nurture Yourself

Many people nurture themselves with food when they need support or to express feelings. Awareness of this behavior is key. The practice of mindfulness described is Chapter 3 can help people identify feelings when they are about to eat, while eating, and afterward. Many people eat when they are bored, anxious, lonely, angry, or sad. Some people eat when feeling excitement or joy.

After identifying *when* and *why* they eat, people can identify habit patterns and make mindful, healthy choices. Instead of eating chocolate cake after a rough day, a person can choose a hot bath. Encouraging people to find truly enjoyable, comforting treats to replace eating is key for success. Group participants can develop their own list of comforts and be encouraged to practice them mindfully. They can avoid denying themselves food when they are hungry and be aware of when they eat for comfort.

Weight Control

The health and economic impact of the increasing numbers of overweight and obese people in the U.S. population is a major public health concern. Medical researchers have estimated that the direct costs of medical treatment for obesity and chronic diseases resulting from obesity, based on 1995 U.S. dollar value, are approximately $70 billion annually.[4] Clinicians leading wellness programs have an opportunity to help address this major health problem and to coach participants in weight-control strategies.

Assessing Body Weight

One common way to assess weight is to determine body mass index (BMI) (Figure 6-1). BMI reflects the relationship between body weight and body stature. As weight increases in proportion to height, the risk of disease increases. An optimal BMI is within the range of 19 to 25. It is important to note, however, that many physically active and healthy individuals have a BMI over 25. Although it is a broadly recognized and clinically useful standard, the BMI method of weight assessment has limitations when assessing individuals with exceptionally large muscle mass. A highly muscular person may have a BMI greater than 25 and yet be within a healthy weight range. Having a weight within the goal range of 19 to 25 BMI does not necessarily assure good health.[1]

Weight Proportion

Where weight is carried on the body has health implications. Excess adipose or fat tissue found in the trunk or abdomen is associated with an increased risk of hypertension, hypercholesterolemia, and diabetes. These elevated risks are not found in people who carry excess weight in the extremities.

Weight Loss

Weight loss is a common struggle in our culture. Although many people begin diets and lose weight, they fail to maintain the weight loss. Successful weight loss requires the active involvement of people in developing and committing to lifestyle changes. People cannot maintain excessively restrictive diets, deny their hunger, and/or participate in excessive amounts of physical activity as a lifestyle. Motivation strategies, coaching, meal planning, mindfulness, physical exercise, as well as minimizing eating in response to stress and emotions all may be needed for people to successfully achieve the lifestyle changes required to keep the weight off.

Eating every 3 to 4 hours and not skipping meals helps prevent overeating or choosing less nutrient-dense food later in the day. Practicing the mindful eating exercise described in Chapter 3 as well as identifying hunger signals versus appetite signals can help by minimizing eating in response to stress or emotions.

Unintended Weight Loss

Underweight individuals are at higher risk for disease caused by weaker immune systems, compromised nutrition and nutritional deficiencies, and increased risk of bone fractures. The bottom line is that eating more calories is necessary for weight gain. Eating a balanced diet is still important; however, nutrient limitations such as restricted sugar should not necessarily be enforced until a healthy body weight is achieved.

Body Mass Index Table

	Normal						Overweight					Obese										Extreme Obesity														
BMI	**19**	**20**	**21**	**22**	**23**	**24**	**25**	**26**	**27**	**28**	**29**	**30**	**31**	**32**	**33**	**34**	**35**	**36**	**37**	**38**	**39**	**40**	**41**	**42**	**43**	**44**	**45**	**46**	**47**	**48**	**49**	**50**	**51**	**52**	**53**	**54**
Height (inches)	**Body Weight (pounds)**																																			
58	91	96	100	105	110	115	119	124	129	134	138	143	148	153	158	162	167	172	177	181	186	191	196	201	205	210	215	220	224	229	234	239	244	248	253	258
59	94	99	104	109	114	119	124	128	133	138	143	148	153	158	163	168	173	178	183	188	193	198	203	208	212	217	222	227	232	237	242	247	252	257	262	267
60	97	102	107	112	118	123	128	133	138	143	148	153	158	163	168	174	179	184	189	194	199	204	209	215	220	225	230	235	240	245	250	255	261	266	271	276
61	100	106	111	116	122	127	132	137	143	148	153	158	164	169	174	180	185	190	195	201	206	211	217	222	227	232	238	243	248	254	259	264	269	275	280	285
62	104	109	115	120	126	131	136	142	147	153	158	164	169	175	180	186	191	196	202	207	213	218	224	229	235	240	246	251	256	262	267	273	278	284	289	295
63	107	113	118	124	130	135	141	146	152	158	163	169	175	180	186	191	197	203	208	214	220	225	231	237	242	248	254	259	265	270	278	282	287	293	299	304
64	110	116	122	128	134	140	145	151	157	163	169	174	180	186	192	197	204	209	215	221	227	232	238	244	250	256	262	267	273	279	285	291	296	302	308	314
65	114	120	126	132	138	144	150	156	162	168	174	180	186	192	198	204	210	216	222	228	234	240	246	252	258	264	270	276	282	288	294	300	306	312	318	324
66	118	124	130	136	142	148	155	161	167	173	179	186	192	198	204	210	216	223	229	235	241	247	253	260	266	272	278	284	291	297	303	309	315	322	328	334
67	121	127	134	140	146	153	159	166	172	178	185	191	198	204	211	217	223	230	236	242	249	255	261	268	274	280	287	293	299	306	312	319	325	331	338	344
68	125	131	138	144	151	158	164	171	177	184	190	197	203	210	216	223	230	236	243	249	256	262	269	276	282	289	295	302	308	315	322	328	335	341	348	354
69	128	135	142	149	155	162	169	176	182	189	196	203	209	216	223	230	236	243	250	257	263	270	277	284	291	297	304	311	318	324	331	338	345	351	358	365
70	132	139	146	153	160	167	174	181	188	195	202	209	216	222	229	236	243	250	257	264	271	278	285	292	299	306	313	320	327	334	341	348	355	362	369	376
71	136	143	150	157	165	172	179	186	193	200	208	215	222	229	236	243	250	257	265	272	279	286	293	301	308	315	322	329	338	343	351	358	365	372	379	386
72	140	147	154	162	169	177	184	191	199	206	213	221	228	235	242	250	258	265	272	279	287	294	302	309	316	324	331	338	346	353	361	368	375	383	390	397
73	144	151	159	166	174	182	189	197	204	212	219	227	235	242	250	257	265	272	280	288	295	302	310	318	325	333	340	348	355	363	371	378	386	393	401	408
74	148	155	163	171	179	186	194	202	210	218	225	233	241	249	256	264	272	280	287	295	303	311	319	326	334	342	350	358	365	373	381	389	396	404	412	420
75	152	160	168	176	184	192	200	208	216	224	232	240	248	256	264	272	279	287	295	303	311	319	327	335	343	351	359	367	375	383	391	399	407	415	423	431
76	156	164	172	180	189	197	205	213	221	230	238	246	254	263	271	279	287	295	304	312	320	328	336	344	353	361	369	377	385	394	402	410	418	426	435	443

Source: Adapted from *Clinical Guidelines on the Identification, Evaluation, and Treatment of Overweight and Obesity in Adults:The Evidence Report.*

Figure 6-1 Body Mass Index Table.
(Source: National Heart, Lung and Blood Institute.)

Guidelines for weight gain include the following:

- Choose enjoyable foods.
- Drink fluids with calories or nutrients such as juice and smoothies rather than tea, coffee, or even water.
- If approved by a physician, drink alcohol before you eat to stimulate the appetite.
- Make the atmosphere comfortable and inviting to eat.
- Eat a little more food than usual every time you eat.

Behavior Change

Achieving sustained weight loss is very difficult for most people. Many will change eating patterns for a few weeks and lose weight, only to return to old eating habits and regain the lost pounds. For others, just the thought of dieting is alienating. Many people associate changing eating habits with deprivation and being "bad" when they eat their favorite foods.

Distinguishing Between Appetite and Hunger

Identifying *why* we are eating can be very important when trying to achieve or maintain a healthy weight. Hunger is the physiological need for food. When hungry, the stomach may growl or the head may become light. These physiological signs indicate that the body needs food. Appetite is the psychological desire for food. These are cues other than the physiological need to eat. For example, a person may eat when feeling tired after a long day at the office or worried about a child's illness. Many people eat when they experience an appetite related to psychological desires rather than physiological hunger. First, observing physical sensations and feelings before, during, and after eating raises awareness. Learning to check in regularly to identify feelings and physical sensations helps people identify if and how often they eat for reasons other than hunger.

Hunger Scale

Self-monitoring has been shown to be helpful for both weight loss and maintenance of weight loss. Observing food intake, physical activity, hunger, feelings, stress levels, and body weight are all examples of beneficial self-monitoring.

Many people do not pay attention to their bodies. They do not notice the signs of hunger or the signs of being full. Without the former, they do not eat until they are ravenous and then eat anything in sight. Without sensing fullness, they continue to eat long after their physiological need for food is met.

A simple technique to help people become aware of hunger is the hunger scale. On the hunger scale, "1" is ravenous. This is when physiologically the body is screaming for food. Under these conditions, a person would eat foods otherwise considered undesirable because of extreme hunger. We want to avoid ever being at a "1" on the hunger scale. When approaching this level of hunger, judgment regarding what to eat is more likely to "impaired."

On the other end of the scale, a rating of "10" would mean eating until a person is so uncomfortable it is difficult to move. This can be thought of as "Thanksgiving full." If regularly eating to this fullness, a person is probably not eating in response to hunger but for other reasons. Learning to differentiate between physical hunger and appetite or emotional or stress eating is imperative for many people.

Building Skills

Teaching people the mindful body scan exercise described in Chapter 3 provides this key skill of body awareness. Applying body awareness to the experience of eating, people can observe their experience before a meal. Observing present moment sensations of hunger, emotions, and thinking about food, people gain insight into what drives their eating: Are they truly hungry? Are they eating out of habit or boredom? Or are other things going on? Are they experiencing unpleasant emotions and seeking to comfort or numb the experience through food?

People can continue to apply mindful awareness to their experience while eating a meal. By becoming aware of the colors, textures, and flavors in food, people can discover greater satisfaction in smaller amounts of food. They can also stop eating at the first sign of being full rather than continue eating unconsciously. They sometimes recognize a relationship between foods and physical symptoms, as the following case example illustrates:

Case Example 6.1.

Janette was a 52-year-old woman diagnosed with lupus, high blood pressure, and fibromyalgia. Her doctor recommended that she take The Wellness Program to help her manage her high stress levels that might be contributing factors to her elevated blood pressure and pain. When she began eating mindfully, she noticed that certain foods exacerbated her symptoms. When she ate citrus, chocolate, or beef, her symptoms of fatigue and pain worsened. Listening to and trusting herself, Janette decided to omit these foods and observe her body's response. Her pain decreased significantly. To her pride and delight, she was able to eliminate the three to four ibuprofen pills she had previously taken daily from her medication regimen.

Once skills of awareness are established, realistic nutrition and dietary goals can be chosen. Just as with any other lifestyle change, establishing realistic and achievable goals is necessary for success. In a group setting, participants can be asked to identify long-term eating and activity goals, and, week by week, establish short-term steps toward achieving those goals.

When changing eating habits, keep in mind the following:

- Identify realistic and achievable changes.
- Include favorite foods.
- Be aware of the easy availability of foods in grocery stores and restaurants.
- Avoid constant hunger.
- Balance physical activity with food requirements.

Consulting with a Dietitian

Coaching and assistance from a registered dietitian may help achieve weight loss or weight gain in the long term. Dietitians are trained in lifestyle changes, coaching, meal planning, recipe adaptations and resources, supporting changes, identifying barriers, and working with a multidisciplinary team to help clients meet their goals. To find a registered dietitian in your area, go to: www.eatright.org and conduct a search for a dietitian practicing in your city and with the expertise you are looking for. Interview the dietitian about his or her expertise and comfort with the area you are interested in and how he or she might work with you.

Introducing Nutrition and Healthy Eating to a Group

Nutrition is a broad topic. Participants often have many questions as well as a wide range of experiences with nutrition and eating. People often have information and experiences with food that can be helpful to other group members. The following class structure is one framework for any clinician to use to introduce the topic of food and nutrition. Clinicians can also survey the group to identify the specific interests and needs of group members. If clinicians do not have the necessary training and experience in nutrition, they can invite a registered dietitian to the class to discuss these specific interests and needs.

1. Ask the group members to define *nutrition* or *nourishment*. Write the definitions on a blackboard.
2. Reflect back to the group any patterns of responses and how "nourishment" can sometimes be mistaken for "nurturing." Guide the group into a discussion of emotional eating or eating in response to appetite rather than hunger and offer the following definitions:
   - Appetite is eating for psychological reasons related to feelings or stress.
   - Hunger is eating in response to physical needs.
3. Ask the group to share how they know they are truly hungry (e.g., stomach growl, headache, irritability).
4. Ask the group to share experiences of eating when not physically hungry but eating because of emotions or stress.
5. Discuss how knowing the difference between the two reasons for eating and bringing awareness to eating and meals is an essential first step. One way to begin this practice is to journal or make a note by asking the question before eating: How am I feeling? Am I hungry? How do I know I am hungry? What am I hungry for? People often realize that they do not know what it feels like to be physically hungry. Others may observe that they regularly go from hunger lows to sugar or caffeine highs.

If your group includes those who are trying to gain weight or eat more calories, this framework can be used. Participants can be encouraged to pay attention to what hunger feels like and what happens when responding to it with a balanced meal.

Summary

Obesity and nutrition-related chronic diseases are on the rise in the United States. Good nutrition is essential to sustain life, promote health, and prevent many diseases. The basic concepts of nutrition include whole foods, variety, balance, moderation, adequacy, and nutrient density. Although these basic nutritional concepts are clearly defined, eating habits are highly personal and influenced by multiple factors. Helping people identify an optimal and achievable diet requires awareness of these factors and the skill to respond with sensitivity to vulnerabilities many people experience while discussing food and eating habits. It requires flexibility and creativity. Identifying issues related to nutrition, hunger, and appetite in a group setting can lead to an informative discussion and an improved understanding of nutritional concepts and eating practices. Building awareness through mindful eating practices can offer the first step toward improved nutritional practices. If a group would benefit from specific nutrition and weight management guidance, a clinician without training in nutrition can invite a dietitian to participate in a discussion of health, nutrition, mindful eating practices, and weight management.

References

1. Whitney EN, Rolfes SR. *Understanding Nutrition* 8th ed. Belmont, Calif: Wadsworth Publishing Co., 1999.
2. Duyff RL. *The American Dietetic Association's Complete Food and Nutrition Guide.* Minneapolis: Chronimed Publishing, 1998.
3. Roehl E. *Whole Food Facts, the Complete Reference Guide.* Rochester, Vt: Healing Arts Press, 1996.
4. Colditz GA. Economic costs of obesity and inactivity. *Med Sci Sports Exerc* 1999;31(11 Suppl):S663–S667.

Annotated Bibliography

Tribole E, Resch E. *Intuitive Eating.* New York: St Martins Mass Market Paper, 1996. Developing a healthy relationship with food is a difficult task in our food-crazed, body-conscious culture. Escape the diet mentality and practice the nondieting principles focused on establishing a comfortable and enjoyable relationship with food and physical activity. By eating intuitively or practicing mindful eating, the dieting and food-related issues begin to disappear and making peace with food blossoms.

Duyff RL. *The American Dietitic Association's Complete Food and Nutrition Guide.* Minneapolis: Chronimed Publishing, 1998. This guide is a comprehensive wealth of information and an easy-to-read resource on the latest subjects related to food and nutrition from weight management to food allergies. User-friendly charts, suggestions, and fun nutrition tidbits are included throughout the book, offering practical, creative ways to improve our dietary choices for everyone from the picky eater to the too-busy-to-cook person. Nutrition and health myths are explored, as well as meal planning, cooking, and shopping tips.

III Exercise

Chapter 7 Fitness

This chapter examines the role of exercise in the treatment of chronic pain and disease, reviews the elements of fitness and principles of training, and provides guidelines for leading group exercise.

Exercise and Chronic Pain, Disease, and Aging

Epidemiological evidence from the U.S. Centers for Disease Control and Prevention indicates that only 15% of adults in the United States participate in regular moderate physical activity, and 40% of adults are not active at all.[1] Certain segments of the population are more sedentary than others. Specifically, sedentary behavior is more prevalent among women (43% of women versus 36% of men), older adults (65% of adults 65 to 74 years of age versus 34% of adults 25 to 44 years of age), and ethnic minorities (52% of African Americans and 54% of Hispanics versus 38% of Caucasians). Less education and less income are associated with increases in sedentary behavior. Forty-six percent of individuals with a high school education report no leisure time activity, whereas 24% of college graduates report being sedentary. Sixty-five percent of those with an annual income of less than $15,000 are sedentary compared with 48% of those with an annual income of more than $50,000. The Healthy People 2010 Initiative, coordinated by the U.S. Office of Disease Prevention and Health Promotion, establishes an ambitious goal of decreasing sedentary behavior across all segments of the adult population to 20% and increasing the number of adults participating in regular moderate physical activity to 30%.[2]

Because most American adults are sedentary and significant health gains are made with low to moderate increases in activity, all health care professionals have the responsibility to promote exercise. A group wellness program provides an ideal opportunity for providing exercise guidelines and instruction and encouraging the habit of exercise. Whether promoting a walking program, a stretching routine, or a comprehensive fitness workout, a wellness program is a key resource for people with chronic conditions to develop the habit of safe and appropriate exercise to maximize physical and mental health and function.

Considerable medical evidence identifies the role of exercise in the prevention and treatment of several common medical conditions, including cardiovascular disease, cancer, chronic pain, diabetes, obesity, osteoporosis, rheumatological conditions, and musculoskeletal pain. Regular exercise also has an important role in healthy aging. Mainly citing review articles, evidence for the role of exercise in the prevention and treatment of these conditions is highlighted in the following sections. The intent is to provide an introduction to the role of exercise in these common medical conditions and to inspire clinicians to include an exercise component in a wellness program serving these populations. For a more thorough examination of exercise for chronic disease populations, see the annotated bibliography at the end of this chapter.

Cardiovascular Disease

Physical inactivity is an independent risk factor for cardiovascular disease (CVD). A meta-analysis of research examining the relationship between physical activity and heart disease concluded that sedentary people have a nearly two-fold increased risk of CVD compared to active individuals.[3] In addition, exercise has significant benefits for those already diagnosed with CVD. In an extensive review of the medical literature examining the role of exercise in the treatment of CVD, authors Lear and Ignaszewski cite the benefits of exercise as an improved CVD risk factor profile, slower disease progression, and reduced morbidity and mortality.[4] In addition, when exercise is combined with a rigorous and comprehensive lifestyle intervention that includes a vegetarian diet, smoking cessation, yoga, and group psychological support, regression of disease has been documented.[5]

Cancer

Moderate physical activity is associated with a decreased risk of colon and pancreatic cancers and breast cancer in postmenopausal women.[6-9] In a review of studies examining health behavior changes in people following a cancer diagnosis, Pinto et al found that conclusions regarding the role of exercise during or following cancer treatment are significantly limited by weak research design.[10] Most studies use very small sample sizes and focus only on the short-term adoption of exercise with either no or limited follow-up. The authors of this review suggest that individuals with cancer should be encouraged to exercise for general health benefits.

Chronic Musculoskeletal Pain

Chronic pain is often accompanied by physical and psychological factors that complicate rehabilitation. These factors may include decreases in flexibility, strength, and aerobic conditioning and changes in psychological status including fear of activity and re-injury, increases in depression and anxiety, and decreases in self-esteem and self-confidence. Limited evidence suggests that exercise is effective in treating chronic neck pain.[11,12] Two systematic reviews of the medical literature confirm that exercise is an effective form of treatment for chronic low back pain.[12,13] The most effective type of exercise (flexion, extension, stretching, strengthening, or aerobic conditioning) remains a subject of controversy.[13-16] Because the causes of back pain vary, the one-size-fits-all approach to exercise commonly used in research may never result in a definitive answer to the question "Which type of exercise is best for chronic low back pain?" Interventions that combine exercise with a cognitive behavioral approach or back education program have been shown to decrease disability and increase function.[17-19]

Diabetes

Exercise has not been shown to improve glucose control in people with Type 1 diabetes.[20] Through regular exercise, however, these individuals can reduce insulin resistance and gain other health benefits, such as reduced risk of CVD. In individuals with Type 2 diabetes, exercise is a significant component of disease management.[21-23] Regular exercise reduces insulin resistance, improves glycemic control, and helps people achieve and maintain a healthy weight range. Regular exercise can lower blood pressure and improve blood lipid profile, decreasing the risk of CVD. In addition, moderate exercise, as a component of a comprehensive lifestyle intervention, has been shown to prevent or delay the onset of diabetes in individuals at high risk for the disease.[24]

Geriatrics

The aging process results in a decline in several physiological parameters, including cardiorespiratory capacity, motor performance, bone density, and neurological status. These decreases may not be caused by the aging process alone, but may be strongly influenced by the adoption of a sedentary lifestyle. Regular exercise may slow or reverse these decreases.[25-27] Endurance exercise training results in improved glucose tolerance and insulin sensitivity, lower blood pressure, improved plasma lipoprotein lipid profiles, and reduced body fat. Because CVD is the major cause of death in older adults, the decrease in CVD risk factors is a major health benefit of exercise in the senior population.

Resistance training in the elderly has been shown to prevent bone mineral density loss and reduce insulin resistance.[28] In addition, research suggests that resistance exercise in older adults improves function, reduces risk factors for falls, and improves walking endurance,[29] increases spontaneous activity level,[30] and improves mood and physical self-efficacy.[31] The group exercise format may be especially important in an older adult population to reduce isolation and loneliness and promote overall satisfaction with life.[32]

HIV/AIDS

Researchers in the field of HIV/AIDS have begun to examine the role of exercise in disease management. Both aerobic and resistive exercise appear to be safe and beneficial for adults living with HIV/AIDS. Regular aerobic exercise has been shown to improve cardiovascular fitness, improve psychological status, and decrease fatigue.[33,34] Resistance training has been associated with increased muscle mass and muscle strength.[35]

Obesity

The prevalence of obesity in the United States has increased 75% in the last 15 years.[36] Obesity, defined as a body mass index (BMI) of 30 kg/m^2 or greater, affects 25% of women and 20% of men. An additional 25% of women and 40% of men have a BMI of 25 to 29.9 kg/m^2 and are overweight. People who are obese or overweight have an increased risk for high blood pressure, heart disease, osteoarthritis, Type 2 diabetes, and some types of cancers. Although weight is influenced by genetic, metabolic, hormonal, and lifestyle factors, the combination of a sedentary lifestyle and high-fat diet is the most likely cause of the increased incidence of obesity.

Regular physical activity prevents or delays the weight gain that often accompanies aging.[37] For the obese and overweight, successful long-term maintenance of weight loss requires participation in regular moderate to vigorous physical activity.[38] Maintaining weight loss is also enhanced by participation in weekly follow-up group behavioral treatment.[39]

Osteoporosis

Exercise has an important role in the prevention and treatment of osteoporosis and prevention of falls.[40,41] A physically active lifestyle may reduce the risk of hip fracture later in life by as much as 50%.[42] Because more than 90% of hip fractures are caused by falls, fall prevention is an important goal when developing an exercise program for people who have already been diagnosed with osteoporosis. Programs that include strength, balance, and weight-bearing aerobic training lower the risk of falls.[43] In addition, resistance exercises that strengthen back extensor muscles reduce new vertebral deformities in people with osteoporosis.[44] In a study of the long-term effect of back-strengthening exercises on vertebral fractures in healthy postmenopausal women, the relative risk for compression fractures at 8 years post-exercise intervention was significantly reduced in the exercise group compared to the control group.[45]

Rheumatological Conditions

When people with osteoarthritis, rheumatoid arthritis, and fibromyalgia engage in appropriate regular exercise, research demonstrates consistently favorable outcomes on a variety of measures.

Osteoarthritis

People with osteoarthritis (OA) are less active and less fit than their peers without the disease.[46,47] Flexibility, strength, and aerobic exercise have been shown to produce positive outcomes in people with OA, including decreased joint pain and impairment, decreased disability and increased function, and improved health status.[48,49] Aerobic exercise has been shown to improve aerobic capacity and general health status without exacerbating symptoms in people with OA.[49,50]

Rheumatoid Arthritis

Regular exercise is important to promote health status and physical function in people with rheumatoid arthritis (RA). Exercise programs designed to increase flexibility, muscle strength, and aerobic capacity have been shown to improve physical function without exacerbating pain or accelerating disease progression.[51,52] During an acute flareup of symptoms, a conservative approach of isometric strengthening and gentle flexibility exercises has been the traditional treatment; however, a preliminary study examining the role of dynamic muscle strengthening against resistance and a conditioning bicycle training program in patients hospitalized with active disease demonstrated improvements in strength and function without adverse consequences on disease activity.[53]

Evidence suggests that when exercise is combined with a comprehensive self-management program, patients with OA and RA experience significant and sustained reductions in pain and disability and reduced health care costs.[54]

Fibromyalgia

A comprehensive meta-analysis of fibromyalgia interventions concluded that optimal treatment for fibromyalgia includes exercise, relaxation, and behavioral strategies.[55] Research has demonstrated that women with fibromyalgia are significantly below average on measures of flexibility, strength, and aerobic capacity.[56] These measures improve with training. Participation in regular exercise programs has been shown to improve cardiorespiratory capacity, flexibility, strength, body pain, tender points, and psychological status in this patient population.[57-60] In addition, patients with fibromyalgia frequently report dyspnea, and the greater their dyspnea, the lower their exercise capacity.[61,62] Accordingly, instruction and continual emphasis on diaphragmatic breathing with daily activities and exercise are important.

Exercise and Mental Health

An analysis of four surveys of household populations in the United States and Canada demonstrated a strong association between physical activity and enhanced mental health.[63] Physical activity was positively associated with positive mood, general well-being, and lower levels of depression and anxiety. In addition to enhancing mental health in the general population, exercise may decrease depressive and anxious symptoms in individuals suffering from mild to moderate depression and anxiety.[64,65] Exercise may also have a role to play in treating major depressive disorder (MDD). In a study examining the role of exercise in treating MDD, an exercise intervention of three supervised aerobic exercise sessions per week for 16 consecutive weeks was as effective as an antidepressant intervention in reducing depressive symptoms.[66] At 10 months follow-up, those who participated in the exercise group were less likely to experience a relapse of depression than those who received medication.[67]

Both physical and psychological mechanisms have been proposed to explain improvements in mental health resulting from participation in regular exercise.[64] One theory suggests that exercise increases self-efficacy and self-confidence and promotes feelings of independence and success. As previously sedentary people experience mastery of physical activity, they may extend the feeling of control and success into other areas of their lives. Physiological mechanisms have also been proposed. One suggests that aerobic exercise enhances aminergic synaptic transmission, which is thought to be otherwise impaired in depressive disorders. A second hypothesis suggests that extended exercise activates endorphin secretion, reducing pain and promoting a euphoric state. Additional research is needed to determine the specific mechanisms that result in mood improvement with exercise.

Developing an Exercise Program

A group wellness program may be designed for a general population or for a patient population with a specific diagnosis. The type, intensity, frequency, and duration of exercise in a group wellness program will be specific to the population the program serves. Physical therapists and exercise physiologists can draw on their education and experience to design and guide the exercise component of a wellness program. A clinician without training and experience in exercise treatment in chronically ill populations should not attempt to provide exercise instruction. In these circumstances, a clinician can invite a physical therapist or exercise physiologist to participate in the development and delivery of the exercise instruction. This collaboration with an expert ensures participant safety, and the appropriate type and intensity of exercise is performed.

Screening for exercise activity is required for participant safety. According to guidelines provided by the American College of Sports Medicine, men older than 40 and women older than 50 should receive a medical evaluation before participation in a *vigorous* exercise program.[68] In addition, adults should see a physician before initiating *any* exercise program if they suffer from a chronic disease, an undiagnosed symptom, shortness of breath, irregular heartbeat, acute thrombosis, infection or fever, undiagnosed weight loss, joint swelling, pain, irregular gait, bleeding or detached retina, recent eye surgery or laser treatment, or a hernia.

The type of medical clearance required before participation in a *low-* or *moderate-intensity* exercise program remains controversial. In many health care settings, adults enrolling in a group exercise program have medical conditions requiring regular visits to a physician and should receive a physician evaluation and referral before enrollment. The Revised Physical Activity Readiness Questionnaire (Figure 7-1) sets minimal standards for adult participation in low to moderate exercise and is a useful preliminary screening tool for exercise involvement.[68,69] If there is any question or doubt about an individual's fitness to participate in a group exercise program, the clinician should refer the individual to a physician for evaluation.

Figure 7-1 Physical Activity Readiness Questionnaire (revised 1994). (© *Canadian Society for Exercise Physiology, Inc.*)

Physical Activity Readiness Questionnaire - PAR-Q (revised 1994)

PAR-Q & YOU

(A Questionnaire for People Aged 15 to 69)

Regular physical activity is fun and healthy, and increasingly more people are starting to become more active every day. Being more active is very safe for most people. However, some people should check with their doctor before they start becoming much more physically active.

If you are planning to become much more physically active than you are now, start by answering the seven questions in the box below. If you are between the ages of 15 and 69, the PAR-Q will tell you if you should check with your doctor before you start. If you are over 69 years of age, and you are not used to being very active, check with your doctor.

Common sense is your best guide when you answer these questions. Please read the questions carefully and answer each one honestly: check Yes or No.

YES	NO	
☐	☐	1. Has your doctor ever said that you have a heart condition and that you should only do physical activity recommended by a doctor?
☐	☐	2. Do you feel pain in your chest when you do physical activity?
☐	☐	3. In the past month, have you had chest pain when you were not doing physical activity?
☐	☐	4. Do you lose your balance because of dizziness or do you ever lose consciousness?
☐	☐	5. Do you have a bone or joint problem that could be made worse by a change in your physical activity?
☐	☐	6. Is your doctor currently prescribing drugs (for example, water pills) for your blood pressure or heart condition?
☐	☐	7. Do you know of any other reason why you should not do physical activity?

If you answered

YES to one or more questions

Talk with your doctor by phone or in person BEFORE you start becoming much more physically active or BEFORE you have a fitness appraisal. Tell your doctor about the PAR-Q and which questions you answered YES.

- You may be able to do any activity you want–as long as you start slowly and build up gradually. Or, you may need to restrict your activities to those which are safe for you. Talk with your doctor about the kinds of activities you wish to participate in and follow his/her advice.
- Find out which community programs are safe and helpful for you.

NO to all questions

If you answered NO honestly to all PAR-Q questions, you can be reasonably sure that you can:

- start becoming much more physically active–begin slowly and build up gradually. This is the safest and easiest way to go.
- take part in a fitness appraisal–this is an excellent way to determine your basic fitness so that you can plan the best way for you to live actively.

DELAY BECOMING MUCH MORE ACTIVE:

- if you are not feeling well because of a temporary illness such as a cold or a fever–wait until you feel better; or
- if you are or may be pregnant–talk to your doctor before you start becoming more active

Please note: If your health changes so that you then answer YES to any of the above questions, tell your fitness or health professional. Ask whether you should change your physical activity plan.

Informed Use of the PAR-Q: The Canadian Society for Exercise Physiology, Health Canada, and their agents assume no liability for persons who undertake physical activity, and if in doubt after completing this questionnaire, consult your doctor prior to physical activity.

You are encouraged to copy the PAR-Q but only if you use the entire form

Note: If the PAR-Q is being given to a person before he or she participates in a physical activity program or a fitness appraisal, this section may be used for legal or administrative purposes.

I have read, understood and completed this questionnaire. Any questions I had were answered to my full satisfaction.

NAME ______________________

SIGNATURE ______________________ DATE ______________________

SIGNATURE OF PARENT ______________________ WITNESS ______________________
or GUARDIAN (for participants under the age of majority)

© Canadian Society for Exercise Physiology
Société canadienne de physiologie de l'exercice

Supported by: 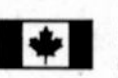 Health Canada Santé Canada

Overview of Fitness

The following overview of fitness identifies the benefits of exercise and basic guidelines for training. For the physical therapist and exercise physiologist, this will be a review. For other clinicians, it will offer a framework for understanding the components of fitness and fundamental elements of a fitness program. For a more comprehensive examination of the components of fitness, the reader is referred to the annotated bibliography at the end of this chapter. Flexibility, strength, and endurance training are components of any comprehensive exercise program. The principles of training apply to any exercise program.

Principles of Training

Overload, specificity, reversibility, and initial values are key principles of exercise training.[70] *Overload* is the application of a physical demand on the system that exceeds the normal load experienced in daily living. An exercise program must progressively overload the system to achieve training gains. Overload can be achieved by increasing frequency, duration, and/or intensity.

Specificity refers to the distinctive physical adaptations that occur as a result of training. These adaptations are localized to the site loaded and determined by the specific mode of exercise performed. For example, strength gains resulting from isometric exercise are limited to the muscle length and joint range at which the exercise is performed and do not carry over to other joint positions or to isotonic activities.

Any gains achieved through an exercise training program are lost when the training program is terminated. This is the principle of *reversibility* or regression. The *initial fitness* at baseline dictates the magnitude of benefit gained by exercise training, with the greatest improvement occurring in those with the lowest initial fitness levels.

Flexibility

Flexibility is the range of motion (ROM) of a joint or series of joints.[71,72] Stretching exercises, which are performed to increase flexibility, fall into three categories: static stretching, ballistic stretching, and proprioceptive neuromuscular facilitation (PNF). Of these three types, static stretching is most easily taught in a group and poses the least risk of muscle soreness or injury.

Static stretching requires maintaining a muscle in a stretched position for 30 to 60 seconds. Body positioning that is comfortable for the individual and ensures complete relaxation of the stretched muscle is required. When performing static stretching, the individual self-regulates the stretch and minimizes the risk of injury caused by overstretching. Static stretching is also associated with minimal muscle soreness and requires low energy expenditure.[71]

Ballistic stretching requires performing rapid bouncing movements at the end range of a stretched muscle and is not recommended because it can lead to muscle soreness and injury.[72] *PNF stretching* techniques are based on principles of neurophysiology, and although effective in improving flexibility, they are not easily taught in a group setting. A second person or props are often required to perform the techniques, and without individual guidance and feedback, participants may be at risk of injury.

Benefits of Stretching[73-82]

The benefits of muscle stretching include the following:

- Improved ROM
- Reduced muscle tension/increased muscle relaxation
- Improved self-worth and subjective well-being
- Decreased pain in individuals with chronic pain conditions
- Improved ease of performing activities of daily living

Muscle Stretching and Injury Prevention

Most research examining the relationship between muscle stretching and injury has used athletes or relatively young, healthy populations as study subjects. These sport-related studies suggest that stretching before exercise does not reduce the risk of injury in an athletic population.[83-87] The relationship between stretching programs and injury in seniors and in populations with various medical disorders remains unexamined.

Factors Influencing Flexibility

Several factors influence flexibility, including gender, age, and temperature. In general, women are more flexible than men.[88] As we age, we lose flexibility because of decreased elasticity of soft tissue and limited physical activity. Lower-extremity joints show a greater decline in flexibility than do upper-extremity joints.[89-91] Increased temperature promotes increased flexibility by increasing the extensibility of tendon and joint capsule collagen.[71]

Duration and Frequency of Static Stretch

Research on the relationship between duration and frequency of static stretch and joint ROM provides important evidence for selecting stretching guidelines.[73-76] Stretch duration may need to increase with increasing age to achieve ROM improvements. Guidelines to hold each stretch for 30 seconds in the general population and for 60 seconds in a senior population are recommended. Stretching 3 to 5 days per week will result in improved flexibility, whereas stretching once a week is necessary to maintain flexibility gains.

Guidelines for Stretching (**Figure 7-2**)

1. Assume a comfortable posture and proper alignment for the desired stretch.
2. Bring awareness to and relax the muscle to be stretched.
3. Breathe deeply. Avoid shallow breathing or holding the breath.
4. Gradually move into the stretch, allowing for a low to moderate stretch sensation. To minimize the risk of injury, avoid an extreme or uncomfortable stretch position.
5. Hold the muscle stretch for 30 to 60 seconds. Do not bounce. Continue to breathe deeply during this time.
6. Slowly return to the initial resting posture.

Strength Training

Muscle strength is the maximum force or tension generated by a muscle or muscle group.[92] For functional purposes, it is the capacity of skeletal muscle to create force to stabilize and mobilize the musculoskeletal system to achieve functional movement.[93]

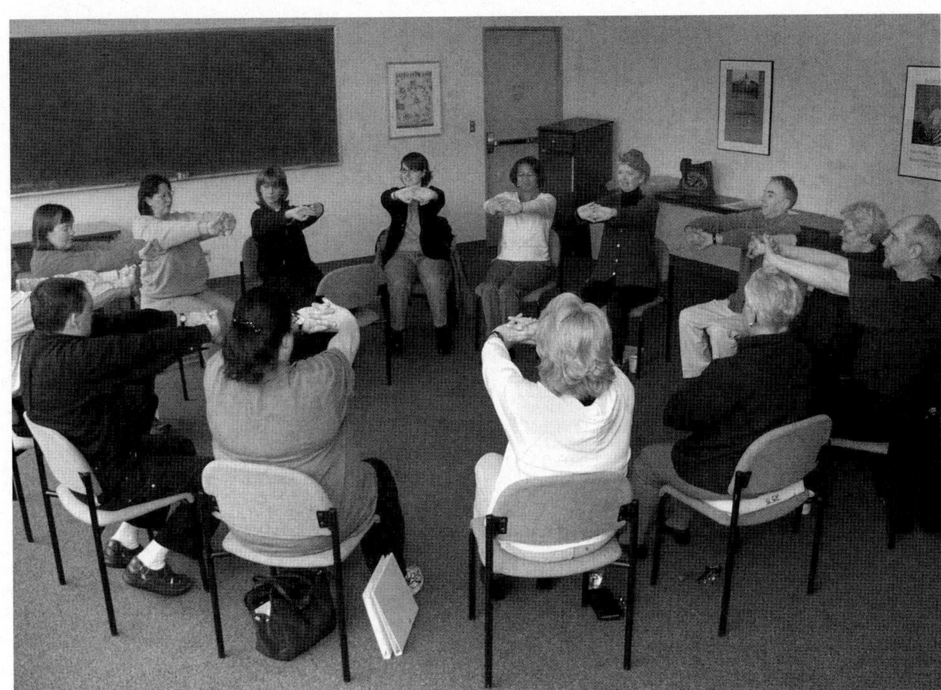

Figure 7-2 Clinician guides stretching exercises.

The Benefits of Strength Training[93-95]

The benefits of strength training include the following:

- Enhanced ability to perform activities of daily living
- Injury prevention
- Increased bone mass important in the prevention and treatment of osteoporosis
- Control of body weight through increased lean tissue mass and decreased percentage of fat
- Improved balance and coordination
- Improved self-image and self-esteem

Factors Influencing Muscle Strength

Multiple factors influence muscle strength, including age, inactivity, and inflammation.[93] Muscle strength decreases with age. The number of motor neurons decline with age, leading to a loss of muscle mass. In addition, sensory and motor conduction velocity and axonal transport slow. The resulting decrease in motor neuron recruitment and in frequency of action potentials slows reaction time and diminishes the ability of elderly individuals to quickly build maximal force.

An extended period of decreased physical activity results in a loss of muscle strength. The severity of the loss depends on the duration and extent of the inactivity. A decrease in muscle mass of 6% to 40% occurs with 4 to 6 weeks of bedrest.[96] With extended inactivity, both the aerobic and the anaerobic capacity of muscle are compromised because of structural and metabolic changes. In addition to strength losses, coordination is also compromised because of decreased neuromuscular activity and sensory input.

The symptoms of pain and effusion accompanying an inflammatory process can decrease strength. The mechanical deformation of tissue caused by joint effusion can inhibit muscle function.

Guidelines for Strength Training

The specifics of frequency, duration, and intensity for strengthening exercise remain controversial. There is no magic formula that assures optimal strength improvements in all individuals. The American College of Sports Medicine recommends the following guidelines for adults:[97]

- Isotonic exercises targeting eight to ten different major muscle groups should be performed.
- A training intensity of 40% to 60% of one repetition maximum (RM) is sufficient for developing muscle strength in most individuals. An intensity of 60% to 80% will produce more rapid gains. Although training intensities of 80% to 100% of 1 RM produce the fastest strength gains, there is a greater risk of overtraining and injury at these higher levels.
- At least one set of 8 to 15 repetitions of each exercise to the point of volitional fatigue should be performed. Single-set programs are less time consuming than multiple-set programs and may promote program adherence. They also produce health and fitness gains similar to multiple-set programs.
- Exercises should be performed at least twice per week. Because most individuals require 48 hours to recover from a typical strength training session, rest time between exercise sessions is important. When training at very low loads, as in some therapeutic circumstances, more frequent training sessions may be tolerated.
- Breathing should be maintained throughout the performance of all strength training exercises. Individuals should exhale during the concentric contraction and inhale during the eccentric contraction. If someone has difficulty with this breathing sequence, he or she should be instructed to breathe at a comfortable pattern throughout the exercise. Holding the breath is to be avoided because it may induce elevations in blood pressure.

Although 1 RM is a standard reference for resistance training, in the group setting it may be more practical, convenient, and safe to initially have participants move against gravity and then progress to the lightest weight available. Once able to tolerate the light weight for 12 to 15 repetitions, they can progress to a heavier weight and return to eight repetitions. The weight progression can occur in 1- to 2-pound increments. Alternately, resistive elastic bands can be used, applying similar principles.

A variety of resistance training machines are available. These machines offer isotonic, variable resistance, or isokinetic training. Many machines are designed to protect the lower back and provide overall stability, minimizing the risk of falls or injury. Although resistance training machines have grown in popularity in recent years, free weights and resistive elastic bands provide a convenient and cost-effective method for strength training. In addition, they are easily used in a group setting and adaptable to a home program.

Aerobic Training

Aerobic means requiring oxygen for energy production. During aerobic exercise, the cardiorespiratory system delivers adequate oxygen to meet the oxygen needs of large muscle groups exercising in a continuous fashion. Maximum oxygen consumption (VO_{2max}) represents the maximum rate at which oxygen can be used by the body for energy production and is the best indicator of the functional capacity of the cardiorespiratory system. Examples of aerobic exercise include swimming, brisk walking, jogging, and cycling.

Adaptations to Aerobic Exercise

Several physiological adaptations occur with regular aerobic training. They include improvements in maximum oxygen consumption, cardiac adaptations, peripheral adaptations, respiratory adaptations, and changes in fuel utilization.[98,99]

1. *Maximum oxygen consumption.* VO_{2max} increases with endurance training. Healthy subjects demonstrate a 10% to 30% increase in VO_{2max}, with the greatest improvements occurring in those who are least fit at baseline.
2. *Cardiac adaptations.* Maximum cardiac output, the product of stroke volume and heart rate, increases with aerobic training. With training, stroke volume increases during maximal and submaximal exercise and at rest. During exercise, heart rate increases in proportion with exercise intensity until the maximal heart rate is reached. Maximal heart rate is unchanged with aerobic training. Training decreases heart rate at submaximal exercise intensities and at rest. Resting heart rates in sedentary people average 70 to 80 beats per minute, whereas those in highly trained athletes average 40 beats per minute.
3. *Peripheral adaptations.* Both structural and metabolic changes enhance oxygen extraction in endurance-trained muscle. The number of capillaries around each muscle fiber increases 20% to 30%. This increase in capillary density contributes to a significant increase in the efficient exchange of gasses, nutrients, and waste products between the blood and muscle tissue. In addition, improved endurance increases the number and size of mitochondria and their respiratory enzyme activity. The oxidative capacity of muscle is also enhanced by increases in muscle myoglobin. Myoglobin transports oxygen entering a muscle to the mitochondria. Any increase in myoglobin increases oxygen delivery.
4. *Respiratory adaptations.* Adaptations of the respiratory system are observed primarily during exercise and minimally at rest. Endurance training may slightly lower the respiratory rate at rest and at low-intensity exercise. At moderate- to high-intensity exercise levels, the respiratory rate for a fixed workload can decrease by 20% to 30% below pretraining levels.
5. *Fuel utilization.* In trained individuals, the rate of carbohydrate metabolism decreases and fatty acid oxidation increases.

Benefits of Endurance Training[100]

In addition to the aforementioned physiological adaptations, the benefits of endurance training include the following:

- Decreased fatigue with daily activity
- Decreased risk of mortality from all causes
- Decreased risk of coronary artery disease, colon cancer, hypertension, non-insulin-dependent diabetes, and osteoporosis
- Decreased risk of anxiety and depression
- Enhanced mood and sense of well-being

Factors Influencing Endurance

Several factors influence endurance, including initial level of fitness, age, gender, and genetics.[98] The magnitude of adaptations to endurance training is greatest among those who are the least fit at baseline. Maximal heart rate declines with age independent of activity level. VO_{2max} typically peaks at 15 to 20 years of age and then gradually declines at a rate of 10% per decade. The age-related decline in VO_{2max} can be slowed through regular endurance training.

VO_{2max} levels for men and women are similar until puberty. Beyond puberty, the average VO_{2max} levels in women are 70% to 75% of those in men. Adaptations to endurance exercise are the same between the sexes, with men and women showing similar cardiorespiratory responses to training. Genetics plays a role in determining VO_{2max} capacities. The extremely high VO_{2max} capacities of elite endurance athletes are thought to be attributable to genetics.

Endurance Exercise Guidelines

The elements of an endurance exercise session are warmup, conditioning period, and cooldown.[94,100] A 5- to 15-minute warmup and cooldown period decreases the risk of ischemic and dysrhythmic cardiac events. In addition, the cooldown period assists in clearing exercised muscle of metabolic waste. An endurance activity performed at 50% of training intensity is an appropriate warmup or cooldown activity.

The conditioning activity should be performed for 20 to 60 minutes. For individuals with medical or age-related limitations, shorter sessions of 10 to 15 minutes repeated two or three times per day may be necessary.

An exercise intensity of 55% to 80% of maximum heart rate is needed to achieve cardiorespiratory improvements. Intensity varies with baseline fitness level.

Figure 7-3 Borg Scale for Rating Physical Exertion (RPE). (For correct usage of the scale, the user must go to the instruction and administration given by Borg in the text *Borg's Perceived Exertion and Pain Scales*; Champaign, Ill: Human Kinetics, 1998.)

BORG SCALE OF PERCEIVED EXERTION	
6	
7	Very, Very Light
8	
9	Very Light
10	
11	Fairly Light
12	
13	Somewhat Hard
14	
15	Hard
16	
17	Very Hard
18	
19	Very, Very Hard
20	

Sedentary individuals show improved cardiorespiratory fitness at training intensities of 55% to 64% of maximum heart rate. Already active adults require higher intensity levels of 65% to 80% of maximum heart rate to achieve cardiorespiratory fitness gains.

Rating Perceived Exertion

Identifying a percentage of maximum heart rate is to be used only as a guideline in establishing exercise intensity. An exerciser's perception of exertion levels that feel challenging but also comfortable is key. Teaching people to pay attention to their subjective experience of exercise intensity reinforces the skills of body awareness, encourages levels of exertion that are healthy and appropriate, and minimizes the risk of injury. The Borg Scale for rating perceived exertion (Figure 7-3) is a tool commonly used by clinicians to train people to pay attention to and rate how vigorously they feel they are exercising.[101] On this scale, 6 represents no exertion, whereas 20 represents a person's maximum effort. A strong linear relationship exists between Borg's rate of perceived exertion (RPE) levels and exercising heart rate. Aerobic fitness training occurs at levels of 11 or "fairly light" in sedentary individuals to 14 or "hard" in already active individuals.[102] For more information about the Borg scale and its appropriate use, the reader is referred to the text, *Borg's Perceived Exertion and Pain Scales* by G. Borg.[101]

Additionally, the talk test is another simple, practical, and commonly used strategy for the subjective evaluation of exercise intensity. For an exercise to achieve an aerobic training level, talking requires more effort than when at rest, but it is not impossible for a person. An individual can carry on a conversation during the activity if necessary.

Leading Group Exercise

A group wellness program offers an opportunity to introduce people to exercise options that are safe, fun, and appropriate for their medical needs and limitations. People often have misconceptions about exercise and can be confused about the type and intensity of exercise that is right for them. Some people are afraid of exercise. Others are impulsive and have poor judgment about exercise. Some may adopt the same attitude toward exercising as an adult with a chronic problem as they had as an adolescent participating in high school athletics. They may compete with others and push themselves more than is appropriate and cause an injury. People in a group often compare themselves to others, try to keep up with the next person, or try to impress the teacher. It is helpful to bring these tendencies to the group's attention. Clinicians can invite participants to express their perceptions of exercise and any concerns they have about beginning an exercise program. They can correct misunderstandings, introduce people to their exercise options, answer questions, and provide instruction in self-monitoring strategies. They can remind participants of the importance of listening to their own bodies and to meet both their abilities and limits with acceptance and respect. Because many chronic diseases are characterized by periods of symptom exacerbation, some participants may benefit from coaching to accommodate exercises and exercise levels to how they feel on a daily basis.

I like to remind people that although there are many similarities, each body in the room is truly unique. Just as when wind blows through a grove of trees, each tree moves differently, so too, when performing any exercise, for each person, the experience will be different. No two will be alike. The greatest gains in people's physical ability and well-being will occur by paying attention to their own bodies.

The group setting creates exercise instruction challenges that are different from those faced in an individual treatment session. The greatest of these challenges is ensuring participant safety and accurate exercise performance with less opportunity for individual attention and feedback. One strategy to meet this challenge is to provide general exercise guidelines to the group before *each* exercise session. Top among these guidelines is the importance of safety. Instruct participants to perform all activities at their own comfort level and to avoid any movement that results in pain or undue discomfort. Especially when beginning an exercise program, it is prudent to "start low and go slow."

To ensure safety and accurate performance of each movement, clinicians should clearly describe an exercise and identify which muscle groups are active. The exercise should be demonstrated and key elements of body alignment and body mechanics should be explained. Participants should always be invited to ask questions if they feel uncertain or confused.

Just because clinicians have made a point in a clear and straightforward manner, they cannot assume to have been heard and understood. People sometimes experience lapses in their attention or are so convinced of their own knowledge that they tune out the instructor. Clinicians must be willing to repeat instructions.

If, for any reason, participants are unable to perform a specific stretch or strengthening exercise, it may be possible for the clinician to modify the movement to meet individual limitations. If it is not possible to accommodate the movement, participants can be asked to rest or to perform a different movement within their ability.

If you are unfamiliar with group settings and exercise instruction, you may wish to take several group exercise classes for the experience of being a participant and to observe how different instructors lead exercise. Another option is to assist an experienced clinician who already provides a program.

Every clinician must remember that teaching exercise in a wellness program is much more than step-by-step instructions to perform movement. It requires coaching people to adopt exercise as a regular habit. This is no easy task. As one of my colleagues commented, "I wonder why most of my training was not in the psychology of behavior change!" The subject of helping people adhere to an exercise program is covered in Chapter 9.

Summary

The prevalence of sedentary behavior in the U.S. population poses a major health concern, increasing the risk of many chronic conditions, including CVD, hypertension, diabetes, and certain cancers, in the majority of the population. All health care providers have a responsibility to encourage people to exercise. Regular exercise has a key role in the prevention and treatment of many common medical conditions. In addition, exercise promotes healthy aging and enhances mental health. A comprehensive fitness program includes stretching, strengthening, and endurance exercise. When offering instruction in a group format, a clinician must emphasize participant safety and provide an exercise program that is appropriate to the abilities, needs, and goals of a group. Those clinicians who are not trained and experienced in exercise treatment for people with chronic conditions can invite a physical therapist or exercise physiologist to take an active role in the design and delivery of an exercise program.

References

1. Surgeon General's Report on Physical Activity in the U.S. (Referenced from the Web) www.cdc.gov/nccdphp/sgr/contents.
2. Healthy People 2010. (Referenced from the Web) www.health.gov/healthpeople.
3. Berlin JA, Colditz GA. A meta-analysis of physical activity in the prevention of coronary artery disease. *Am J Epidemiol* 1990;132:612-628.
4. Lear SA, Ignaszewski A. Cardiac rehabilitation: a comprehensive review. *Curr Control Trials Cardiovasc Med* 2001;2(5):221-232.
5. Ornish D, Scherwitz LW, Billings JH et al. Intensive lifestyle changes for reversal of coronary heart disease. *JAMA* 1998;280(23):2001-2007.
6. Thune I, Furberg AS. Physical activity and cancer risk: dose-response and cancer, all sites and site-specific. *Med Sci Sport Exer* 2000;23(6 Suppl): S530-S550.
7. Michaud DS, Giovannucci E, Willett WC et al. Physical activity, obesity, height and the risk of pancreatic cancer. *JAMA* 2001;286(8):967-968.
8. Carpenter CL, Ross RK, Paganeni-Hill A, Bernstein L. Lifetime exercise activity and breast cancer risk among post-menopausal women. *Br J Cancer* 1999;80(11):1852-1858.
9. Friedenreich CM, Bryant HE, Courneya KS. Case-control study of lifetime physical activity and breast cancer risk. *Am J Epidemiol* 2001;154(4):336-347.
10. Pinto BM, Eakin E, Maruyama NC. Health behavior changes after a cancer diagnosis: what do we know and where do we go from here? *Ann Behav Med* 2000;22(1):38-52.
11. Bronfront G, Evans R, Nelson B et al. A randomized clinical trial of exercise and spinal manipulation for patients with chronic neck pain. *Spine* 2001;26(7):788-797.
12. Mior S. Exercise in the treatment of chronic pain. *Clin J Pain* 2001;17(4):S77-S85.
13. van Tulder M, Malmivaara A, Esmail R, Koes B. Exercise therapy for low back pain: a systematic review within the framework of the Cochran Collaboration Back Review Group. *Spine* 2000;25(21):2784-2796.
14. McKenzie R. Re: van Tulder et al. Exercise therapy for low back pain. *Spine* 2001;26(16):1829-1831.
15. May S. Re: Exercise therapy for low back pain: a systematic review within the framework of the Cochran Collaboration Back Review Group. *Spine* 2001;26(16):1829.
16. Donelson R. Re: van Tulder et al, Exercise therapy for low back pain. *Spine* 2001;26(16):1827-1829.
17. Frost H, Moffett JA, Moser JS, Fairbank JCT. Randomised controlled trial for evaluation of fitness programme for patients with chronic low back pain. *BMJ* 1995;310:151-154.
18. Glomsrod B, Lonn JH, Soukup MG et al. "Active back school," prophylactic management for low back pain: three-year follow-up of a randomized, controlled trial. *J Rehab Med* 2001;33(1):26-30.

19. Hodselman AP, Jaegers SM, Goeken LN. Short-term outcomes of a back school program for chronic low back pain. *Arch Phys Med Rehabil* 2001;82(8):1099-1105.
20. Wasserman DH, Zinman B. Fuel homeostasis. In Ruderman N, Devlin JT (eds), *Health Professional's Guide to Diabetes and Exercise*. Alexandria, Va: American Diabetes Association, 1995; 29-47.
21. Creviston T, Quinn L. Exercise and physical activity in the treatment of type 2 diabetes. *Nurs Clin N Am* 2001;36(2):243-271.
22. Albright A, Franz M, Hornsby G et al. Exercise and type 2 diabetes. *Med Sci Sports Exerc* 2000;32(7):1345-1360.
23. Eriksson J. Exercise in the treatment of type 2 diabetes: an update. *Sports Med* 1999;27(6):381-391.
24. Knowler WC, Barrett-Connor E, Fowler SE et al. Reduction in the incidence of type 2 diabetes with lifestyle intervention or metformin. *N Engl J Med* 2002 Feb 7;346(6):393-403.
25. Mazzeo R, Cavanagh P, Evans WJ. Exercise and physical activity in older adults: ASCM position stand. *Am Sci Sports Exerc* 1998;30(6):992-1008.
26. Mazzeo RS, Tanaka H. Exercise prescription for the elderly: Current recommendations. *Sports Med* 2001;31(11):809-818.
27. Christmas C, Anderson RA. Exercise and older patients: guidelines for the clinician. *J Am Geriatr Soc* 2000;48(3):318-324.
28. Hurley BF, Roth SM. Strength training in the elderly. *Sports Med* 2000;30(4):249-268.
29. Ades PA, Ballor DL, Ashikaga T et al. Weight training improves walking endurance in healthy elderly persons. *Ann Int Med* 1996;124(6):568-572.
30. Evans WJ. Effects of exercise on body composition and functional capacity of the elderly. *J Gerontol A Biol Sci Med Sce* 1995;50 Spec No:147-150.
31. Tsutsumi T, Don BM, Zaichkowsky DL et al. Physical fitness and psychological benefits of strength training in community dwelling older adults. *Appl Human Sci* 1997;16(6):257-266.
32. McAuley E, Blissmer B, Marquez DX et al. Social relations, physical activity and well-being in older adults. *Prev Med* 2000;31(5):608-617.
33. Nixon S, O'Brien K, Glazier RH, Wilkins AL. Aerobic exercise interventions for people with HIV/AIDS. *Cochrane Database Syst Rev* 2001;(1):CD001798.
34. Smith BA, Neidig JL, Nickel JT et al. Aerobic exercise: effects on parameters related to fatigue, dyspnea, weight and body composition in HIV-infected adults. *AIDS* 2001;15(6):693-701.
35. Bhasin S, Storer TW, Javanbkht M. Testosterone replacement and resistance exercise in HIV-infected men with weight loss and low testosterone levels. *JAMA* 2000;383(6):763-770.
36. Leermakers EA, Dunn AL, Blair SN. Exercise management of obesity. *Med Clin N Am* 2000;84(2):419-440.
37. DiPietro L, Kohl HW III, Barlow CE et al. Physical fitness and the risk of weight gain in men and women: The Aerobics Center Longitudinal Study. *Med Sci Sports Exerc* 1997:29;S115.
38. McGuire MT, Wing RR, Klem ML et al. Long-term maintenance of weight loss: do people who lose weight through various weight loss

methods use different behaviors to maintain their weight? *Int J Obes Relat Med Disord* 1998;22:572-577.

39. Wadden TA, Foster GD. Behavioral treatment of obesity. *Med Clin N Am* 2000;84(2):441-461.
40. Marcus R. Role of exercise in preventing and treating osteoporosis. *Rheum Dis Clin N Am* 2001;27(1):131-141.
41. Hertel KL, Trahiotis MG. Exercise in the prevention and treatment of osteoporosis. *Nurs Clin N Am* 2001;36(3):441-453.
42. Joakimsen RM, Magnus JH, Fonnebo V. Physical activity and predisposition for hip fractures: a review. *Osteoporos Intl* 1997;7(6): 503-513.
43. Gardner MM, Robertson MC, Campbell AJ. Exercise in preventing falls and fall related injuries in older people: a review of randomized controlled trials. *Br J Sports Med* 2000;34:7-17.
44. Sinaki M, Mikkelsen BA: Post-menopausal spinal osteoporosis: flexion versus extension exercises. *Arch Phys Med Rehabil* 1982;65:593-596.
45. Sinaki M, Wahner HW, Wollan P et al. Stronger back muscles reduce the incidence of vertebral fractures: a prospective 10 year follow-up of post-menopausal women. *Bone* 2002;30(6):836-841.
46. Fisher NM, Pendergast DR. Reduced muscle function in patients with osteoarthritis. *Scan J Rehab Med* 1997;29:213-221.
47. Minor MA, Hewett JE, Webel RR et al. Exercise tolerance and disease related measures in patients with rheumatoid arthritis and osteoarthritis. *J Rheumotol* 1988;15:905-911.
48. Minor MA. Exercise in the treatment of osteoarthritis. *Rheum Dis Clin North Am* 1999;25(2):397-415.
49. Exercise prescription for older adults with osteoarthritis pain: consensus practice recommendations. A supplement to AGS clinical practice guidelines on the management of chronic pain in older adults. *J Am Geriatric Soc* 2001;49(6):808-823.
50. O'Grady M, Fletcher J, Ortiz S. Therapeutic and physical fitness exercise prescription for older adults with joint disease. *Rheum Dis Clin North Am* 2000;26(3):617-646.
51. Van de Ende CH, Vliet Vlieland TP, Munneke M, Hazes JM. Dynamic exercise therapy in rheumatoid arthritis: a systematic review. *Br J Rheumatol* 1998;37(6):677-687.
52. Hakkin A, Sokka T, Kotanieme A, Hannonen P. A randomized two-year study of the effects of dynamic strength training on muscle strength, disease activity, functional capacity, and bone mineral density in early rheumatoid arthritis. *Arthritis Rheum* 2001;44(3):515-522.
53. Van de Ende CH, Breedveld FC, le Cessie S et al. Effect of intensive exercise on patients with active rheumatoid arthritis: a randomized clinical trial. *Ann Rheum Dis* 2000:59(8):615-621.
54. Lorig KR, Mazonson PD, Holman HR. Evidence suggesting that health care education for self-management in patients with chronic arthritis has sustained health benefits while reducing health care costs. *Arthritis Rheum* 1993;36(4):439-446.
55. Rossy LA, Buckelew SP, Dorr N et al. A meta-analysis of fibromyalgia treatment interventions. *Ann Behav Med* 1999;21(2):180-191.

56. Mannerkorpi K, Burckhardt CS, Bjelle A. Physical performance characteristics of women with fibromyalgia. *Arthritis Care Res* 1994;7(3):123-129.

57. Jentoft ES, Kvalvik AG, Mengshoel AM. Effects of pool-based and land-based aerobic exercise on women with fibromyalgia/chronic widespread muscle pain. *Arthritis Rheum* 2001;45(1):42-47.

58. Martin L, Nutting A, MacIntosh BR. An exercise program in the treatment of fibromyalgia. *J Rheumatol* 1996;23(6):1050-1053.

59. Meiworm L, Jakob E, Walker UA et al. Patients with fibromyalgia benefit from aerobic endurance exercise. *Clin Rheumatol* 2000;19(4):253-257.

60. Sandstrom MJ, Keefe FJ. Self-management of fibromyalgia: the role of formal coping skills training and physical exercise training programs. *Arthritis Care Res* 1998;11(6):432-447.

61. Caidahl K, Lurie M, Bake B et al. Dyspnoea in chronic primary fibromyalgia. *J Intern Med* 1989;226(4):265-270.

62. Lurie M, Caidahl K, Johansson G et al. Respiratory function in chronic primary fibromyalgia. *Scan J Rehabil Med* 1990;22(3):151-155.

63. Stephens T. Physical activity and mental health in the United States and Canada: evidence from four population surveys. *Prev Med* 1988;17(1): 35-47.

64. Paluska SA, Schwenk TL. Physical activity and mental health: current concepts. *Sports Med* 2000;29(3):167-180.

65. Meyer T, Broocks A. Therapeutic impact of exercise on psychiatric diseases: guidelines for exercise testing and prescription. *Sports Med* 2000;30(4):269-279.

66. Bleumenthal JA, Babyak MA, Moore KA et al. Effects of exercise training in older patients with major depression. *Arch Int Med* 1999;159: 2349-2356.

67. Babyak M, Bleumenthal JA, Herman S et al. Exercise treatment for major depression: maintenance of therapeutic benefit at 10 months. *Psychosom Med* 2000;62:633-638.

68. Johnson EP (ed). *ASCM's Guidelines for Exercise Testing and Prescription.* Philadelphia: Lippincott Williams & Wilkins, 2000, pp. 22-32.

69. Thomas S, Reading J, Shephard RJ. Revision of the Physical Activity Readiness Questionnaire (PAR-Q). *Can J Sport Sci* 1992;17:338-345.

70. Durstine JL, Davis PG. Specificity of exercise training and testing. In Franklin BA (ed), *ASCM's Resource Manual for Guidelines for Exercise Testing and Prescription* 4th ed. Philadelphia: Lippincott Williams & Wilkins, 2001, pp. 484-491.

71. Krivickas L. Training flexibility. In Frontera W (ed). *Exercise in Rehabilitation Medicine.* Champaign, Ill: Human Kinetics, 1999, pp. 83-102.

72. Fredette D. Exercise recommendations for flexibility and range of motion. In Roitman J (ed), *ASCM's Resource Manual for Guidelines for Exercise Testing and Prescription* 4th ed. Philadelphia: Lippincott Williams & Wilkins, 2001, pp. 468-477.

73. Roberts J, Wilson K. Effect of stretching duration on active and passive range of motion in the lower extremity. *Br J Sports Med* 1999;33:259-263.

74. Bandy W, Irion J. The effect of time on static stretch on the flexibility of the hamstring muscles. *Phys Ther* 1994;74(9):845-850.

75. Bandy W, Irion J, Briggler M. The effect of time and frequency of static stretching on flexibility of the hamstring muscle. *Phys Ther* 1997;77: 1090-1096.

76. Feland J, Myrer J, Schulthies S. The effect of duration of stretching of the hamstring muscle group for increasing range of motion in people aged 65 years or older. *Phys Ther* 2001;81(5):1100-1117.

77. Carlson C, Collins F, Nitz A et al. Muscle stretching as an alternative relaxation procedure. *J Behav Ther Exp Psychiat* 1990;21(1): 29-38.

78. Carlson C, Curran S. Stretch-based relaxation training. *Patient Educ Couns* 1994;23(1):5-12.

79. McAuley E, Blissmer B, Marquez D et al. Social relations, physical activity, and well-being in older adults. *Prev Med* 2000;31:608-617.

80. Moore T. A workplace stretching program: physiologic and perception measurements before and after participation. *AAOHN J* 1998;46(12): 563-568.

81. King AC, Pruitt LA, Phillips W et al. Comparative effects of two physical activity programs on measured and perceived functioning and other health-related quality of life outcomes in older adults. *J Gerontol Med Sci* 2000;55A(2):M74-M83.

82. Sugano A, Nomura T. Influence of water exercise and land stretching on salivary cortisol concentrations and anxiety in chronic low back pain patients. *J Physiol Anthropol* 2000;19(4):175-180.

83. Gleim G, McHugh M. Flexibility and its effects on sports injury and performance. *Sports Med* 1997 Nov;24(5);289-299.

84. Shrier I. Should people stretch before exercise? *West J Med I* 2001;174(4):282-283.

85. Shrier I. Stretching before exercise: an evidence based approach. *Br J Sports Med* 2000;34(5):324-325.

86. Shrier I. Stretching before exercise does not reduce the risk of local muscle injury: a critical review of the clinical and basic science literature. *Clin J Sports Med* 1999;9:221-227.

87. Pope R, Herbert R, Kirwan J et al. A randomized trial of pre-exercise stretching for prevention of lower limb injury. *Med Sci Sports Exer* 2000;32:271-277.

88. Bell RD, Hoshizaki TB. Relationships of age and sex with range of motion of seventeen joint actions in humans. *Can J Appl Sport Sci* 1981 Dec; 6(4):202-206.

89. Escalante A, Lichtenstein MJ, Harzuda HP. Determinants of shoulder and elbow flexion range: results from the San Antonio Longitudinal Study of Aging. *Arth Care Res* 1999 Aug;12(4):277-286.

90. Grimston SK, Nigg BM, Hanley DA et al. Differences in ankle joint complex range of motion as a function of age. *Foot Ankle* 1993 May; 14(4):215-222.

91. Roach MK, Miles TP. Normal hip and knee active range of motion: the relationship to age. *Phys Ther* 1991 Sep;71(9):656-665.

92. DiNubile NA. Strength training. *Clin Sports Med* 1991;10(1):33-62.

93. Harris BA, Watkins MP. Adaptations to strength conditioning. In Frontera W (ed), *Exercise in Rehabilitation Medicine.* Champaign, Ill: Human Kinetics, 1999, pp. 71-81.
94. Pollock ML, Gaesser GA, Janus D et al. The recommended quantity and quality of exercise for developing and maintaining cardiorespiratory and muscular fitness and flexibility in healthy adults. *Med Sci Sports Exerc* 1998;30(6):975-991.
95. Bryant CX, Peterson JA, Graves JE. Muscular strength and endurance. In Roitman J (ed), *ASCM's Resource Manual for Guidelines for Exercise Testing and Prescription* 4th ed. Philadelphia: Lippincott Williams & Wilkins, 2001, pp. 460-467.
96. Bloomfield SA. Changes in musculoskeletal structure and function with prolonged bed rest. *Med Sci Sports Exerc* 1997 Feb;29(2):197-206.
97. Feigenbaum MS, Pollock ML. Prescription of resistance training for health and disease. *Med Sci Sports Exerc* 1999;31(1):38-45.
98. Hoffman MD. Adaptations to endurance exercise training. In Frontera W (ed), *Exercise in Rehabilitation Medicine.* Champaign, Ill: Human Kinetics, 1999, pp. 55-70.
99. Franklin BA, Roitman JL. Cardiorespiratory adaptations to exercise. In Roitman J (ed), *ASCM's Resource Manual for Guidelines for Exercise Testing and Prescription* 4th ed. Philadelphia: Lippincott Williams & Wilkins, 2001, pp. 160-166.
100. Holly RG, Shaffrath JD. Cardiorespiratory endurance. In Roitman J (ed), *ASCM's Resource Manual for Guidelines for Exercise Testing and Prescription* 4th ed. Philadelphia: Lippincott Williams & Wilkins, 2001, pp. 449-467.
101. Borg G. *Borg's Perceived Exertion and Pain Scales.* Champaign, Ill: Human Kinetics, 1998.
102. Huddelson J. Exercise. In Edelman CL, Mandle CL (eds), *Health Promotion Throughout the Lifespan* 5th ed. St. Louis: 2002, Mosby, p. 335.

Annotated Bibliography

Durstine LJ (ed). *ASCM's Exercise Management for Persons with Chronic Diseases and Disabilities.* New York: Human Kinetics, 1998. Written and edited by leading authorities in the field, this text offers evidence-based exercise recommendations for cardiovascular and pulmonary diseases, metabolic diseases, immunological and hematological diseases, orthopedic and neuromuscular disorders, and cognitive, emotional, and sensory disorders. This is a succinct reference for the health care professional working with people with chronic conditions.

Franklin B. *ASCM's Guidelines for Exercise Testing and Prescription* 4th ed. Philadelphia: Lippincott Williams & Wilkins, 2001. This book is considered the "gold standard" for exercise guidelines for cardiac and pulmonary patients. Contributing authors include experts from the fields of physiology, cardiology, pulmonary medicine, physical therapy, nursing, fitness, and epidemiology. This text presents procedures for health screening, exercise testing, and exercise prescription. It offers a succinct examination of strategies to promote successful exercise adherence and additional behavioral changes. The legal concerns of licensed and nonlicensed exercise professionals are addressed. The ACSM certification examinations are based on the knowledge, skills, and abilities covered in this text. A concise, practical volume presenting current information in an accessible form, this text is an important resource for any health care professional engaged in exercise treatment of chronically ill populations.

National Heart, Lung and Blood Institute, National Institutes of Health. *Clinical Guidelines on the Identification, Evaluation and Treatment of Overweight and Obesity in Adults: the Evidence Report.* Washington, DC, 1998. NIH Publication No. 98-4083. This comprehensive report is based on a systematic review of published scientific literature examining weight control and chronic disease. It reviews the application and effectiveness of weight control strategies and recommends weight control interventions. Clear, concise, and informative, this is an excellent resource for the health care professional offering weight management programs. This text can be ordered on the Web at www.nhlbi.nih.gov/guidelines/obesity/ob_home.htm.

Roitman J (ed). *ASCM's Resource Manual for Guidelines for Exercise Testing and Prescription* 4th ed. Philadelphia: Lippincott Williams & Wilkins, 2001. This text is an authoritative manual on exercise guidelines, procedures, and protocols. It is a resource for fitness professionals who are candidates for certification by the American College of Sports Medicine and a companion to the *ACSM's Guidelines for Exercise Testing and Prescription.* It offers a comprehensive examination of exercise physiology and principles of fitness. It addresses the role of exercise programming in treating a range of common chronic diseases and the importance of behavior modification in exercise promotion. It offers a detailed discussion of fitness program management and administration in clinical, corporate, or community settings. This comprehensive manual is a practical and informative resource for a health care professional.

Ruderman N, Devlin JT. *Health Professional's Guide to Diabetes and Exercise.* Alexandria, Va: American Diabetes Association, 1995. Written and edited by leaders in the field, this text provides a comprehensive examination of exercise for people with diabetes. Topics covered include the metabolic benefits of exercise, exercise recommendations for people with diabetes, and guidelines for patients with diabetic complications. This practical, informative, and well-written text is an outstanding resource for the health care professional.

Resources

American College of Sports Medicine
P.O. Box 1440
Indianapolis, IN 46206
www.acsm.org

American Physical Therapy Association
111 North Fairfax Street
Alexandria, VA 22314-1488
Phone: 800-999-2782
www.apta.org

The President's Council on Physical Fitness and Sports
DHHS/OS/OPHS
200 Independence Ave. SW
HHH Building
Washington, DC 20201
Phone: 202-690-9000
www.os.dhhs.gov

Chapter 8 Mindful Movement

Mindful movement combines the principles of mindfulness with movement and exercise. This chapter identifies the role of mindful movement in helping people with chronic medical conditions develop healthy relationships with their bodies and positive attitudes toward exercise. The Alexander Technique, the Feldenkrais Method, T'ai Chi, Ch'i Kung, and yoga are described. Applying principles of mindfulness to standard physical therapy exercises is examined. Walking meditation is introduced as an additional strategy for combining mindfulness and movement.

Principles of Mindful Movement

Western educational models prize the ability to think clearly and rationally. Body awareness is not valued as necessary for success and is neglected in standard educational systems. When attention is given to the body, competition and performance, not awareness, are emphasized. This focus can have unintended negative consequences. One example of the adverse outcome of this approach is the story of my friend's daughter. A straight-A student in academic subjects, she regularly received a C in middle school physical education. Consistently receiving this low grade alienated her from exercise, and she was delighted to attend a high school with no physical education requirement. Because school systems develop the intellect separate from the body and emphasize physical competition and performance, respect for each person's individual physical capacities and limits is neglected. The ability to listen to kinesthetic information, physical sensations associated with emotions, and instinctual and intuitive knowledge available via physical cues is undeveloped. The need and capacity to be at home and at peace in one's body in order to be at home and at peace in the world are not recognized or addressed. Many people come into adulthood alienated from the body, lack skills to listen and respond to the body's kinesthetic cues, and have negative feelings toward exercise.

In addition, the diagnosis of a chronic medical condition can further complicate how people relate to the body. They may feel shame or grief about physical limitations or feel betrayed by the body. They may focus on their physical problems and have no skills to listen to the body as a whole or to parts of the body that are symptom free. Disappointed by their limitations, they may forget to focus on the body's abilities. Rather than exercise within appropriate parameters, they may equate exercise with "no pain, no gain" and falsely conclude that they are better off avoiding exercise. Or they may overextend themselves when they exercise, leading to symptom exacerbation or injury. Once recovered, they return to an exercise program only to repeat this cycle. Mindful movement, with its emphasis on body awareness and the noncompetitive experience of movement, is a perfect strategy to help people feel comfortable in the body and develop a positive attitude toward regular physical activity. Especially in the initial stages of a wellness program, learning to feel at home in the body, to enjoy physical activity, and to build the habit of exercise *are keys to success* and are more important than achieving an improved fitness level.

Mindful movement schools offer exercise formats that actively engage the mind and the body in the experience of movement. They bring mindful awareness *to* movement, building concentration and mind-body awareness as well as fitness. Mindful movement activities are generally performed slowly. The body is met with respect, acceptance, and patience. Judging a movement as good or bad, right or wrong is suspended while an approach of openness, curiosity, and exploration is cultivated. Mindful movement emphasizes the present moment inner experience and does not prioritize achieving any preestablished goal. Awareness of the breath is often a component of these activities. Improved fitness levels become the natural outcome of this combination of an inward focus on attention and movement.

The philosophy of mindful movement is similar to that of a gardener working in a garden. When a gardener plants a seed, something in the seed carries the knowledge of how to root, stalk, and blossom. The gardener's job is to cooperate with nature's intelligence, providing the right light, water, and nutrients. Mindful movement takes a similar approach, acknowledging and cooperating with the body's intelligence. It does not impose a rigid external agenda on the body. Paying attention to and working with the capacity for movement already present within the body are emphasized.

This inward focus of attention combined with movement promotes an experience of self-confidence, self-control, and self-mastery. It offers a therapeutic response to feelings of helplessness and being out of control that often accompany the experience of chronic illness. Participants pay close attention to the sensations arising with each movement and meet their experience with acceptance. Based on these observations, they choose to increase or decrease the intensity or explore variations of the movement. These shifts in effort occur moment by moment and can be very small. Vigorously pushing or forcing a movement in any way is discouraged. Observing breathing patterns and choosing diaphragmatic breathing often accompanies these activities. This approach promotes self-awareness and self-management. It builds skills to regulate inner responses to physical symptoms as well as external circumstances. With a regular practice of mindful movement, people experience improvement in flexibility and strength.

Mindful movement may also promote skills to self-regulate the body's stress reaction.[1] Increased sympathetic nervous system activity results in physiological changes, which are detailed in Chapter 4. These changes include increased respiratory rate and decreased tidal volume associated with shallow, rapid breathing. Muscle tension in the upper back and shoulders also increases as the body assumes a guarded stance, bracing in the face of a perceived threat. Because mindful movement promotes the psycho-neuro-physiological pathways for self-regulating breathing patterns and muscle tension levels, an individual develops the skills to shift from shallow breathing to diaphragmatic breathing and from muscle tension to muscle relaxation.

There are several schools of mindful movement. Two Western and two Eastern schools are described in the following sections. These movement schools were selected because they are commonly known in the health care field, are generally taught in group settings, and are referenced in the medical literature. For any clinician interested in introducing these movement practices in a group setting, I encourage 3 or more years of study and practice in the movement discipline before taking on the challenging responsibility of teaching.

Western Schools of Mindful Movement

The Alexander Technique and the Feldenkrais Method are two schools of movement emphasizing mind-body awareness that have roots in Europe and the United States. Commonly taught in a group format, they offer clinicians models for exercise that draw on the principles of mindfulness.

The Alexander Technique

FM Alexander (1865-1955) was a Shakespearean actor who recovered from recurring hoarseness by exploring the relationship between his neck tension and posture and his voice quality.[2] Once he was able to align his head and neck and relax his neck musculature, he no longer suffered from a loss of voice. He applied this awareness and re-education model to musculoskeletal problems experienced by other performers and those in a variety of occupations. Alexander felt that unconscious and automatic movement and posture habits could be corrected through a process that actively engaged the mind and body. By bringing awareness to unhealthy movement patterns and introducing more beneficial patterns, conscious choices are made to establish more healthy movement patterns.

Alexander developed four core instructions that guide a person toward a more beneficial alignment and improved movement pattern. These instructions are: (1) release the neck so the head balances forward and up; (2) allow the torso to lengthen and widen; (3) allow the legs to release away from the torso; and (4) release the shoulders out to the sides. During an Alexander lesson, the student contemplates and integrates these four instructions while the teacher provides verbal guidance and light touch to help students experience new movement and alignment. Diaphragmatic breathing is emphasized in all activities.

The Alexander Technique is commonly taught in schools for the performing arts. Very few studies have been conducted examining the role of the Alexander Technique in the treatment of chronic medical conditions or of older adults.[3-7] These studies use small sample sizes and focus only on a short-term intervention with limited follow-up. Further research is warranted to determine the therapeutic benefits of the Alexander Technique.

The Feldenkrais Method

Moshe Feldenkrais (1880-1967), an electrical engineer and judo practitioner, developed an approach to movement based on his background in physics and judo and his study of anatomy, physiology, and the Alexander Technique.[2,8] Feldenkrais believed in the capacity of the individual to learn new movement patterns, regardless of age or fitness levels. He developed a learning system that emphasizes the functional awareness of the individual in the environment. This method explores the functional activities of rolling, bending, turning, sitting, and walking. Through a series of movement sequences, parts of the body that have been out of awareness are brought to attention. Students become conscious of automatic neuromuscular habit patterns, and alternative options for moving are explored. The Feldenkrais Method emphasizes a process of inquiry rather than achieving a predetermined solution. Awareness and attitude are more important than the specific physical movement.

There are two formats for teaching the Feldenkrais Method. They are Awareness Through Movement (ATM) and Functional Integration (FI). ATM is taught in groups and involves a practitioner verbally guiding the participants through movement sequences. FI is taught individually. In addition to verbal instruction, the FI practitioner gently touches the student to provide feedback and introduce new movement possibilities.

Preliminary research suggests that the Feldenkrais Method may have a beneficial role in the treatment of Parkinson's disease, multiple sclerosis, and back pain and may improve range of motion.[9-12] These results must be considered cautiously because the studies use very small sample sizes and focus only on the short-term adoption of exercise with either no or limited follow-up. Further research examining the application of the Feldenkrais Method in the care of people with chronic medical conditions and older adults is warranted.

Eastern Schools of Mindful Movement

T'ai Chi Ch'uan, Ch'i Kung, and yoga are ancient traditions from Eastern cultures that integrate mind, body, and spirit into the experience of movement. Commonly taught in a group format, they offer clinicians additional models for exercise that apply the principles of mindfulness to movement.

T'ai Chi Ch'uan and Ch'i Kung

T'ai Chi Ch'uan is a Chinese martial art that promotes the harmonious integration of mind, body, breath, and spirit. T'ai Chi Ch'uan translates as "Grand Ultimate Fist" and is considered one of the three primary schools of Chinese internal martial arts. It originated in the late Ming (1368-1644) and was formalized in the early Qing (1644-1911) dynasties.[2,13] Many family styles developed over the centuries. The Chen, Yang, Sun, and Wu (originated by Quan You), and Wu (originated by Hao) schools are considered the five primary schools of T'ai Chi Ch'uan. In 1956, a meeting of T'ai Chi masters convened by the Chinese National Council of Sports and Physical Education produced a simplified T'ai Chi short form that conveys the central components of the long form of several of these traditional schools. This popular simplified short form is actively promoted among the Chinese population and throughout the world.

The cultivation of chi (qi) is fundamental to this practice. Chi is considered to be the innate life energy found in all living systems. Good health reflects a balanced and free circulation of chi, whereas poor health indicates an imbalance and stagnation of chi. T'ai Chi movements, performed in a continuous, slow, and flowing manner, stimulate and promote both the circulation of blood and chi, thus encouraging healing, well-being, and longevity. Breathing and mental focus are emphasized throughout all movements.

T'ai Chi is a form of mindful movement that has gained the attention of medical researchers investigating aerobic training and fall prevention in older adults. T'ai Chi can be an aerobic activity. The short form may produce cardiorespiratory changes consistent with light aerobic exercise, and the more vigorous long form may produce changes consistent with moderate aerobic exercise.[14] Research suggests that regular T'ai Chi practice results in cardiovascular training effects, including an increase in VO_{2max} and a decrease in blood pressure.[14-19] It may also delay the decline in cardiorespiratory function in older adults.[16]

T'ai Chi also offers a promising approach for fall prevention and improved functional status in the elderly. Preliminary research indicates that a T'ai Chi practice intervention contributes to improved postural stability and balance, increased lower-extremity muscular strength and endurance, and decreased frequency of falls.[15, 20-25] Although these results are very promising, they lack long-term follow-up analysis.

Ch'i Kung (qigong) is a practice that predates T'ai Chi Ch'uan. Tracing its similar Chinese roots back 5000 years, Ch'i Kung is not a martial art, but a system of health and meditation. In both the moving and meditative forms, Ch'i Kung cultivates and balances the internal energy (ch'i), blood flow, and the relationship among the internal organs.

Translated loosely as "the study or practice of ch'i," Ch'i Kung, like acupuncture, emphasizes unblocking meridians—the energy pathways throughout the body—to benefit health. Currently there are approximately 7000 different forms and styles of Ch'i Kung practiced throughout the world. Ch'i Kung has been shown to benefit blood pressure in a very small sample of healthy subjects.[26]

Yoga

Yoga is an ancient Indian discipline traditionally practiced for the purpose of self-realization.[25] The Sanskrit word *yoga* means to yoke or to bind together. It reflects a joining of the mind and body and of the individual self with the transcendent self. The mind and body are brought into harmony, and insight is achieved through physical postures called *asanas* and breathing exercises. Practicing these postures and breathing exercises develops physical strength, flexibility, and endurance, as well as builds mental concentration, emotional stability, and inner calm. In the West, the degree to which the spiritual aspects of yoga are integrated into yoga instruction depends on the teacher. Some teach yoga solely as a form of physical exercise similar to calisthenics, free of any association with spiritual growth. Other teachers introduce spiritual concepts and instruct their students with an appreciation for a larger spiritual framework. Although generally taught in a class format, yoga instruction can also be offered individually.

There are several schools of yoga.[26,27] They include the following main schools:

- *The Iyengar school.* The Iyengar school is perhaps the most well-known and popular in the United States. Close attention is paid to detailed elements of each posture, such as the specific placement of the hands and feet and the alignment of the pelvis and spine. The pace of Iyengar yoga is generally slow to moderate.
- *The Ashtanga school.* Ashtanga yoga, sometimes called power yoga, is a more rigorous yoga practice, requiring a rapid and flowing progression from posture to posture. This practice is a high-intensity aerobic workout designed to increase heat and achieve a cleansing and detoxification effect.
- *The Viniyoga school.* Viniyoga is an individualized yoga practice in which postures are chosen and modified to address the specific needs of the student. The importance of the breath and the coordination of the breath with movement are emphasized.
- *The Kundalini school.* The goal of Kundalini yoga is to awaken and circulate the Kundalini, or the life energy stored at the base of the spine. This energy is directed through the body's chakras or energy centers through a practice of breathing, chanting, postures, and meditation.
- *The Kripalu school.* Kripalu yoga emphasizes an internal and contemplative focus, initially holding postures for short durations and primarily building body awareness. Next, postures are held for longer periods while concentration and detachment are developed. Finally,

students of Kripalu yoga are asked to develop their own rhythm and flow of movement.

- *The Integral school.* Integral yoga is an integrative practice that emphasizes incorporating the yoga principles of ease, peace, and usefulness into daily life. Ease in the body, peace in the mind, and usefulness in the community are the guiding themes of integral yoga. Integral yoga classes follow a structured format of postures, deep relaxation, breathing exercises, and meditation.

Within these schools of yoga, some instructors offer classes in restorative yoga, gentle yoga, and therapeutic yoga. These classes are generally very low intensity and emphasize stretching and relaxation postures. On completing a wellness program that includes yoga, a clinician may recommend to those participants who want to continue with yoga that they begin with a restorative, gentle, or therapeutic yoga class rather than a beginner class. The intensity of beginner classes varies with the instructor's view of "beginner" and can sometimes be too rigorous for people with chronic conditions. Clinicians should encourage participants to speak privately with an instructor before class to discuss medical concerns and limitations.

Preliminary research suggests that yoga may have a therapeutic role in treating osteoarthritis, carpal tunnel syndrome, and asthma.[28-32] These studies use very small sample sizes and focus only on the short-term adoption of yoga with either no or limited follow-up.

Introducing Schools of Mindful Movement into Group Programs

A health care clinician with extensive training in a mindful movement discipline may want to integrate this exercise form into a wellness program (Figure 8-1). Ideally, the clinician would be a physical therapist. Realistically, many non-physical therapist clinicians, trained in these disciplines, offer classes attended by people with chronic medical problems. One successful example is the employment of health care practitioners who are also experienced yoga teachers, offering yoga instruction in the Dean Ornish Program, a comprehensive treatment program for people with heart disease.

Non-physical therapist clinicians must recognize that working with a group of people with chronic medical problems is vastly different from teaching healthy adults. For example, spinal forward flexion from a standing position is a movement commonly performed in yoga, yet this movement results in the temporary increase in force load and intradiscal pressures in the lumbar spine and should be avoided, especially by back pain patients. A participant with vertebral osteoporosis needs to avoid all spinal flexion exercises to prevent increasing anterior load on vertebral bodies and increasing the risk of fracture. This information is included in a physical therapist's education but may not be part of the training or experience of practitioners from other disciplines. Even for an experienced physical therapist, teaching exercises in a group format can present significant challenges when group member physical ability varies. Working closely with a physical therapist on program development and exercise instruction to ensure the safe and appropriate exercise for a patient population is strongly recommended for clinicians who are not trained in exercise instruction.

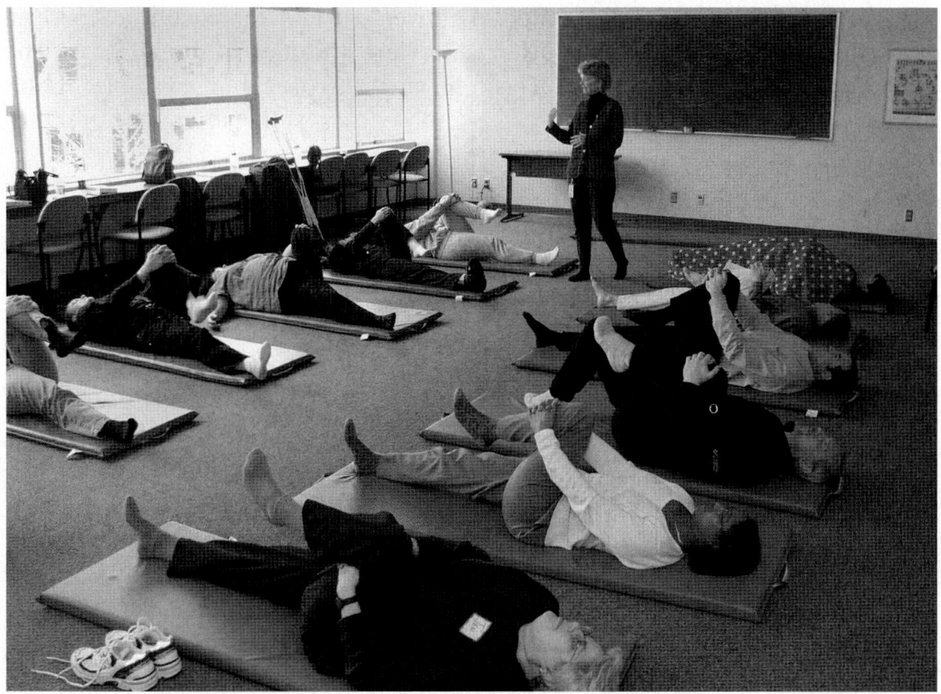

Figure 8-1 Clinician guides mindful movement.

Mindful Movement and Physical Therapy Exercise Instruction

A physical therapist can teach a particular school of mindful movement and/or combine the principles of mindful movement with therapeutic exercise instruction. Combining the principles of mindful movement with therapeutic exercise instruction requires providing participants not only with guidance on the mechanics of exercise but also with coaching on *how* to listen to the body during movement. This approach differs from the traditional method of exercise instruction in the following four ways:

1. Mindful movement emphasizes an *inward focus of attention*, building mind-body awareness and developing concentration in addition to performing a physical activity. Traditional exercise instruction mainly focuses on the mechanics of exercise performance.
2. Mindful movement emphasizes the *present moment process* and an individual's unique experience of movement. There is no focus on an ideal goal. Although physical therapy exercise instruction attends to the proper performance of an exercise in the present moment, achieving a predetermined goal is usually an important component of the instruction.
3. Mindful movement focuses on the *quality and nuances of a movement*. Although traditional exercise instruction also focuses on the quality of movement, additionally there is much greater focus on the quantity of movement, such as number of repetitions a weight is lifted or the length of time a person walks.
4. Mindful movements are *generally guided and performed more slowly* than traditional exercise.

To combine principles of mindful movement and therapeutic exercise in a group class, a physical therapist can review attitudes of mindfulness and their application to movement. The following exercise is an example of this review:

We will be performing a series of movements. As we move through each of them, I want you to keep a few key principles in mind. First, allow your awareness to rest fully with your present moment experience. If your mind wanders at any time, simply note this and gently and firmly guide your attention back to your breathing and your body.

Meet your body with acceptance and respect. This is necessary to prevent injury as well as to build the mind-body relationship. When we are in a group, we often push ourselves more than we would otherwise. We either try to keep up with our neighbor or try to impress the instructor. When this happens, we disconnect our attention from what is truly going on in our body and put attention on someone outside of ourselves. Because we are no longer paying attention to the signals from our own body, we cannot respond appropriately to them. Body awareness is lost, and we miss the opportunity to be engaged in our experience in that moment. So whether your energy level feels high or low, a joint feels flexible or stiff, or a muscle strong or weak, meet your body with acceptance and respect.

Meeting your body with acceptance and respect requires not judging it as good or bad, right or wrong. For example, if you observe that your left shoulder is more flexible than your right, you might have the tendency to think your left shoulder is somehow "better" than your right. Try to avoid making these judgments. Instead, experiment with letting it be neither good nor bad. It simply is. If you were looking at a tree, you might notice that some branches are longer and others are shorter. This is just the way things are. Bring this same understanding to your body.

Move in a manner that is comfortable for you. Do not strain or push yourself aggressively. Listen to your body moment to moment. Imagine how a plant unfolds from a seed, extending its roots downward, its stalk upward, responding to an inner impulse. You might think of your body like a seed, in each moment unfolding from your own inner impulses.

Building strength and flexibility requires challenging the body at its present limits. You will experience some discomfort as you do this; however, overdoing it places you at risk for injury, so "start low and go slow." If any movement causes pain that you feel is beyond the normal discomfort that comes with challenging your limits, stop the movement and assume a position that is comfortable for you.

After reviewing the important principles of mindfulness, a physical therapist can introduce any therapeutic exercise applying the principle of mindful movement. For example, applying mindful movement principles to cervical side bending, a therapist might guide as follows:

Observing your breath. Breathing in and breathing out. Bringing present moment awareness to your neck and shoulders. Do the right and left sides feel the same or are there differences? Just notice. Now, with awareness, gently drop your right ear toward your right shoulder, experiencing a gentle stretch along the left neck and shoulder. Observing this sensation with acceptance, openness, and curiosity. You might also notice how other parts of your body feel as you perform this movement, noticing your face, torso, and legs. Breathe in a deep and calm manner. Allowing your left neck and shoulder to soften. Relaxing into the stretch only to the degree that feels comfortable for you. You can imagine breathing into the stretch and out from the stretch. And now, with awareness, slowly returning your head to the midline. Once again, noticing how both shoulders feel.

Now, gently drop your left ear toward your left shoulder, experiencing a gentle stretch along the right neck and shoulder. The right side might feel similar or different compared to the left. Breathe in a deep and calm manner. Allowing your right neck and shoulder to soften. Relaxing into the stretch only to the degree that feels comfortable for you. Observing present moment sensations. You can imagine breathing into the stretch and out from the stretch. Listening with openness and curiosity. And now, with awareness, slowly returning your head to the midline. Once again, noticing how both shoulders feel.

Mindful Walking

Mindful walking is a strategy that integrates mindful awareness and movement. When we walk, the mind is often elsewhere. We are often thinking of where we are going and what will happen when we get there. Rarely do we pay attention to the experience of an individual footstep. Mindful walking involves paying attention, moment by moment, to the experience of walking without any focus on an intended destination. When walking mindfully, the intent is to bring full awareness to the present moment experience of each step.

This practice, also know as *walking meditation*, involves focusing attention on the sensation of the feet touching and leaving the ground and the sensations of the legs swinging through space. The focus of attention can include the sensations of breathing, the rotation of the torso that occurs with each step, and the entire body moving through space. No particular place of focus is "better" than any other; however, when beginning the practice, paying attention to the sensations of the feet touching the ground is helpful for developing concentration. The key is to pay attention to the here and now experience of walking.

To reinforce that there is no particular place to get to, it is useful to walk in a large circle or to walk back and forth along a 12- to 15-foot line. The traditional pace of walking meditation is very slow. Each step is coordinated with the breath: breathing in, left foot step; breathing out, right foot step.

If mindful walking is new to you, you may want to practice in your living room, bedroom, or a secluded hallway to avoid the self-conscious feelings that can occur when walking slowly in public. It is common to take a few steps and suddenly find your mind somewhere else or commenting on your experience. Thoughts such as "I should be doing laundry" or "What am I doing this for?" can occur. When this happens, just as when practicing other mindful strategies, simply notice your thinking and return your awareness to your present moment experience and the sensation of your foot touching the ground.

Walking slowly is wonderful for becoming familiar with the practice of walking meditation and building present moment concentration. Mindful walking can also be adapted to walking at faster speeds and into activities of daily life. Any period spent walking can be an opportunity to practice mindful walking. You can practice present moment awareness when walking from your front door to your car, from the bus stop to your office, or when you take out the trash. I practice walking meditation each time I walk the long sky bridge from the physical therapy department to the cardiac rehabilitation center. I am often in a hurry to teach a class or see a patient, yet the practice of mindful walking connects me with a feeling of inner ease and calm.

I have found that people with balance problems, including patients with multiple sclerosis or cerebellar disorders, feel unsteady when walking slowly. When they apply mindfulness to walking at a pace they experience as comfortable, however, they often describe increased gait stability.

Summary

Mindful movement is a form of exercise that integrates the principles of mindful awareness and the experience of movement. A present moment, inward focus of attention is emphasized, building mind-body awareness and mental concentration in addition to fitness. There are many schools of mindful movement, including the Alexander Technique, the Feldenkrais Method, T'ai Chi, and yoga. A clinician including mindful movement in a group program should first have extensive personal experience with the practice of mindful movement. To ensure the safe and appropriate exercise for a patient population, a non-physical therapist clinician should work closely with a physical therapist on program development and exercise instruction. A physical therapist can teach a mindful movement discipline or combine pertinent elements of mindful movement with therapeutic exercise. Mindful walking is another practice that combines principles of mindful awareness with movement.

References

1. Taylor M. Putting the movement system back in the patient: An example of wholistic physical therapy. *Orthopedic Practice* 2000;2(12):15-20.
2. Cotter A. Western movement therapies. *Phys Med Rehab Clin N Am* 1999;10(3):603-615.
3. Stallibrass C. An evaluation of the Alexander Technique for management of disability in Parkinson's disease: a preliminary study. *Clin Rehab* 1997;11(1):8-12.

4. Dennis RJ. Functional reach improvement in normal older women after Alexander Technique instruction. *J Gerontol A Biol Sci Med Sci* 1999;54(1):M8-M11.
5. Elkayam O, Ben Itzhak S, Avrahami E et al. Multidisciplinary approach to chronic back pain: prognostic elements of the outcome. *Clin Exp Rheumatol* 1996;14(3):281-288.
6. Prentice C, Canty AM, Janowitz I. Back school programs: the pregnant patient and her partner. *Occup Med* 1992;7(1):77-85.
7. Austin JH, Ausubel P. Enhanced respiratory muscular function in normal adults after lessons in proprioceptive musculoskeletal education without exercises. *Chest* 1992;102(2):486-490.
8. Shafarman S. *Awareness Heals: the Feldenkrais Method for Dynamic Health*. Reading, Mass: Perseus Books, 1997, pp. 1-4.
9. Schenkman M, Donavan J, Tsubota J et al. Management of individuals with Parkinson's disease: rationale and case studies. *Phys Ther* 1989;69(11):944-955.
10. Johnson SK, Frederick J, Kaufman M et al. A controlled investigation of bodywork in multiple sclerosis. *J Altern Complement Med* 1999;5(3):237-243.
11. Lake B. Acute back pain. Treatment by the application of Feldenkrais principles. *Aust Fam Physician* 1985;14(11):1175-1178.
12. Dunn PA, Rogers DK. Feldenkrais sensory imagery and forward reach. *Percept Mot Skills* 2000;91(3 Pt 1):755-757.
13. Wolf SL, Coogler C, Xu T. Exploring the basis for T'ai Chi Ch'uan as a therapeutic exercise approach. *Arch Phys Med Rehabil* 1997;78(8):886-892.
14. Li JX, Hong Y, Chan KM. T'ai chi: physiological characteristics and beneficial health effects. *Br J Sports Med* 2001;35(3): 148-156.
15. Hong Y, Li JX, Robinson PD. Balance control, flexibility and cardiorespiratory fitness among older t'ai chi practitioners. *Br J Sports Med* 2000;34(1):29-34.
16. Lai JS, Lan C, Wong MK et al. Two-year trends in cardiorespiratory function among older T'ai Chi Ch'uan practitioners and sedentary subjects. *J Am Geriatr Soc* 1995; 43(11):1222-1227.
17. Lan C, Chen SY, Lai JS et al. The effect of T'ai Chi on cardiorespiratory function in patients with coronary artery bypass surgery. *Med Sci Sports Exerc* 1999;31(5):634-638.
18. Lan C, Lai JS, Chen SY et al. Twelve month T'ai Chi training in the elderly: its effects on health and fitness. *Med Sci Sports Exerc* 1998;30(3):345-351.
19. The effects of aerobic exercise and T'ai Chi on blood pressure in older people: results of a randomized trial. *J Am Geriatric Soc* 1999;47(3):277-284.
20. Wong AM, Lin YC, Chou SW et al. Coordination exercise and postural stability in elderly people: effect of T'ai Chi Ch'uan. *Arch Phys Med Rehabil* 2001;82(5):608-612.
21. Tse SK, Bailey DM. T'ai Chi and postural control in the well elderly. *Am J Occup Ther* 1992;46(4):295-300.

22. Lan C, Lai JS, Chen SY et al. T'ai Chi Ch'uan to improve muscular strength and endurance in elderly individuals: a pilot study. *Arch Phys Med Rehabil* 2000;81(50):604-607.
23. Li F, Harmer P, McAuley E et al. An evaluation of the effects of T'ai Chi exercise on physical function among older persons: a randomized controlled trial. *Ann Behav Med* 2001;23(2):139-146.
24. Wolf SL, Barnhart HX, Kutner NG. Reducing frailty and falls in older persons: an investigation of Tai Chi and computerized balance training. Atlanta FICSIT Group. Frailty and injuries: cooperative studies intervention techniques. *J Am Ger Soc* 1996;44(5):599-600.
25. Hain TC, Fuller L,Weil L et al. Effects of T'ai Chi on balance. *Arch Otolaryngol Head Neck Surg* 1999;125(11):1191-1195.
26. Lee MS, Kim BG, Huh HJ et al. Effect of Qi-training on blood pressure, heart rate and respiration rate. *Clin Physiol* 2000;20(3):173-176.
25. Carrico M. *Yoga Journal's Yoga Basics: the Essential Beginner's Guide to Yoga for a Lifetime of Health and Fitness.* New York: Henry Holt and Co., 1997, pp. 3-4.
26. Farrell SJ, Marr Ross AD, Sehgal KV. Eastern movement therapies. *Phys Med Rehab Clin N Am* 1999;10(3):617-629.
27. Carrico M. *Yoga Journal's Yoga Basics: the Essential Beginner's Guide to Yoga for a Lifetime of Health and Fitness.* New York: Henry Holt and Co., 1997, pp. 32-37.
28. Garfinkel M, Schumacher HR. Yoga. *Rheum Dis Clin N Am* 2000;26(1):125-132.
29. Garfinkel MS, Schumacher HR, Husain A et al. Evaluation of a yoga based regimen for treatment of osteoarthritis of the hands. *J Rheumatol* 1994;21(12):2341-2343.
30. Garfinkel MS, Singhal A, Katz W et al. Yoga-based intervention for carpal tunnel syndrome: a randomized trial. *JAMA* 1998;280(18):1601-1603.
31. Vedanthan PK, Kesavalu LN, Murthy KC et al. Clinical study of yoga techniques in university students with asthma: a controlled study. *Allergy Asthma Proc* 1998;19(1):3-9.
32. Jain SC, Uppal A, Bhatnagar SO et al. A study of response pattern of non-insulin dependent diabetics to yoga therapy. *Diabetes Res Clin Pract* 1993;19(1):69-74.

Annotated Bibliography

Mindful movement disciplines cannot be learned from reading texts. They require personally experiencing movement positions and sequences with mindful attention. That said, these books offer the interested clinician the basic philosophy, framework, and movements taught within each discipline.

Carrico M. *Yoga Journal's Yoga Basics: the Essential Beginner's Guide to Yoga for a Lifetime of Health and Fitness.* New York: Henry Holt and Co., 1997.
Mara Carrico has taught yoga for more than 25 years. In collaboration with the editors of *Yoga Journal*, she offers a clear, concise look at the roots of yoga, describes several schools of hatha yoga, and describes breathing exercises,

yoga postures, and basic yoga routines. The ideal introduction to yoga is a class taught by an experienced teacher. This book is the next best thing.

Cohen KS. *The Way of Qigong: the Art and Science of Chinese Energy Healing.* New York: Random House, 1999. Acclaimed Qigong master and China scholar, Kenneth Cohen, offers an excellent introduction to the Chinese practice of Qigong. He presents a history of Qigong and describes the Chinese model of body energy, disease, and healing. He offers a rationale for the practice of Qigong, describes basic movements that promote the harmony of the mind and body, and suggests additional readings. This book is considered a classic in its field and offers a rich and educational examination of Chinese energy healing.

Huang CA. *Essential T'ai Ji.* Berkeley, Calif: Ten Speed Press, 2001. Chungliana Al Huang is an internationally recognized T'ai Chi master, public speaker, and leader in promoting mind-body wellness in business, education, and health fields. Drawing from his training and experience in martial arts, calligraphy, and Eastern philosophy, he skillfully articulates Eastern concepts in a manner accessible to a Western mind. In this text, he provides an elegant and basic introduction to T'ai Chi and describes elementary T'ai Chi movements. His book *Embrace Tiger, Return to Mountain*, also published by Ten Speed Press, offers a more detailed examination of T'ai Chi. T'ai Ji is a contemporary translation of T'ai Chi.

MacDonald G, MacDonald G. *The Complete Illustrated Guide to the Alexander Technique: a Practical Program for Health, Poise and Fitness.* Rockport, Mass: Element Books, 1998. Glynn and Glenn MacDonald, accomplished instructors of the Alexander Technique, introduce the basic principles and practices of this movement discipline and present simple exercises for building awareness, releasing tension, and increasing ease of movement. This text is a wonderful introduction to the Alexander Technique.

Shafarman S. *Awareness Heals: the Feldenkrais Method for Dynamic Health.* Reading, Mass: Perseus Books, 1997. Steven Shafarman is a certified Feldenkrais practitioner who received extensive training in this movement discipline from its founder, Moshe Feldenkrais. Shafarman describes the Feldenkrais Method, discusses its benefits, and offers six basic Feldenkrais lessons to build breath, body, and movement awareness. His clear, straightforward writing style combined with the breadth of his knowledge and expertise in the field make this an excellent introduction to the Feldenkrais Method.

Chapter 9 Adherence to Exercise

The benefits of exercise will only be realized with long-term participation in regular physical activity. This chapter examines factors influencing exercise adherence and guidelines for adopting these factors in the design of a wellness program to optimize adherence. Social learning theory is reviewed as a model for promoting exercise adherence.

Factors Influencing Exercise Adherence

The best exercise program is of no use if people do not do it. Unfortunately, low rates of adherence to exercise are common. Of those people beginning an exercise program, 40% to 60% quit within the first 6 months.[1] For clinicians to effectively promote a lifetime habit of regular exercise, understanding factors that influence exercise adherence and strategies to improve long-term exercise participation are essential.

The choice to adopt an exercise program and remain physically active can be understood as a complex interaction of personal, environmental, and program factors, disease characteristics, and the practitioner-client relationship.

Personal Factors

In addition to demographic factors, such as age and ethnicity (noted in Chapter 7), several personal variables influence participation in physical activity. Individuals who are nonsmokers, who are more fit at baseline, and who have a history of being physically active are more likely to remain consistent with an exercise program.[2-8] Positive beliefs about the benefits of exercise, self-reported motivation, and inner determination are also correlated with increased exercise adherence.[2,6,9-11]

Individuals who are under minimal to moderate stress are more likely to demonstrate increased exercise adherence, whereas those with high stress levels are less likely to be consistent with regular exercise.[12-15] It is hypothesized that people experiencing high levels of stress are unable to make the time for an exercise program, whereas those under less stress may find exercise an effective stress-relieving strategy.

In general, obese individuals are less active and less likely to be successful adhering to an exercise program than are healthy-weight individuals.[13]

Environmental Factors

Environmental factors influencing exercise adherence include social support and surrounding physical conditions. Social support increases adherence to an exercise program.[16-18] Social support may come from several sources, including clinicians, family and friends, co-workers, and fellow participants in a group exercise program. Specifically, spouses play a significant role in adherence. Those individuals whose spouses are neutral or unsupportive are much more likely to drop an exercise program.[19] The availability of home exercise equipment and the proximity of exercise facilities are also associated with increased exercise adherence.[20]

Program Factors

Several characteristics of exercise programs are correlated with adherence. Programs that enable participants to set their own exercise goals foster higher rates of exercise participation than those in which the clinician establishes goals without participant input.[21] Increased adherence is associated with moderate exercise rather than high-intensity programs.[4, 21-24] Injuries, which interrupt an exercise program and lead to dropout, are less common in lower-intensity programs.[4] Within aerobic programs, walking is associated with higher adherence rates than other forms of aerobic activity.[1] Providing participants with printed materials in addition to verbal recommendations enhances adherence.[25]

Participants are more likely to adhere to a regular exercise program if exercises are easy to accommodate into daily life.[4,10,26] Rarely have researchers examined the role of the number of exercises or time required to perform an exercise program and adherence. Common sense might suggest that a large number of exercises may prove unmanageable and be associated with decreased adherence, whereas fewer exercises may be associated with increased adherence. In one preliminary study examining the effect of the number of home exercises on adherence and performance in adults older than 65 years of age, those individuals who were assigned two exercises were more consistent with self-reported home practice than those who were assigned eight exercises.[27]

Although group programs may help people establish the habit of exercise, home-based exercise programs are associated with greater long-term adherence.[13,17,22,26,28] Home-based programs may be more convenient for participants because they are able to exercise at any time of day and do not need to travel to a gym or other facility.

Programs that tailor treatment to at least some of the specific needs of the individual or group are more likely to be successful in promoting adherence than a single one-size-fits-all approach.[29]

Disease Characteristics

In a study of exercise adherence in physical therapy, the disease suffered by the patient and its characteristics were examined.[30] Patients with trauma or postoperative conditions were more likely to follow through on exercises than those with other kinds of illnesses. The degree of disability showed a strong relationship to adherence. People whose disease caused a greater degree of disability adhered to a home exercise program with greater consistency than those who were less disabled by their medical condition. Also, people who believed they could be cured exercised more consistently than those who believed their condition was chronic.

Practitioner-Client Relationship

In a study of short-term adherence to exercise prescribed by a physical therapist, people who received positive feedback and reported that their physical therapist was satisfied with their exercising were more adherent than those who did not know if their therapist valued their adherence to their exercise program.[30] People were also more likely to be adherent if their physical therapist asked them to state their needs and ideas, monitored their exercise performance, and encouraged them to exercise at home.

In a study examining the role of physician-patient interaction on adherence to general treatment among arthritis patients, those patients who perceived their doctor as personable were more likely to follow through on their treatment program than those who found their physician more businesslike.[31] Individuals who rated their communication with their physician as good and who felt their physician spent enough time with them were more likely to adhere to their treatment program than those who rated their communication as poor and who felt their physician did not spend adequate time with them.

Enhancing Exercise Adherence

Keeping in mind that adherence is the result of the complex interaction of multiple variables, clinicians can incorporate appropriate elements from each influencing factor into the overall design of a wellness program.

Personal Factors

Clinicians can have a positive impact on participant belief systems by teaching about the benefits of exercise and connecting these benefits to the goals and activities that are personally relevant to participants. If participants do not recognize the personal benefits of exercise, they will be less likely to participate in regular physical activity. Whether it is having the strength and stamina to lift a grandchild or climb a mountain, cope with pain, or decrease the risk of disease, making the connection between the benefits of exercise and the goals important to participants will promote adherence.

Uncovering misperceptions and unrealistic attitudes about exercise among participants is necessary for promoting exercise adherence. One common misperception held by sedentary people and first-time exercisers is that exercise must be painful in order to be beneficial. Clarifying the health benefits of light to moderate activity is needed to promote exercise in this group. Exercise needs to feel good, not painful, for people to remain active.

Another group requiring special attention are those who bring an all-or-nothing approach to exercise. They must "give their all" in order to be personally satisfied. Moderation is a foreign concept and is often misconstrued as failure. This attitude leads people to overextend themselves and increase their risk of injury. They must be helped to understand moderation not as failure but as the most skillful means to achieve their health goals and minimize injury or symptom exacerbation.

In addition, assessing and addressing stress levels of participants is necessary to promote exercise adherence. If individuals experience mild to moderate stress levels, emphasizing the stress-reduction benefits of regular exercise can be helpful. If participants are under high stress levels, additional stress management strategies may be required in order to attain adherence. See Chapter 4 for a detailed discussion of stress.

Environmental Factors

Because social support is consistently associated with increased exercise adherence, clinicians can promote support in a group by creating a comfortable group atmosphere in which ideas and experiences are safely shared and mutual encouragement among participants is readily expressed. With the agreement of participants, a phone or email list can be provided, enabling people to be in contact between classes. A buddy system can be established, pairing participants and asking that they check in with one another at least once between class meetings.

In addition, clinicians can foster spousal support for a participant's exercise program when possible. A spouse can be educated about the value of exercise, encouraged to exercise with the participant, and coached to actively create time in the family's schedule for exercise. The family can be encouraged to become flexible, accommodating the participant's exercise program.

Clinicians also play an important role in supporting participants by developing collaborative relationships and providing positive feedback, pointing out progress, and reminding participants of the personal benefits of regular activity. The power of a positive word in the world of a first-time exerciser should never be underestimated. The following story of a participant in my class is a good reminder of an instructor's influence:

Example 9.1.

Amelia was a 53-year-old woman who was overweight and experienced chronic hip and back pain caused by osteoarthritis. On completing The Wellness Program, she enrolled in a community-based gentle yoga class. When I met her several months later, she commented to me: "One of the reasons I continue in my yoga class is every now and then Denise (the teacher) says to me, 'That looks beautiful, Amelia.' No one has ever said that about how I move. It helps me to feel good about myself and my body."

Clinicians should avoid emphasizing a participant's limitations. It is important to meet people where they are and build on their abilities. Focusing on people's poor fitness levels can cause them to feel discouraged and contribute to a decision to quit an exercise program. Encouraging people to accept their bodies as they are and build on their strengths can have powerful outcomes, as the following example demonstrates:

Example 9.2.

Sandy was a 28-year-old woman who enrolled in The Wellness Program to learn pain management techniques to help cope with chronic migraine headaches. During a discussion about exercise, she described a recent meeting with a personal trainer to develop an appropriate exercise program. The personal trainer made so many comments about how weak and out of shape she was that she never went back. She commented, "If you're made to feel crummy about yourself and your body, you're not exactly inspired to do much else except sit around and feel worse. And you're especially not going to want to spend any more time with the person who brought up all these negative feelings in the first place!"

Sandy was eager to improve her health, and she built her confidence in her body and ability to exercise through the gentle yoga component of The Wellness Program. Two months after she completed the program, I received the following email from her: "I've been taking a yoga class with Denise at Seattle Yoga Arts. She is fantastic. I especially like the non-competitive atmosphere and the wide range of skill levels in the classes as well as the emphasis on not straining or hurting yourself. Today I even did a handstand—who would've thought???"

Teachers of mindful movement schools described in Chapter 8 who offer gentle movement classes or classes specifically for people with chronic conditions serve as a wonderful resource for program graduates. Also, given that exercise adherence is associated with proximity of an exercise facility, providing people with practical information about community-based facilities and programs can promote adherence. A list of programs sponsored by such organizations as the YMCA, YWCA, Arthritis Foundation, American Heart Association, and Multiple Sclerosis Society, as well as facilities such as community walking paths, gyms, and pools, can be a valuable resource for people.

Providing a resource list for those interested in purchasing home exercise equipment, exercise CDs, DVDs, or videos is also valuable to promote adherence.

Program Factors

Several program components can be tailored to enhance exercise adherence:

- Programs should enable participants to actively work with clinicians to choose activities and set realistic goals. Clinicians and participants should collaborate in a climate of mutual respect and open communication in selecting goals and activities that are personally meaningful to the participants and that fit their lifestyles.[25,32]
- The exercise program should be convenient. The more effort it takes to prepare for exercise, the greater the potential for dropout. For example, the need to drive a long distance to a pool or gym and change clothing may eventually lead to dropping the activity. Simply putting on a pair of walking shoes and stepping out the front door may make it easy to remain in a habit of regular exercise.
- Some individuals prefer groups. They value the professional guidance and social support they receive in a group. For individuals with chronic disease or who may otherwise feel isolated, the opportunity to meet other people and share experiences has tremendous value. For many people, the group experience serves as a powerful introduction to developing the habit of safe and regular exercise. For others, a group may be necessary to achieve adherence, as with older adults who experience forgetfulness or mental confusion and require the professional supervision available in a group.
- The number of exercises and time required to perform them must be appropriate and easily accommodated into a person's daily activities.
- A moderate-intensity program is preferable to a high-intensity program. For sedentary people, first-time exercisers, and people with chronic conditions that include symptoms of pain or fatigue, clinicians should start with a low-intensity program and gradually increase the intensity in small increments. Many people in these populations have negative feelings and attitudes toward exercise and their bodies. These negative feelings are reinforced if they start a program that significantly increases their symptoms, results in injury, or is unrealistic and leads to an experience of failure. Clinicians must create a pleasant atmosphere and develop a program that maximizes chances of success. They need to avoid letting their own knowledge and enthusiasm for exercise lead to a misjudgment and the creation of an exercise program that is too ambitious and unrealistic for a first-time exerciser. Helping people to have fun and develop the habit of exercise is the priority. A more rigorous program may need to be sacrificed for a simpler one that participants enjoy and easily achieve. *In the initial stages of a group wellness program,*

helping people establish the habit of exercise is more important than the rapid achievement of improved fitness measures.

- Opportunities to generalize training can be created by providing guidelines and handouts for exercising between class meetings. For example, a clinician teaching a weekly osteoporosis class can provide handouts describing the exercises and recommendations for performing them at home on two additional occasions between each class meeting. The clinician can provide positive feedback when participants are successful with their home program and troubleshoot problems as they arise. This approach helps establish the habit of exercising at home. When the program ends, the participants are already in the habit of doing the exercises at home.

Disease Characteristics

Although a clinician has no influence on the characteristics of a disease, people suffering from chronic diseases may specifically benefit from patient education about the benefits of exercise. The person who believes he or she will recover full function through exercise has a powerful reason to adhere to the exercise program. A strong effort must be made with people with chronic disease to make the case for maximizing function, decreasing pain, and minimizing limitations and other complications through regular exercise.

Practitioner-Client Relationship

Patient-centered care, emphasizing participant perceptions, needs, ideas, and goals, is a central factor of enhancing adherence.[25,32] Establishing a respectful, caring, and collaborative relationship that enables participants to feel comfortable expressing their beliefs, feelings, and experiences is necessary to promote adherence. A one-sided businesslike approach promoting the clinician's medical expertise and agenda will decrease chances for success. Clinicians must avoid the temptation to promote an exercise program that is consistent with their own knowledge and passion for exercise, but that is overly ambitious and not in line with participant goals and needs. They must strive to understand the participants' circumstances, develop appropriate exercise programs, and provide positive feedback whenever possible.

They can reinforce the healthy choices made by participants and the positive consequences of these behaviors. They can point out progress, even when improvements are small. The real problems and major challenges people face when they try to change their habits or lifestyles can be discussed. Clinicians can actively inquire about the kinds of obstacles participants experience and avoid judging people for nonadherent behavior. They can ask: "What gets in your way of being consistent with your exercise program?" This approach enables people to be honest and forthcoming with their concerns. It helps clinicians develop an exercise program that is realistic for participants. Clinicians should attempt to stand in the participants' shoes and view problems through their eyes. From this perspective, different exercise options and solutions can be sought through a process of mutual investigation and cooperation.[25,32]

Relapse Prevention

Inevitably, people who begin an exercise program will experience a disruption in their exercise routines. This may be the result of several factors, including holiday activities, travel, family responsibilities, or illness. Clinicians need to address the likelihood of a disruption in an exercise program in advance. For some people, any break in an exercise routine becomes an excuse to stop altogether. For others, catastrophic self-statements such as "I knew I couldn't do it" and "I always fail" undermine any motivation to return to exercise. Clinicians should let people know that disruptions in an exercise routine are normal and are not reasons to stop exercising or to become self-judging. They can provide participants with a relapse prevention plan that includes the following:

1. Acknowledging disruptions in routine with an attitude of understanding and acceptance
2. Reviewing the reasons for exercising and why exercise is personally beneficial
3. Establishing realistic goals for returning to activity
4. Contacting other group members for support and positive reinforcement

Through acknowledging relapse prevention guidelines, clinicians provide additional tools participants need to successfully develop the lifelong habit of exercise.[32]

Social Learning Theory

Although no single theory of human behavior effectively explains why people adhere to an exercise program, social learning theory offers a context to understand how interacting factors influence behavior change and offers a framework for improving adherence.[1]

Social learning theory views human behavior as a function of the interaction among environmental, behavioral, and cognitive factors.[19] These factors interact to influence a person's sense of self-efficacy. Self-efficacy is the belief that one is able to perform a specific behavior necessary to achieve a desired goal. Social learning theory suggests that people will engage in activities that they believe are within their capabilities and will lead to positive outcomes. Building self-efficacy specific to exercise may increase the likelihood of successfully maintaining an exercise program.[33-37]

Strategies that enhance self-efficacy include those that build self-confidence, self-trust, and mastery of health-promoting behaviors. Specific strategies that improve self-efficacy are (1) skills mastery, (2) modeling, (3) reinterpretation of physiological signs and symptoms, and (4) persuasion.[38]

Skills Mastery

Skills mastery is achieved by helping people identify and successfully perform health-enhancing behaviors. It includes breaking activities down into small, realistic, and achievable tasks. The key to skills mastery is achieving success. People often need help setting realistic exercise goals. Many have the tendency to overdo it. Rather than master the activity, they leave themselves vulnerable to pain, injury, and an experience of failure. The success experienced when a person achieves an exercise goal reinforces the habit of regular exercise.

Modeling

Modeling provides an opportunity for people to see others engage in health-enhancing behaviors. Groups provide a rich opportunity for modeling. A participant who observes a peer making healthy choices can find the inspiration and develop confidence to do the same.

Modeling also enables people to see themselves as experienced experts. They recognize their own breadth of knowledge and insight and the valuable role they have in helping others. Participants can often provide ideas and inspiration to each other that a health care professional cannot offer.

Reinterpretation of Physiological Signs and Symptoms

People may have beliefs and attitudes about disease and health that actually limit their ability to improve or engage in health-promoting activities. How people perceive their bodies and talk to themselves has a powerful influence on their behavior. Teaching people how to listen to their bodies and appropriately interpret signs and symptoms is an important step. Coaching people to develop realistic, health-enhancing beliefs and attitudes helps them achieve their health goals.

Persuasion

Persuasion simply involves verbally encouraging an individual to adopt a certain behavior and is a strategy commonly used by clinicians to enhance self-efficacy. Just as in skills mastery, participant success with the recommended activity is important.

By applying these four strategies, clinicians can increase participants' self-efficacy for exercise and the chances for maintaining an exercise program. Even for an experienced and creative clinician, getting people to stick to an exercise program can be a challenge. It is essential to remember that clinicians can only do their best to understand a person and presenting medical condition, provide an appropriate exercise program, and work with a person to overcome obstacles to regular exercise. The final responsibility of adherence always rests with the participant.

Summary

Multiple variables interact to influence a person's adherence to an exercise program. These variables include personal, environmental, and program factors, disease characteristics, and the client-practitioner relationship. Knowledge of these factors provides clinicians with practical information and insight helpful to promote exercise adherence. Social learning theory offers a context to understand the role these interacting factors play in behavior change and offers a framework for improving adherence through increasing self-efficacy for exercise.

References

1. Robison JI, Rogers MA. Adherence to exercise programmes: recommendations. *Sports Med* 1994;17(1):39-52.
2. Jette AM, Rooks D et al. Home-based resistance training: predictors of participation and adherence. *Gerontologist* 1998 Aug;38(4):412-421.
3. Martin KA, Bowen DJ et al. Who will adhere? Key issues in the study and prediction of adherence in randomized controlled trials. *Control Clin Trials* 2000;21:195S-199S.

4. King AC, Haskell WL et al. Group- vs. home-based exercise training in healthy older men and women: a community-based clinical trial. *JAMA* 1991;226(11):1535-1542.
5. Stentsrom CH, Arge B, Sundbom A. Home exercise and compliance in inflammatory rheumatic diseases—a prospective clinical trial. *J Rheum* 1997;24:470-476.
6. Resnick B, Spellbring A. Understanding what motivates older adults to exercise. *J Gerontol Nsg* 2000;26(3):34-42.
7. Culos-Reed SN, Rejeski J et al. Predictors of adherence to behavior change interventions in the elderly. *Control Clin Trials* 2000;21:200S-205S.
8. Minor MA, Brown JD. Exercise maintenance of persons with arthritis after participation in a class experience. *Health Educ Q* 1992;20(1):83-95.
9. Caserta MS, Gillett PA. Older women's feelings about exercise and their adherence to an aerobic regimen over time. *Gerontologist* 1998;38(5):602-605.
10. Campbell R, Evans M et al. Why don't patients do their exercises? Understanding non-compliance with physiotherapy in patients with osteoarthritis of the knee. *J Epidemiol Comm Health* 2001;55:132-138.
11. Welsh MC, Labbe EE, Delaney D. Cognitive strategies and personality variables in adherence to exercise. *Psychol Reports* 1991;68:1327-1335.
12. Klonoff EA, Annechild A, Landrine H. Predicting exercise adherence in women: the role of psychological and physical factors. *Preventive Med* 1994;23:257-262.
13. King AC, Kiernan M et al. Can we identify who will adhere to long-term physical activity? Signal detection methodology as a potential aid to clinical decision making. *Health Psych* 1997;16(4):380-389.
14. Stetson BA, Rahn JM et al. Prospective evaluation of the effects of stress on exercise adherence in community-residing women. *Health Psychol* 1997;16(6):515-520.
15. Oman RF, King AC. The effect of life events and exercise program format on the adoption and maintenance of exercise behavior. *Health Psychol* 2000;19(6):605-612.
16. Stahl T, Rutten A et al. The importance of social environment for physically active lifestyle - results from an international study. *Soc Sci Med* 2001;52:1-10.
17. Olka RK, King AC, Young DR. Sources of social support as predictors of exercise adherence in women and men ages 50 to 60 years. *Women's Health: Re Gender, Behav and Policy* 1995;1(2):161-175.
18. Eyler AA, Brownson RC et al. Physical activity social support and middle- and older-aged minority women: results from a US survey. *Soc Sci Med* 1999;49(6):781-789.
19. Wallace JP, Raglin JS, Jastremski CA. Twelve month adherence of adults who joined a fitness program with a spouse vs. without a spouse. *J Sports Med Phys Fitness* 1995;35(3):206-213.
20. Sallis JF, Johnson MF et al. Assessing perceived physical environmental variables that may influence physical activity. *Es Q Exerc Sport* 1997;68(4):345-351.
21. Marcus BH, Dubbert P et al. Physical activity behavior change: issues in adoption and maintenance. *Health Psychol* 2000;19(1):S32-S41.

22. King AC, Taylor CB, Haskell WL. Effects of differing intensities and formats of 12 months of exercise training on psychological outcomes in older adults. *Health Psychol* 1993;12(4):292-300.

23. Laitakari J, Ilkka V, Pekka O. Is long-term maintenance of health-related physical activity possible? An analysis of concepts and evidence. *Health Educ Res* 1996;11(4):463-477.

24. Pate RR, Pratt M et al. Physical activity and public health. *JAMA* 1995;273(5):402-407.

25. Jensen GM, Lorish CD. Promoting patient cooperation with exercise programs. *Arthritis Care and Res* 1994;7(4):181-189.

26. Jakicic JM, Winters C et al. Effects of intermittent exercise and use of home exercise equipment on adherence, weight loss, and fitness in overweight women. *JAMA* 1999;282(16):1554-1560.

27. Henry K, Rosemond C, Eckert L. Effect of number of home exercises on compliance and performance in adults over 65 years of age. *Phys Ther* 1999;79:270-277.

28. Oman RF, King AC. Predicting the adoption and maintenance of exercise participation using self-efficacy and previous exercise participation rates. *Amer J Health Promot* 1998;12(3):154-161.

28. Marcus BH, Bock BC et al. Efficacy of an individualized, motivationally-tailored physical activity intervention. *Ann Behav Med* 1998;20(3):174-180.

30. Sluijs EM, Kok GJ, van der Zee J. Correlates of exercise compliance in physical therapy. *Phys Ther* 1993;73(11):771-782.

31. Feinberg J. The effect of patient-practitioner interaction on compliance: a review of the literature and application in rheumatoid arthritis. *Patient Educ Counsel* 1988;11:171-187.

32. Marcus BH, King TK, Clark MM et al. Theories and techniques for promoting physical activity behaviours. *Sports Med* 1996;2(5):321-331.

33. Clark N, Dodge J. Exploring self-efficacy as a predictor of disease management. *Health Educ Behav* 1999 Feb;26(1):72-89.

34. Holden G. The relationship of self-efficacy appraisals to subsequent health related outcomes: a meta-analysis. *Soc Work Health Care* 1991;16(1):53-93.

35. Jensen M, Turner J, Romano J. Self-efficacy and outcome expectancies: relationship to chronic pain coping strategies and adjustment. *Pain* 1991;44:263-269.

36. Arnstein P, Caudill C, Mandle C. Self-efficacy as a mediator of the relationship between pain intensity, disability and depression in chronic pain patients. *Pain* 1999;80:483-491.

37. McAuley E, Bane S, Mihalko S. Exercise in middle-aged adults: self-efficacy and self-presentational outcomes. *Prevent Med* 1995;24: 319-328.

38. Lorig K. *Patient Education: a Practical Approach.* Thousand Oaks, Calif: Sage Publications, 1996, pp. 198-206.

IV Program Development

Chapter 10 Sample Eight-Week Wellness Program

This chapter provides practical ideas for the structure of an eight-session wellness program. It identifies individual class purposes and objectives and offers sample handouts. This material offers an initial framework for a wellness program. Ultimately, your program must be built on your interests, expertise, and the specific needs of the population you are serving. The handout material in this chapter can be photocopied for use in a wellness program without the additional permission of the author or publisher.

Class 1

Purposes:

1. To introduce group members to each other
2. To introduce group members to the basic principles of body awareness
3. To provide group members with an experience of breathing exercises
4. To provide group members with an experience of progressive relaxation or mindful body scan

Objectives: By the end of the class, group members will be able to:

1. Identify three ways in which body awareness influences their health or symptoms
2. Describe and demonstrate the difference between shallow breathing and diaphragmatic breathing
3. Have an introductory understanding of and skill level in applying diaphragmatic breathing to symptom and stress management
4. Be comfortable enough with progressive relaxation or mindful body scan to begin a daily home program of the exercise guided with instructions on a CD or cassette tape

Class Plan:

Group member introductions

Raisin-eating exercise

Introduction to body awareness

Breathing exercises

Progressive relaxation or mindful body scan

Discuss home program

Class 2

Purposes:

1. To create a supportive and safe environment where members are comfortable sharing their experiences, ideas, and feelings

2. To review and reinforce principles of body awareness and their direct application to daily life and symptom management
3. To provide basic information about the role of stress in health and the body's reaction to stress
4. To demonstrate the difference between an automatic physical habit reaction and a conscious physical response to a stressful situation

Objectives: By the end of the class, group members will be able to:

1. Provide a functional definition of stress
2. Describe the body's fight-or-flight reaction and specifically identify how they personally experience this physical reaction
3. Describe how body awareness applies to choosing a conscious, skillful response to symptoms or other stressful situations
4. Be comfortable enough with the relaxation or mindful body scan exercise to include it in a daily home program of the exercises guided with instructions on a CD or cassette tape

Class Plan: Breathing exercises

Group discussion

Define stress

Describe the fight-or-flight response

Examine the role of awareness in consciously responding to stress rather than automatically reacting

Relaxation or mindful body scan exercise

Discuss home program

Class 3

Purposes:

1. To promote adherence to the home program
2. To introduce the benefits of stretching and strengthening exercise
3. To introduce the principles and benefits of mindful movement
4. To provide group members with a positive experience of their bodies and exercise through a guided mindful movement emphasizing stretching

Objectives: By the end of the class, group members will be able to:

1. Identify any personal obstacles to adhering to their home program and strategies to overcome these obstacles
2. Define the benefits of stretching and identify those benefits that are personally meaningful
3. Define the principles and benefits of mindful movement and identify those benefits that are personally meaningful
4. Be comfortable enough with a mindful stretching program to include the program, guided with written instructions or on a CD or cassette tape, as a component of the home program. If, for any reason, the stretching program performed in the group is not appropriate for an individual, that group member will be able to apply the mind-body awareness principles of mindful movement to whatever individually designed exercise program the group member already performs. If the group member is

unable to perform the mindful movement program and does not have an alternative existing exercise program, a recommendation to seek physical therapy for an individualized program will be discussed.

Class Plan: Breathing exercises

Group discussion

Adherence discussion

The benefits of stretching and strengthening

The principles and benefits of mindful movement

Mindful movement exercise emphasizing stretching with closing brief relaxation or mindful body scan exercise

Discuss home program

Class 4

Purposes:

1. To review and reinforce the value of stretching and strengthening exercises and mindful movement
2. To introduce the role of attitudes and beliefs in health
3. To introduce steps to identify maladaptive attitudes and beliefs and to develop constructive attitudes and beliefs
4. To provide members with a positive experience of their bodies and exercise through a guided mindful movement program emphasizing strengthening

Objectives: By the end of the class, group members will be able to:

1. Identify the role of attitudes and beliefs in health
2. Identify how thinking habits influence symptoms and vice versa
3. Know steps to change unrealistic, distorted thinking to more realistic, clear thinking
4. Be comfortable enough with a mindful movement strengthening program to include the program, guided with written instructions or with a CD or cassette tape, as a component of their home program. If, for any reason, the strengthening program performed in the group is not appropriate for an individual, that group member will be able to apply the principles of mindful movement to whatever individually designed exercise program the group member already performs.

Class Plan: Breathing exercises

Group discussion

Describe the role of attitudes and beliefs in health

Challenging negative and distorted attitudes and beliefs

The value of mindful movement for stretching and strengthening

Mindful movement exercise emphasizing strengthening with closing brief relaxation or mindful body scan exercise

Home program guidelines

Class 5

Purposes:

1. To expand the mindful movement program to include exercises to be done in a chair
2. To acknowledge the real difficulties and challenges people face when living with a chronic medical condition
3. To introduce the direct application of class material to dealing with life's difficulties and challenges
4. To help group members identify and develop their inner capacities, based on program material, to skillfully manage difficulties and challenges

Objectives: By the end of the class, group members will be able to:

1. Apply principles of awareness to examine physical, mental, and emotional reactions to a problem situation or challenging circumstance
2. Identify a component of their habit reaction to one challenging circumstance that increases distress
3. Develop a strategy to skillfully respond to a challenging circumstance that decreases distress
4. Be comfortable enough with mindful movement performed in a chair to include the program as a component of their home program if appropriate

Class Plan: Breathing exercises

Mindful movement in a chair

Group discussion

Addressing difficult and challenging situations

Responding to difficult and challenging situations guided imagery

Discuss home program

Class 6

Purposes:

1. To continue instruction in mindful movement for stretching and strengthening
2. To identify the personal meaning of nutrition and nourishment and how that meaning may influence behaviors and feelings about food
3. To introduce the concept of eating in response to hunger versus appetite
4. To introduce mindful eating practice
5. To identify the nutritional challenges group members have when managing chronic illness and physical limitations

Objectives: By the end of the class, group members will be able to:

1. Have increased experience and self-confidence performing mindful movement for stretching and strengthening
2. Describe the difference between hunger and appetite and the applications of these to nourishment
3. Describe personal hunger signs and use the hunger scale to evaluate hunger

4. Identify one personal challenge to nourishing the body with wholesome nutrition and one strategy to meet that challenge

Class Plan: Group sharing
Hunger scale
Mindful eating exercise
Nutrition concepts
Mindful movement
Discuss home program

Class 7

Purposes:

1. To continue instruction in mindful movement for stretching and strengthening
2. To begin the transition from the weekly group format to program completion and the responsibility to continue with program practices independent of the group setting
3. To introduce principles of positive self-regard
4. To introduce strategies to quiet the inner critic and increase self-worth

Objectives: At the end of the class, group members will be able to:

1. Have increased experience and self-confidence performing mindful movement for stretching and strengthening
2. Identify personal patterns of self-talk that are unkind, critical, and unfriendly and their negative effects on well-being
3. Have skills to develop basic positive self-regard through the practice of self-talk that is kind, forgiving, compassionate, and friendly
4. Acknowledge that the program is coming to an end and "make the program one's own" by choosing to adhere to three program activities during the coming week that have been personally most important and meaningful

Class Plan: Breathing exercises
Group discussion
Developing basic positive self-regard
Beginning to make the program your own
Mindful movement
Discuss home program guidelines

Class 8

Purposes:

1. To summarize the main themes of the program
2. To highlight and reinforce what group members learned and gained during the 8 weeks
3. To identify what group members would like to continue to practice and apply from program material, any obstacles to doing so, and means to overcome obstacles
4. To provide group members with information about additional community-based resources to support adherence

5. To provide an opportunity for group members to share their thoughts and feelings about the program and its coming to an end

Objectives: At the end of the class, group members will be able to:

1. Identify three or more program activities or themes that have been personally meaningful and have contributed to increased well-being
2. Identify at least three components of the program they plan to adhere to following program completion
3. Identify one obstacle to adhering to their home program and two strategies to overcome the obstacle
4. Identify one or more community resources of personal interest to investigate following program completion
5. Have had the opportunity to share with other group members their thoughts and feelings about the program and its ending

Class Plan: Relaxation or mindful body scan

Program summary

What did group members learn and gain?

What would group members most like to maintain?

What are obstacles to adherence and how to overcome them?

Community resources

Closing group sharing

Handouts

Handouts are an important component of any wellness program. Handouts clarify class material, help remind participants of key class concepts, and promote adherence with a home program. This section includes handouts that can be modified or used in the present format in a wellness program without additional permission from the author or publisher.

List of Handouts

Breathing
Mindfulness Meditation
Driving Awareness Activities
The Challenge of Stress
Exercise
The Benefits of Mindful Movement
Changing Maladaptive Thoughts and Stories
Change Your Mind
Addressing Difficulties
Eat to Be Well
The Keys to Nutrition and Wellness
Food Guide Pyramid
Opening the Heart
Strengthening Your Self-Worth
Tips for Living Well
Bibliography

Breathing

A primary muscle responsible for our ability to breathe is the diaphragm. The diaphragm is a domelike muscle that attaches to the lower ribs. When the diaphragm contracts, muscle fibers shorten and its dome shape moves downward, pushing on the abdominal contents. The lower ribs move slightly outward. This action enlarges the lung space inside the chest, and the lungs fill with air. As the diaphragm moves downward on the in breath, it pushes on the abdomen, causing the abdomen to move outward slightly. On the exhalation, the diaphragm relaxes and returns to its resting state. The abdomen gently falls, and ribs return to their original position. This rise and fall of the abdomen and movement of the lower ribs is the signal that the diaphragm is actively involved in breathing. This action of the diaphragm performs approximately 70% to 80% of the work of quiet breathing in a healthy individual. Diaphragmatic breathing also promotes relaxation. Additional muscles that assist in breathing originate from lower vertebrae in the neck and insert into the upper surface of the first and second ribs, and other small muscles run between the ribs. These muscles lift and expand the rib cage during inspiration.

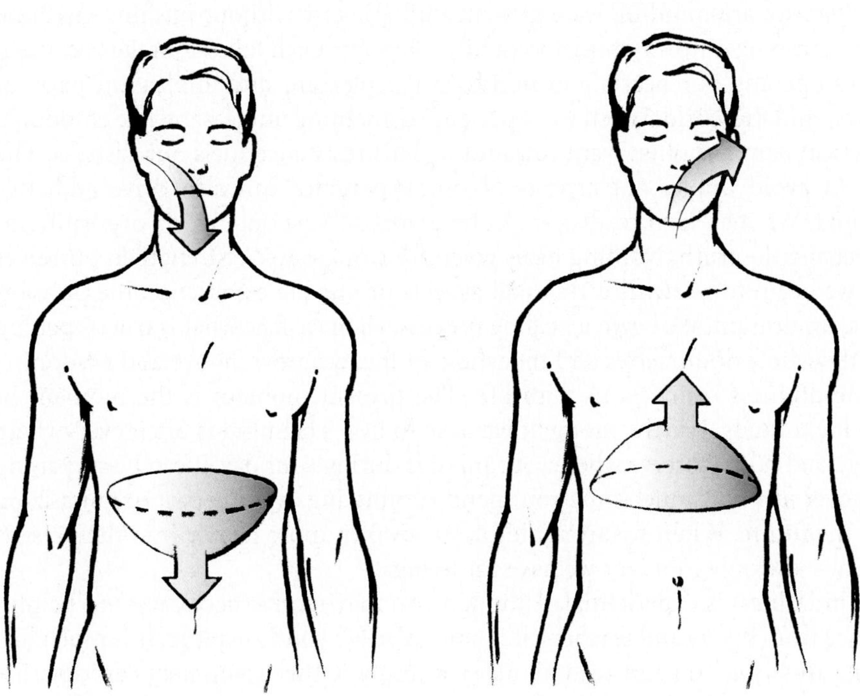

Mindfulness Meditation

Life presents us with many challenges. There are periods in life when we feel as if we were on a roller coaster with sudden highs, lows, and unexpected turns. Even when things are going smoothly, we may experience an underlying tension or worry. To find peace and well-being in the midst of life's changes and uncertainty, we often look outside ourselves. If only I had the right job, a larger income, the right partner, then I would be happy. Even when our desires are met, the joy is often temporary. Our grasping at external solutions to fulfill the search for peace and well-being is ultimately misguided. The true roots of peace are to be found within ourselves. Mindfulness meditation offers an approach to life that helps reveal those roots.

When we are mindful, we are fully aware of our present moment experience. Our attention is receptive to what is happening in the here and now. We meet physical sensations, emotions, and thoughts without judgment. We consciously choose to open our hearts and minds to our experience just as it is. We are not trying to change anything, do anything, or make anything happen. We are not trying to make ourselves or the outside world different. Practicing mindfulness, we meet our experience as it unfolds with patience and acceptance.

When we are mindful, we experience life directly without pushing anything away or grasping onto anything too tightly. This approach takes courage because it requires opening our hearts and minds to the pleasant *and* unpleasant parts of ourselves and the world. When we experience something unpleasant, like emotional or physical pain, we often want to avoid it. This resistance fuels our distress. The desire to avoid unpleasant aspects of our experience can also drive addictive behaviors. We may turn to drugs, alcohol, work, TV, shopping, or overeating to avoid facing the truth. Nothing heals when we run away. We strengthen ourselves when we begin to relate directly to all aspects of our life experience, the pleasant and the unpleasant. We begin a healing process when we face what is true. Opening up to the whole of ourselves and the whole of life, we grow in love and wisdom.

Mindfulness connects us with life. The present moment is the moment in which life unfolds. It is the moment we have to live. The mind is often everywhere but here and now. Observe where your mind is during your day. It can be surprising to discover just how much time you spend ruminating over the past or fantasizing about the future. When we are mindful, we awaken more deeply into the present moment—the only moment we have for living.

Mindfulness is experiential. Although you may receive necessary and helpful guidance from books and teachers, it is a practice for you to explore. It is much like learning to swim. You can read about swimming. Other swimmers can describe swimming to you. Ultimately, in order to swim, you must jump in the water and try it yourself. So too with meditation. The benefit of mindfulness meditation arises out of your own lived experience and investigation. A regular meditation practice helps develop inner confidence, calm, and peace. It is not a solution to life's problems, but mindfulness meditation can help you respond to life's challenges with greater skill, understanding, wisdom, and love.

There is no gift like the present.

Driving Awareness Activities

1. BREATHE.
2. Feel your body in the car seat. Let the car seat hold you, rather than you holding up the car with your muscle tension.
3. Become aware of your shoulder tension. You need some tension in your shoulders to stabilize and control your arm movements, but not a lot. Explore how much tension is needed for this activity. Release unnecessary tension by letting your shoulders sink gently downward.
4. Notice your grip on the steering wheel. Do you tend to drive with a "white-knuckled" tight grasp or a comfortable hold? Explore what amount of tension is needed in your hands and arms to steer the car, and release unnecessary tension.
5. Become aware of the tension you carry in your face. Remember that the facial muscles, especially the jaw muscles, are not required to drive. Relax your face.
6. Play calming music. Avoid talk shows or music that is agitating.
7. Practice present moment attention. When you are driving, just drive. Be right where you are, moment to moment.
8. When you arrive at a stop sign or red light, use this moment to observe your breath and relax your face and shoulders.
9. Recognize the reality of heavy traffic and unskillful drivers. For as long as you continue to drive, you are going to come across traffic tie-ups and poor drivers. You have a choice about how you want to respond to these circumstances. What responses are most healthy for you? Why give traffic power over your well-being? Choose responses that are truly supportive of your well-being.
10. Practice commuter kindness meditation:

    May I reach my destination with ease and safety.
    May all of these people reach their destinations with ease and safety.

The Challenge of Stress

An ingredient of living well is managing stress effectively. Stress is a part of life. Because stress is here to stay, it is to our advantage to make the time to examine it. What is stress? How does it affect us? What are skillful strategies to respond to stress?

Stress is a household word commonly used to describe the pressures and demands we experience in life. Stress itself is not necessarily negative. A certain amount of stress supports and encourages our growth in positive ways. Consider stress as occurring in a continuum. Too little stress, and we are bored and unengaged in life in any meaningful way. Too much stress, and we feel overextended and suffer "burnout." Our physical and mental health can be compromised at either extreme. The middle ground in this continuum is where we are experiencing challenge and change in a manner that keeps us creatively engaged in life.

Although some people may suffer from too little stress, most of us find ourselves trying to cope with too many challenges and changes. When this is the case, it is useful to break stress down into its components and identify what we can change to improve our situation.

The Components of Stress

Stress can be broken down into two components. The first is the situation itself. The second is our reaction to the situation.

Stress = The Situation + Our Reaction

For example, an employer assigns an employee a complex work task to be completed in a brief time frame. The stressful situation is the work assignment with a fast-approaching deadline. The employee's reaction to the assignment can vary considerably. Do her muscles tense or does she remain calm? Is she realistic in her expectations or does she demand perfection? How the employee chooses to see and handle this situation will determine how much stress she experiences.

Sometimes we can change the situation that is triggering the stress. In the previous example, it may be possible to extend the deadline or enlist the help of co-workers. At other times, the situation itself cannot be changed. Examples include experiencing chronic pain or illness, a decision by company owners to downsize the office, or getting stuck in traffic on the way to an important engagement. When we cannot change the situation to reduce our stress, we can look inward and take charge of our response.

Our Response to Stress

Three elements constitute our response to stress: (1) our *physical reaction* or what is happening in the body, (2) our *cognitive reaction* or what we are thinking and our attitude toward the situation, and (3) our *emotional reaction* or what we are feeling. These three responses are interwoven and influence one another.

This section of the class focuses on the body's response to stress. The body is designed to deal with stress that is short in duration and can be resolved by running or fighting. This biologic adaptation, which we share with all other animals, served us well when we were cave dwellers in the Stone Age. This reaction includes increased muscle tension, especially throughout our neck, shoulders, and upper back. We become physically on guard. The body braces in the face of a perceived threat, and we become readied to fight or run. The breath becomes short, shallow, and rapid. We may actually stop breathing for brief periods when we feel stressed. Heart rate increases. Blood pressure rises. Digestion slows as blood is drawn away from the stomach and intestines and is directed to major muscle groups. Hands and feet become cool as blood is directed from the extremities to major muscle groups. We become prepared to fight or run for survival. Through the physical exertion of fighting or running, this reaction is worked out of the body. The body returns to its original state, and the stress itself has been eliminated.

In modern living, our stressors are frequently long term in nature and cannot be resolved by fighting or running away; however, our bodies react as if we lived in the Stone Age. We may also respond to pain with this fight-or-flight reaction. For many of us, this fight-or-flight state becomes a permanent way of life. We are always on guard, in a constant state of alarm, ready to fight or run at any moment. The body was not designed to function in this manner, and this unabated stress reaction can contribute to a loss of well-being.

Controlling Our Physical Reaction to Stress

If we have been in this state of habitual alarm, it is possible to retrain the body to relax. In the moment of feeling stressed, it is possible to change our reaction from the fight-or-flight response to a relaxation response. If we feel pain, rather than tensing the surrounding muscle tissue, it is possible to relax and soften around the discomfort.

The Breath

One resource to shift from the fight-or-flight response to relaxation is our breath. "Breathe." It sounds so simple. Yet when you are under stress or experiencing pain, it is not always easy. You may even catch yourself holding your breath. When you allow yourself to pause and observe your breathing, the physical and cognitive changes that occur can help you respond to stress or pain in a more skillful manner. You decrease the body's stress reaction and evoke a physical relaxation response.

Mindfulness Meditation and Relaxation Exercises

Another strategy to decrease a pattern of chronic fight-or-flight reactivity is the regular practice of mindfulness meditation and/or relaxation exercises. Relaxation exercises include progressive relaxation exercises, autogenic training, relaxation body scan, and mental imagery. These exercises generally feel good. They can leave you feeling refreshed and renewed. The regular practice of some form of meditation or relaxation decreases the stress reaction and helps the body maintain its natural balance and well-being.

Exercise

Regular exercise helps you stay active and maximizes your ability to do the things you like to do. It also promotes a positive mood and general well-being, improves your energy level and self-confidence, and decreases depression and anxiety. Even short periods of gentle or moderate activity can bring significant health gains. Regular exercise can reduce your risk for heart disease by nearly half. It can also reduce your risk for high blood pressure, diabetes, colon and pancreatic cancers, and osteoporosis. It helps you maintain a healthy weight range. Regular exercise can be fun and helps you feel good.

A comprehensive exercise program includes flexibility, strength, and aerobic training. Our capacities in these fitness measures decrease with age and inactivity and can increase with regular exercise, even in the elderly.

Flexibility Training

Flexibility refers to the range of motion of a joint. For example, to reach a product on the top shelf of a grocery store, you need your arm to move freely overhead. A healthy range of motion in your shoulder joint is required to perform this activity.

Stretching exercises performed three to five times per week improve flexibility. Additional benefits of stretching include decreased muscle tension and increased muscle relaxation, decreased pain in individuals with chronic pain conditions, improved ease of performing daily activities, and increased self-esteem and well-being.

Strength Training

Muscle strength is the amount of force generated by a muscle. Muscle strength is needed to stabilize and mobilize your body during activity.

The benefits of strength training include an increased ease in the ability to perform daily activities, improved balance and coordination, decreased risk of falls or injury, increased bone mass important in the prevention and treatment of osteoporosis, maintenance of healthy body weight, and improved self-image and self-esteem.

Aerobic Training

Aerobic means requiring oxygen for energy production. During aerobic exercise, your heart, lungs, and circulatory system deliver oxygen to large muscle groups that are exercising in a continuous fashion. Examples of aerobic exercise include swimming, brisk walking, jogging, and cycling.

The benefits of aerobic training include decreased risk of mortality from all causes; decreased risk of coronary artery disease, colon and pancreatic cancer, hypertension, diabetes, and osteoporosis; decreased risk of depression and anxiety; decreased fatigue with daily activity; maintenance of healthy body weight; and enhanced mood and sense of well-being.

If you have a chronic medical condition, talk with a physical therapist to identify the exercise program that is best for you.

The Benefits of Mindful Movement

A regular practice of mindful movement:

- Increases mind-body awareness
- Builds strength and flexibility
- Cultivates mental equanimity, stability, and well-being
- Reduces muscle tension and increases muscle relaxation
- Increases range of motion
- Promotes circulation
- Prevents injuries
- Feels good

Guidelines for Mindful Movement Practice

- Move into each position slowly and with awareness. Do not rush.
- Postures should be relaxed and sustained. Avoid bouncing or quick, jerky movements.
- Let your awareness be on the process. Accept your body as it is. Experience yourself in a pose with moment-to-moment awareness.
- Start low and go slow. Be gentle. Extend yourself in a pose to a point that is comfortable. Relax and breathe as you hold the pose. Particularly with stretching poses, you may find that after holding a pose for about 20 seconds you can move a little farther into the pose, achieving a deeper stretch. Do not push yourself aggressively. Move gradually. Listen to your body.
- BREATHE. Let your breath be steady and calm. If you find yourself holding your breath, be sure you are not trying too hard or pushing the movement too aggressively. Your breath should be comfortable and relaxed. Ease up and back off the pose if necessary.
- Remember that you are the authority. Only you know what it feels like inside your body and what is best for you. Do not push yourself in any way that increases pain. Do not perform any movement that, for any reason, you feel is not right for you or puts you at risk of injury or a flareup of your symptoms.

Changing Maladaptive Thoughts and Stories

Life happens. Then we tell ourselves stories *about* what happened. Sometimes these stories are negative, unrealistic, and distorted. We start to believe what we are thinking even when there may be little factual basis for our ideas. The mind, caught in maladaptive thinking patterns, is like a distorted mirror in a circus fun house. Just as the mirror grossly alters an image, the mind, clouded with distorted thinking, grossly alters our perception of reality. Unfortunately, we make choices and adopt behaviors based on these maladaptive views that often compound our distress.

Dr. Martin Seligman of the University of Pennsylvania examined the health of people who adopted negative and pessimistic thinking patterns when faced with negative life events and compared them with those who choose a positive outlook when faced with the same events. Pessimists blamed themselves for negative events. They saw one negative circumstance as reflecting a pattern of defeat affecting many aspects of their lives. If one situation was negative, they concluded that their whole life was negative. In contrast, optimists did not blame themselves for negative events and kept them in perspective. They saw a negative event as limited in duration and believed a solution was possible. Dr. Seligman found that those individuals with highly pessimistic thinking patterns had a higher risk of becoming depressed and of experiencing physical symptoms. Optimistic thinking appeared to be associated with better mental and physical health.

The first step in changing maladaptive thinking is to recognize it when it happens. Once you have observed your thinking, acknowledge it for what it is. It is just thinking. It is just a story you are telling yourself. Remember, thoughts are just thoughts. They are not who you are and not evidence of reality. You can use mental imagery to detach yourself from the compulsive pull of a thought by considering it to be like a weather pattern floating in the clear blue sky of your mind. Sometimes, just stepping back from a thought and observing it can result in a new insight or new perspective. Other times, it offers you an opportunity to reflect, examine the situation, and choose a more realistic or healing way of thinking. You can ask yourself questions that promote your control of your thinking and encourage you to think in new ways, such as the following:

Is this a story I want to give more of my time and energy to?
Is this a healing story?
Is there another way of talking to myself that would be more healing, realistic, or comforting?

Observing and changing thinking patterns does not deny or minimize the genuine difficulties and suffering you face. Rather, it is a strategy to address difficult situations with greater mental insight and skill. Wellness and well-being, in the face of life's joys and sorrows, is a complex process involving the dynamic interaction of physical, mental, emotional, spiritual, social, and environmental factors. Learning to observe your thoughts and change distorted thinking patterns is one of many tools in an expanding toolbox for dealing with difficult circumstances.

Change Your Mind

1. *All-or-nothing thinking.* You assess people and/or situations to be black and white, all good or all bad. Alternately, you remain open to the whole spectrum. Rarely are things in life all good or all bad. You are sensitive to the whole picture, with its many shades of gray.
2. *Focusing exclusively on the negative.* This is "the cup is half empty" viewpoint. You place your attention on what is negative, unwanted, or unpleasant. If your life was a garden, you would water the weeds. Alternately, you see the whole picture and keep a negative event, quality, or problem in context.
3. *Discounting the positive.* You reject or diminish positive experiences. Alternately, you affirm the positive. You fully acknowledge and let yourself be nourished by the good things that happen. In your life's garden, you water the seeds of joy.
4. *Jumping to conclusions.* You conclude the worst when there is no evidence to support your judgment.
   - *Mind/emotion reading.* You assume someone is reacting negatively to you without checking it out. Alternately, you seek clarification. Check out your impressions. You gather information and are open to the process.
   - *Fortune telling.* You assume things will turn out poorly. Alternately, you live in the present and are open to the outcome. You address the situation in the present and refrain from predicting a negative future. None of us knows what tomorrow may bring.
5. *Making "should" statements.* You tell yourself someone or something "should" be a certain way. "Should" statements often reflect unrealistic, idealized expectations of ourselves, other people, and life. We can create anger, anxiety, and distress when we try to mold the world to our perfect ideas and concepts. Alternately, you choose priorities and accept limits. You identify what is true, realistic, and important to you. You weigh the costs and benefits of participation in activities and make choices that are consistent with your well-being and priorities. You let go of those things over which you have no control. Remember, sometimes less is more.
6. *Labeling and name-calling.* Labels are harmful terms that make constructive communication, understanding, and insight impossible. Alternately, you seek understanding. You keep in mind that people are doing the best they can. You recognize that all people suffer and have difficulties and develop compassion for yourself and others.
7. *Personalization and blame.* You assume responsibility for a negative situation that is not totally in your control. You blame others for circumstances that are not totally within their control. Alternately, you assume appropriate responsibility. You identify that which is in your control and let go of that which is not. You take responsibility for that which you can control.

These seven thinking habits were adapted from a comprehensive examination of this subject found in Burns D: *Feeling Good: the New Mood Therapy.* New York: William Morrow and Co., 1999.

Addressing Difficulties

Every life has difficulties. No one is immune from them. We have no choice about this situation. Life presents us with all sorts of problems and challenges. Our choice is in our *response.*

What are our habitual responses to life's inevitable difficulties? We may blame or judge the outside world. "It's all their fault," we lament. Or we may blame or judge ourselves. "I failed. It's all my fault." We may turn to our favorite addiction to numb or avoid the distress we feel. We may completely deny our difficulties, desperately claiming there is nothing the matter. Or we may completely indulge our problems, painting a scenario of doom and gloom. These responses contribute to even more suffering. We can get stuck in our unskillful responses for days, weeks, months, and sometimes years or an entire lifetime.

The question we face is: What is the wisest and most skillful way to respond to life's inevitable difficulties? There are no simple answers to this question; however, as we reflect, experiment, and learn about life and ourselves, we can grow in understanding, wisdom, and compassion and in our experience of connectedness with other people.

Sometimes when we stop and examine a problem or difficult situation, it feels as if our suffering were increasing because we are no longer fleeing into habit patterns that numb us from the truth. Although distraction can be a helpful coping tool at times, nothing heals or is solved by constantly running away. It takes courage to whole-heartedly examine a difficult circumstance. Often when we do, we gain new insight and understanding and sometimes discover new ways of responding that decrease our distress.

Examining a Difficult Situation

Identify a situation you find difficult, unpleasant, or challenging.

____

____

____

____

Reflect on how you react to this situation.
How do you talk to yourself about this situation? What are the stories you tell yourself?

____

____

____

____

What happens in your body when you think of this situation? What physical sensations do you experience?

____

____

____

____

What is your emotional reaction to this situation?

____

____

____

____

Every situation has both personal and universal elements. That is, in every situation some things are unique to you. Other things are common to all people. For example, if you have a chronic medical problem, some things about your diagnosis, symptoms, and treatment experience are unique to you. Simultaneously, many other people with your same diagnosis are dealing with similar symptoms and treatment. You share certain aspects of your situation in common with them. Imagine all of the people in your local community who might be facing a situation similar to your own. Imagine all of the people on the planet who might be facing a situation similar to your own. When you think of other people also dealing with this situation, does this influence how you feel or your perspective on your own situation? If so, how?

____

____

____

____

If you think of yourself at 90-years-old looking at this situation, what kind of advice would this senior-self give you?

____

____

____

____

Reflecting on your responses to the previous questions, is there anything you could modify or change about your present response to this situation that would decrease your distress?

If you think of life as a big adult education program and you are majoring in understanding, wisdom, and love, is there some lesson for you in this situation?

Eat to Be Well

Water

Drink water. Water is the *most* essential of all the nutrients. Our bodies may go days, even weeks without food, but not without water. Almost all processes carried out in the body require water. Water is needed for regulating the body's temperature, transporting nutrients, and cushioning joints and body tissues. On average, an adult requires about 8 to 10 cups of water daily, with additional fluids required with physical exertion and hot weather.

Practical ways to ensure adequate water intake include the following:

1. Carry a water bottle with you and drink from it throughout the day.
2. Drink a full glass of water when taking medications.
3. Drink a full glass of water before each meal.
4. Drink a glass of water after urination.
5. Take water breaks instead of coffee or soda breaks.
6. Drink juice or carbonated water for a break.
7. Drink additional water before, during, and after exercise.
8. Eat plenty of fruits and vegetables throughout the day (lettuce is 95% water, watermelon is 92%, and broccoli is 91%).

Connect with Food Sources

Practical suggestions to connect with our food sources:

- Shop at a farmer's market.
- Visit a local farm, orchard, or ranch.
- Grow your own vegetables.
- Start an herb garden.
- Participate in "pick your own" farms and orchards.
- Join a sustainable farm program.
- Participate in urban communal gardening.

Food Combinations

Meal and snack ideas to incorporate a variety of nutrients:

- Natural peanut butter and whole-grain bread
- Low-fat/nonfat milk and cereal
- Low-fat/nonfat yogurt and fruit
- Fruit and low-fat/nonfat cottage cheese
- Hummus or any bean dip and pita with vegetables
- Sandwich with whole-grain bread, lean meat, and vegetables
- Bean or lentil soup and a whole-grain roll

Nurture Yourself

Some ideas to nurture yourself:

- Walk your dog.
- Treat yourself to a movie.
- Listen to your favorite music.
- Read from your favorite book or play a talking book.
- Indulge yourself in a long-distance call to a good friend.
- Reminisce through photo albums.
- Write your thoughts and experiences in a journal.
- Go for a hike at a nearby trail.
- Practice gentle stretching or yoga.
- Renew a lost hobby.
- Write a loved one a letter.

The Keys to Nutrition and Wellness

- Quality, rather than just quantity, of food is important to health and wellness.
- Plant-based foods as the majority of foods eaten helps ensure adequate fiber and nutrient intake without excessive calories, saturated fat, and cholesterol.
- Whole foods rather than processed foods are wellness foods. The less processed a food is, the more nutritious it is to the body. When food is heated, milled, bleached, or exposed to light or air, nutrients are lost. Therefore, the less processed and the more whole food we eat, the more nutrition our body is receiving.
- Healthy and handy snacks and meals are key to maintaining the balance and moderation in our busy daily lives. Grab-and-go healthy snacks such as trail mix, dried fruit and nuts, low-fat/nonfat yogurt, fruit, or a cup of soup can be just what we need to energize us and make it through the day without overeating later or grabbing something less nutritious because of convenience. Keep low-fat, nutritious frozen meals on hand for when you want to eat immediately.
- Eat mindfully. It takes approximately 20 minutes for the body to notify the brain that the stomach is full. We often eat too fast to allow the body to deliver this information and end up overeating. Sometimes we eat so quickly that we are unaware of how much we've eaten until the food is gone. Mindless eating and eating while multitasking is common in the United States as we become busier. Avoid eating on the run or eating while standing or walking. Sit down to eat a meal.
- Calories do count. It is important to realize that no matter where the calories come from, excess calories may lead to weight gain and disease.
- Eating local and seasonal food provides maximum nutrition and contributes to a sense of community and belonging that connects the food source to the consumers.
- Choose to eat foods you enjoy, know how to prepare, and are convenient or fun to prepare.

Food Guide Pyramid

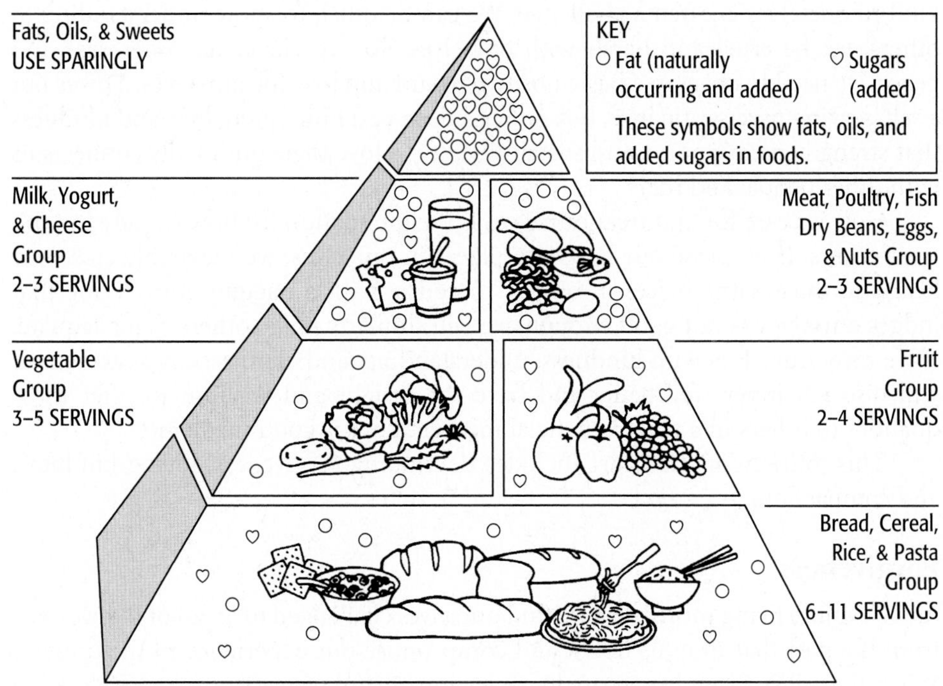

WHAT COUNTS AS A SERVING?

With the Food Guide Pyramid, what counts as a "serving" may not always be a typical "helping" of what you eat. Here are some examples of servings:

Bread, Cereal, Rice, and Pasta
6–11 servings recommended
Examples of one serving:
- 1 slice of bread
- 1 oz. of ready-to-eat cereal
- 1/2 cup of cooked cereal, rice, or pasta
- 3 or 4 small plain crackers

Vegetables
3–5 servings recommended
Examples of one serving:
- 1 cup of raw leafy vegetables
- 1/2 cup of other vegetables, cooked or chopped raw
- 3/4 cup of vegetable juice

Fruits
2–4 servings recommended
Examples of one serving:
- 1 medium apple, banana, or orange
- 1/2 cup chopped, cooked, or canned fruit
- 3/4 cup of fruit juice

Milk, Yogurt, and Cheese
2–3 servings recommended
Examples of one serving:
- 1 cup of milk or yogurt
- 1 1/2 oz. of natural cheese
- 2 oz. of process cheese

Meat, Poultry, Fish, Dry Beans, Eggs, and Nuts
2–3 servings recommended
Examples of one serving:
- 2–3 oz. of cooked lean meat, poultry, or fish
- 1/2 cup of cooked dry beans, 1 egg, or 2 table spoons of peanut butter = 1 oz. of lean meat

How Much Is an Ounce of Meat?
Here's a handy guide to determining how much meat, chicken, fish, or cheese weigh:
1 ounce is the size of a **match box.**
3 ounces is the size of a **deck of cards.**
8 ounces is the size of a **paperback book.**

Food Guide Pyramid. (*From the U.S. Department of Agriculture and the U.S. Department of Health and Human Services.*)

Opening the Heart

Opening our heart to ourselves and to others is a lifelong journey. Learning to be kind to ourselves is often a challenge. We can be quick to show understanding to others, yet be cruel and harsh with ourselves. To experience an inner ease and peace, we need to develop a basic positive regard and love for ourselves. This is not a self-serving narcissistic love, but rather a deep and nourishing love and kindness that strengthens, supports, and sustains us. It is a love that continually connects us with other people and life.

How we care for and treat ourselves is the foundation for how we care for and treat others. If we close our hearts to places in ourselves, we inevitably close our hearts to those same places in others. If we live with a nagging inner critic that judges ourselves as not good enough, we will similarly judge others as inadequate. If we meet ourselves with kindness, understanding, and compassion, however, we will discover inner well-being and have the insight and wisdom to offer these qualities to others in a truly beneficial manner. Love is good medicine.

This journey of the heart includes developing forgiveness, loving kindness, and compassion.

Forgiveness

As we explore living more fully, we find ourselves challenged to let go of old wounds from the past that drag us down and compromise our experience in the present. When the mind is caught repeatedly reviewing hurtful scenes from the past, mental and emotional energy is trapped in the past and not available for living here and now. We are confined to a perception of being a victim and unaware of the depth of the heart's love and wisdom.

Forgiveness is the key to healing wounds from the past. Some people think forgiveness requires condoning a harmful behavior. This is not true. When we forgive someone, we are not showing approval for a harmful behavior. Rather, we are freeing ourselves from the burden and pain of a past experience. When we forgive someone, we are no longer caught in anger, resentment, and the need for revenge. Forgiveness is something we do for ourselves. It is an affirmation of our ability to learn, grow, love, and heal. The harmful behavior remains unacceptable; however, when we forgive, we choose to be released from its negative influence.

Forgiving ourselves for past mistakes is sometimes difficult. Recognize that none of us are given the script "How to be Human and Do It Right the First Time." We learn by trial and error. We all make mistakes. Life is not about *not* making mistakes. Mistakes are a common component of the human experience, so forgiveness is a necessary ingredient in life and in learning to love. The person who experiences forgiveness understands an important dimension of love. It is important to remember that forgiveness is a process. It can take time, especially when we have been deeply hurt by someone's behavior.

Is there something you said or did in the past that needs your forgiveness? What feelings do you presently experience that are tied to this past action? Is there anything that keeps you holding onto this past action and these feelings? Imagine the experience of forgiving yourself for this past action.

Is there someone who caused you harm in the past? What feelings do you presently carry that are tied to this past experience? Is there anything that keeps you holding onto this past experience and feelings? Imagine what it would be like to be free of the burden of these feelings. Recognize that all people suffer. It is out of suffering such as pain, fear, ignorance, or confusion that we cause other people harm. Can you glimpse how this person who hurt you was hurting at the time? Experiment with the feeling of freeing yourself from the negative feelings you carry as a result of this situation through forgiveness.

Loving Kindness

Loving kindness means friendliness. An important component of friendship is understanding. Throughout the day, particularly when we feel stressed, loving kindness means meeting ourselves with understanding and treating ourselves like we would treat a good friend.

Rather than show kindness to ourselves, we often think or act out of unconscious habits and undermine our happiness. We get caught in "shoulds," other people's expectations, trying to please people who will never be satisfied, or doing things just because that is what our parents did. We can be self-judging rather than understanding. Sometimes we create larger-than-life expectations of ourselves and then, failing to meet them, we criticize ourselves as inadequate. We can persist in behaviors that are unkind and sabotage our happiness. When we practice loving kindness, we make the effort to understand our own needs, vulnerabilities, desires, and feelings and respond in a caring manner toward ourselves.

What makes you a good friend? Do you offer these same qualities to yourself? How are you skillful at being friendly toward yourself and bringing yourself happiness? How are you unkind to yourself? Where do you need to bring more loving kindness toward yourself?

Compassion

Compassion is the ability to bear difficulty with an open heart and respond with wisdom and caring. In doing so, our sorrows are lightened. So often we are not compassionate toward ourselves but are our own harshest critics, and cruelest judges. We are often harder on ourselves than we would be toward anyone else in our shoes. So often our fears, insecurities, awkward places, and imperfections need our acceptance and love. When we choose compassion, we choose to open our heart to these places. We accept ourselves just as we are. We stop running from ourselves and choose to be there for ourselves.

What are your self-judging voices? Where do they come from? Where do you close your heart? How does this feel? What part or parts of yourself need your understanding and acceptance? Where do you need to open your heart to yourself, and what would that look or feel like?

For the purposes of reflecting on opening the heart, these comments and questions have focused on how we care for ourselves. Realize that as you are bringing these qualities of forgiveness, loving kindness, and compassion to yourself, you are doing it for everyone. We all benefit. The insight you gain in bringing love to yourself will also deepen your skills in understanding and loving others.

Strengthening Your Self-Worth

Think of your self-worth and inner critic as two seeds in your garden. If you stop watering the inner critic seed, it will no longer grow. If you water the self-worth seed, it *will* grow. To strengthen your self-worth and weaken your inner critic, identify the following:

1. The love you have given and presently give, and the love you have received and presently receive:

2. Your strengths, skills, contributions, and what you like about yourself:

Every day, water the seed of your self-worth by acknowledging the above list. Let the seed of your inner critic dry up.

Tips for Living Well

1. *Recognize your need for renewal.* It is necessary to stop, to pause, and to renew.
2. *Take time out to be alone and listen inwardly.* Stay in touch with yourself. Identify what is important to you and what you want. Make plans and choose actions based on your desires and priorities.
3. *Take control of how you utilize your time and energy.* Prioritize. Say "NO" to those activities you do not want to be involved in. Say "YES" to those things that add to your life and are consistent with your values, wants, and priorities. Remember, sometimes less is more.
4. *Exercise.* Regular exercise enhances physical and emotional health. If you are not on a regular exercise program, find something you enjoy doing and "start low and go slow."
5. *Water the seeds of happiness in your life.* Do something each day that brings you joy. Identify what nourishes you, what adds to your life, and what you love. Make time for these activities.
6. *Modify or let go of excessive demands and unrealistic expectations.* Examine the demands you place on yourself and others. Are they realistic? Remember that the task of humans is wholeness, not perfection.
7. *Create healing stories.* Recognize that your thoughts are just thoughts. They come and go like clouds in the sky. Step back from a storyline that increases your stress. In many situations, it is possible to drop "the story" or to modify it to decrease stress.
8. *Be on your side, not on your case.* Deflate your inner critic and give energy to your inner cheering squad. Cultivate unconditional friendliness toward yourself.
9. *Live more in the present.* Spend less time and mental energy ruminating over the past and worrying about the future. Focus your mind in the here and now. Practice present moment awareness. The present moment is the only moment we have for experiencing life.
10. *Create and nourish a personal support system.* Seek out the company of those you trust and with whom you can be yourself. Build relationships where caring is reciprocal.
11. *Practice effective listening and self-expression skills.* Never underestimate the power of reflective listening. When expressing yourself, use "I" language.
12. *Break your routine.* Do something out of the ordinary. If you always go to the same restaurant, try a new one. Go to a concert or get season tickets to a theater. Take a class in something just for fun. Be a little unpredictable.
13. *At the end of your day, review what went well, what was positive or added to your life.* Cultivate gratitude for the goodness in your day.
14. *Stop and smell the roses.* Remember that many riches of life are found in small things. Sometimes the conditions for happiness are right in front of us.

Bibliography

Living Well with Chronic Pain and Illness

Caudill M. *Managing Pain Before it Manages You*. New York: Guilford Press, 1995.

Fennell P. *The Chronic Illness Workbook: Strategies and Solutions for Taking Back Your Life*. Oakland, Calif: New Harbinger Publications, 2001.

Kabat-Zinn J. *Full Catastrophe Living: Using the Wisdom of Your Body and Mind to Face Stress, Pain and Illness*. New York: Delacorte Press, 1990.

Lorig K, Holman H, Sobel D et al. *Living a Healthy Life with Chronic Conditions*. Palo Alto, Calif: Bull Publishing, 2000.

Spero D: *The Art of Getting Well: a Five-Step Plan for Maximizing Health When You Have a Chronic Illness*. Berkeley, Calif: Hunter House Publishers, 2002.

Taylor S, Epstein R. *Living Well with a Hidden Disability: Transcending Doubt and Shame and Reclaiming Your Life*. Oakland, Calif: New Harbinger Publications, 1999.

Additional Wellness-Related Books

Borysenko J. *Minding the Body, Mending the Mind*. New York: Bantam Books, 1988.

Borysenko J. *Inner Peace for Busy People*. Carlsbad, Calif: Hay House, 2001.

Burns D. *Feeling Good Handbook*. New York: Penguin Books, 1989.

Gunaratana H. *Mindfulness in Plain English*. Boston: Wisdom Publications, 1991.

Kabat-Zinn J. *Wherever You Go, There You Are: Mindfulness Meditation in Everyday Life*. New York: Hyperion, 1994.

Nhat Hanh T. *Peace is Every Step*. New York: Bantam, 1991.

Foster R, Hicks G. *How We Choose to be Happy*. New York: Perigee, 1999.

Ornish D. *Stress, Diet & Your Heart*. New York: Signet, 1984.

Ornish D. *Love & Survival*. New York: HarperCollins, 1998.

Remen R. *My Grandfather's Blessings: Stories of Strength, Refuge and Belonging*. New York: Riverhead Books, 2000.

Rosenberg M. *Nonviolent Communication*. Del Mar, Calif: Puddle Dancer Press, 1999.

Sapolsky R. *Why Zebras Don't Get Ulcers*. New York: WH Freeman and Co., 1998.

Exercise and Mindful Movement

American College of Sports Medicine. *ACSM Fitness Book*. Champaign, Ill: Human Kinetics, 1997.

Carrico M. *Yoga Journal's Yoga Basics: The Essential Beginner's Guide to Yoga for a Lifetime of Health and Fitness*. New York: Henry Holt and Co., 1997.

Cohen KS. *The Way of Qigong: The Art and Science of Chinese Energy Healing*. New York: Random House, 1999.

Huang CA. *Essential T'ai Ji*. Berkeley, Calif: Ten Speed Press, 2001.

Shafarman S. *Awareness Heals: The Feldenkrais Method for Dynamic Health*. Reading, Mass: Perseus Books, 1997.

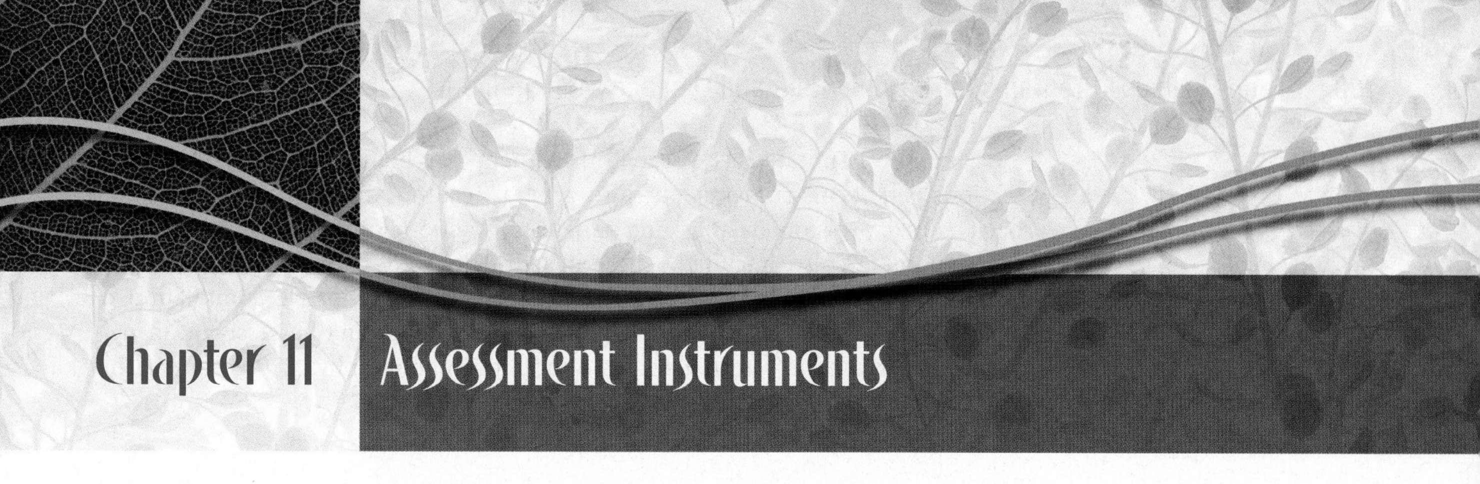

Chapter 11 Assessment Instruments

This chapter discusses assessment instruments appropriate for examining wellness program outcome measures. Qualitative and quantitative assessments are defined, and specific instruments evaluating general health, pain, disability, depression, balance, and patient satisfaction are presented.

Choosing Assessment Instruments

Assessment instruments are used to determine the effectiveness of a wellness program and also provide feedback to participants. Standardized assessment instruments that are reliable and valid are recommended for use in a group program. Assessment instruments measure knowledge, medical status, behavior, attitude, and/or health care utilization.[1] Generic assessment tools apply across a range of medical conditions and patient populations, whereas specific assessment tools are tailored to address questions pertinent to a single medical condition or patient population.

An effective assessment instrument must be simple to administer and easy to analyze. An adequate number of measures or questions is required for an instrument to be valid and sensitive to change with treatment; however, a long and tedious assessment tool is too cumbersome to complete and analyze. A compromise must be achieved between the length and complexity of an assessment tool and its ease of completion and analysis.

The two types of assessment instruments are qualitative and quantitative.[2] Qualitative assessments are used when a health care practitioner desires information that might not be accessed in a quantitative analysis. They examine and attempt to understand the subjective experience of people in depth. Through interviews or focus groups, they explore people's thoughts and feelings to determine how people perceive, explain, or find personal meaning in their circumstances. Qualitative assessments are especially helpful when clinicians are seeking information that is not easily translated into numerical values or pioneering new topics and unsure of what questions need asking. The outcomes of qualitative assessments are presented in detailed, descriptive language.

Quantitative assessments entail the identification, detached observation, and precise measurement of variables that can be statistically examined. They require collecting clinical data or administering questionnaires. They are usually easier to conduct and less time consuming than qualitative assessments and gather information that can be presented as numerical data.

The choice of a specific assessment instrument is determined by the goals of a program and the information sought by the clinician. In some circumstances, a clinician may want to use both qualitative and quantitative assessment instruments.

Several quantitative assessment instruments are highlighted in the following sections. These instruments measure general health, pain, disability caused by back pain, depression, balance, and patient satisfaction. Fitness assessment recommendations are also included. These instruments were chosen because of their common use in research. They do not represent an exhaustive compilation of assessment tools. For a more thorough list and examination of assessment instruments, the reader is referred to the annotated bibliography at the end of this chapter.

General Health

The SF-36 Health Survey (Figure 11-1) is a widely used, multipurpose, 36-question general health assessment tool that provides an eight-scale health profile and physical and mental health summary measures.[3,4] It is a comprehensive, generic measure that can be administered in 5 to 10 minutes. The SF-36 has been determined to be valid and reliable and is widely referenced. It can easily be used in combination with other specific questionnaires that are tailored to an individual medical condition or patient population. Further information about obtaining and using the SF-36 in clinical settings can be found at www.sf-36.com.

Pain

Instruments examining pain measure pain intensity and the multidimensional qualities of pain.

Pain Intensity

Pain intensity is commonly measured by responses to a verbal rating scale (VRS), a visual analogue scale (VAS), and a numeric rating scale (NRS).[5] A VRS provides people with a list of adjectives describing pain intensity from which to choose the adjective most descriptive of their pain severity. Each adjective is assigned a point value. For example, no pain is scored as 0, mild pain as 1, moderate pain as 2, and severe pain as 3. The verbal rating scale is simple to administer and analyze. Although it is a valid instrument for registering pain intensity and has shown sensitivity to treatment, it is not used as frequently as other pain intensity measures in clinical research.

The VAS is a 10-centimeter line with "no pain" at one end of the line and "severe pain" at the other end. Additional points may be added along the line with corresponding adjectives or numbers to indicate levels of pain intensity. A person is asked to mark an "X" on the line that identifies his or her pain level. The VAS is very commonly used in clinical research and has been determined to be a valid scale and sensitive to change with treatment.[5]

The NRS asks people to rate pain on a 0 to 10 scale. No pain is rated 0, whereas severe pain is scored as 10. The NRS has been shown to be valid and sensitive to change resulting from treatment.[5] It is simple to administer and analyze.

The Multidimensional Nature of Pain

No practitioner can precisely know what another person's pain feels like. The McGill Pain Questionnaire (MPQ) (Figure 11-2) attempts to identify and provide

Your Health and Well-Being

This survey asks for your views about your health. This information will help keep track of how you feel and how well you are able to do your usual activities. *Thank you for completing this survey!*

For each of the following questions, please mark an ☒ in the one box that best describes your answer.

1. In general, would you say your health is:

Excellent	Very good	Good	Fair	Poor
☐ 1	☐ 2	☐ 3	☐ 4	☐ 5

2. <u>Compared to one year ago</u>, how would you rate your health in general <u>now</u>?

Much better now than one year ago	Somewhat better now than one year ago	About the same as one year ago	Somewhat worse now than one year ago	Much worse now than one year ago
☐ 1	☐ 2	☐ 3	☐ 4	☐ 5

3. The following items are about activities you might do during a typical day. Does <u>your health now limit you</u> in these activities? If so, how much?

	Yes, limited a lot	Yes, limited a little	No, not limited at all
a. <u>Vigorous activities</u>, such as running, lifting heavy objects, participating in strenuous sports	☐ 1	☐ 2	☐ 3
b. <u>Moderate activities</u>, such as moving a table, pushing a vacuum cleaner, bowling, or playing golf	☐ 1	☐ 2	☐ 3
c. Lifting or carrying groceries	☐ 1	☐ 2	☐ 3
d. Climbing <u>several</u> flights of stairs	☐ 1	☐ 2	☐ 3
e. Climbing <u>one</u> flight of stairs	☐ 1	☐ 2	☐ 3
f. Bending, kneeling, or stooping	☐ 1	☐ 2	☐ 3
g. Walking <u>more than a mile</u>	☐ 1	☐ 2	☐ 3
h. Walking <u>several blocks</u>	☐ 1	☐ 2	☐ 3
i. Walking <u>one block</u>	☐ 1	☐ 2	☐ 3
j. Bathing or dressing yourself	☐ 1	☐ 2	☐ 3

Figure 11-1 *(From Ware JE, Snow KK, Kosinski M. SF-36® Health Survey: Manual and Interpretation Guide. Lincoln, RI: QualityMetric Incorporated, 1993, 2000. Used with permission.)*

4. During the past 4 weeks, have you had any of the following problems with your work or other regular daily activities as a result of your physical health?

	Yes	No
a. Cut down on the amount of time you spent on work or other activities	☐ 1	☐ 2
b. Accomplished less than you would like	☐ 1	☐ 2
c. Were limited in the kind of work or other activities	☐ 1	☐ 2
d. Had difficulty performing the work or other activities (for example, it took extra effort)	☐ 1	☐ 2

5. During the past 4 weeks, have you had any of the following problems with your work or other regular daily activities as a result of any emotional problems (such as feeling depressed or anxious)?

	Yes	No
a. Cut down on the amount of time you spent on work or other activities	☐ 1	☐ 2
b. Accomplished less than you would like	☐ 1	☐ 2
c. Did work or other activities less carefully than usual	☐ 1	☐ 2

6. During the past 4 weeks, to what extent has your physical health or emotional problems interfered with your normal social activities with family, friends, neighbors, or groups?

Not at all	Slightly	Moderately	Quite a bit	Extremely
☐ 1	☐ 2	☐ 3	☐ 4	☐ 5

7. How much bodily pain have you had during the past 4 weeks?

None	Very mild	Mild	Moderate	Severe	Very Severe
☐ 1	☐ 2	☐ 3	☐ 4	☐ 5	☐ 6

8. During the past 4 weeks, how much did pain interfere with your normal work (including both work outside the home and housework)?

Not at all	A little bit	Moderately	Quite a bit	Extremely
☐ 1	☐ 2	☐ 3	☐ 4	☐ 5

(SF-36 Standard, US Version 1.0)

Figure 11-1—Cont'd (For legend see page 191).

9. These questions are about how you feel and how things have been with you during the past 4 weeks. For each question, please give the one answer that comes closest to the way you have been feeling. How much of the time during the past 4 weeks...

	All of the time	Most of the time	A good bit of the time	Some of the time	A little of the time	None of the time
a. Did you feel full of pep?	☐1	☐2	☐3	☐4	☐5	☐6
b. Have you been a very nervous person?	☐1	☐2	☐3	☐4	☐5	☐6
c. Have you felt so down in the dumps that nothing could cheer you up?	☐1	☐2	☐3	☐4	☐5	☐6
d. Have you felt calm and peaceful?	☐1	☐2	☐3	☐4	☐5	☐6
e. Did you have a lot of energy?	☐1	☐2	☐3	☐4	☐5	☐6
f. Have you felt downhearted and blue?	☐1	☐2	☐3	☐4	☐5	☐6
g. Did you feel worn out?	☐1	☐2	☐3	☐4	☐5	☐6
h. Have you been a happy person?	☐1	☐2	☐3	☐4	☐5	☐6
i. Did you feel tired?	☐1	☐2	☐3	☐4	☐5	☐6

10. During the past 4 weeks, how much of the time has your physical health or emotional problems interfered with your social activities (like visiting friends, relatives, etc.)?

All of the time	Most of the time	Some of the time	A little of the time	None of the time
☐1	☐2	☐3	☐4	☐5

11. How TRUE or FALSE is each of the following statements for you?

	Definitely true	Mostly true	Don't know	Mostly false	Definitely false
a. I seem to get sick a little easier than other people	☐1	☐2	☐3	☐4	☐5
b. I am as healthy as anybody I know	☐1	☐2	☐3	☐4	☐5
c. I expect my health to get worse	☐1	☐2	☐3	☐4	☐5
d. My health is excellent	☐1	☐2	☐3	☐4	☐5

Thank you for completing these questions!

Figure 11-1—Cont'd (For legend see page 191).

McGill-Melzack Pain Assessment Questionnaire

Cover sheet:

Patient's name: ______________________________ Age: ________
Hospital No.: ____________________
Clinical category (e.g., cardiac, neurologic, etc.): ______________________
Diagnosis: ______________________________

Analgesic (if already administered):

1. Type: ________________
2. Dosage: ________________
3. Time given in relation to this test: ______________

Patient's intelligence: Circle number that represents best estimate:

1 (low) 2 3 4 5 (high)

This questionnaire has been designed to tell us more about your pain. Four major questions we ask are:

1. Where is your pain?
2. What does it feel like?
3. How does it change with time?
4. How strong is it?

It is important that you tell us how yor pain feels now. Please follow the instructions at the beginning of each part.

Part 1.
Where is your pain?

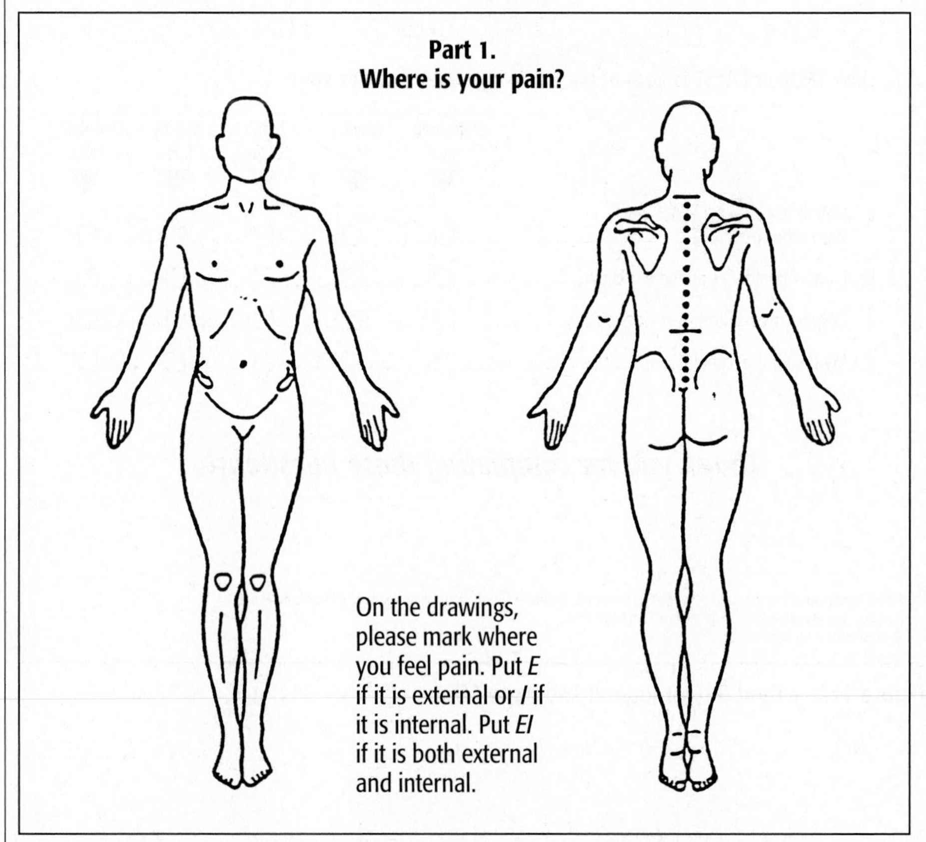

On the drawings, please mark where you feel pain. Put *E* if it is external or *I* if it is internal. Put *EI* if it is both external and internal.

Figure 11-2 *(Reprinted from Melzack R. The McGill Pain Questionnaire: major properties and scoring methods. Pain 1975;1:275-277. With permission from Elsevier Science.)*

Part 2. What does your pain feel like?

Some of the words below should describe your present pain. Circle only those words that best describe it. Use only a *single word* in each appropriate category–the one that applies best. Leave out any category that is not suitable.

1	2	3	4	5
Flickering Quivering Pulsing Throbbing Beating	Jumping Flashing Shooting	Pricking Boring Drilling Stabbing Lancinating	Sharp Cutting Lacerating	Pinching Pressing Gnawing Cramping Crushing
6	**7**	**8**	**9**	**10**
Tugging Pulling Wrenching	Hot Burning Scalding Searing	Tingling Itchy Smarting Stinging	Dull Sore Hurting Aching Heavy	Tender Taut Rasping Splitting
11	**12**	**13**	**14**	**15**
Tiring Exhausting	Sickening Suffocating	Fearful Frightful Terrifying	Punishing Grueling Cruel Vicious Killing	Wretched Blinding
16	**17**	**18**	**19**	**20**
Annoying Troublesome Miserable Intense Unbearable	Spreading Radiating Penetrating Piercing	Tight Numb Drawing Squeezing Tearing	Cool Cold Freezing	Nagging Nauseating Agonizing Dreadful Torturing

Part 3. How does your pain change with time?

1. Which word or words would you use to describe the pattern of your pain?

1	2	3
Continuous Steady Constant	Rhythmic Periodic Intermittent	Brief Momentary Transient

2. What kind of things relieve your pain?

____
____
____
____

3. What kind of things increase your pain?

____
____
____
____

Part 4. How strong is your pain?

People agree that the following five words represent pain of increasing intensity. They are:

1	2	3	4	5
Mild	Discomforting	Distressing	Horrible	Excruciating

To answer each question below, write the number of the most appropriate word in the space beside the question.

1. Which word describes your pain right now? ________
2. Which word describes it at its worst? ________
3. Which word describes it when it is the least? ________
4. Which word descibes the worst toothache you ever had? ________
5. Which word descibes the worst headache you ever had? ________
6. Which word descibes the worst stomachache you ever had? ________

Figure 11-2—Cont'd (See opposite page for legend).

greater insight into the qualitative experience of pain.[6] The MPQ is comprised of 20 groups of single-word pain descriptions, identifying sensory, affective, and evaluative qualities of pain. The words in each group are listed in order of intensity and assigned a numerical value. Respondents are asked to choose the words that describe their feelings and sensations of pain at the present moment. The sum of the values for each pain description selected results in the Pain Rating Index. In addition, the MPQ includes a body diagram, a scale of five adjectives describing

Roland-Morris Disability Questionnaire

Roland/Morris Disability Questionnaire

NAME ______________________ PHONE ______________

DATE __________ TIME __________ SUBJECT CODE ____________

ADMINISTRATION # ______________ ORDER ______________

When your back hurts, you may find it difficult to do some of the things you normally do.

This list contains some sentences that people have used to describe themselves when they have back pain. When you read them, you may find that some stand out because they describe you today. As you read the list, think of yourself *today*. When you read a sentence that describes you *today*, put a check beside the number of the sentence. If the sentence does not describe you, then leave the space blank and go on to the next one. Remember, only check the sentence if you are sure that it describes you *today*.

_____ 1. I stay at home most of the time because of my back.
_____ 2. I change position frequently to try and get my back comfortable.
_____ 3. I walk more slowly than usual because of my back.
_____ 4. Because of my back, I am not doing any of the jobs that I usually do around the house.
_____ 5. Because of my back, I use a handrail to get upstairs.
_____ 6. Because of my back, I lie down to rest more often.
_____ 7. Because of my back, I have to hold onto something to get out of an easy chair.
_____ 8. Because of my back, I try to get other people to do things for me.
_____ 9. I get dressed more slowly than usual because of my back.
_____ 10. I only stand up for short periods of time because of my back.
_____ 11. Because of my back, I try not to bend or kneel down.
_____ 12. I find it difficult to get out of a chair because of my back.
_____ 13. My back is painful almost all the time.
_____ 14. I find it difficult to turn over in bed because of my back.
_____ 15. My appetite is not very good because of my back pain.
_____ 16. I have trouble putting on my socks (or stockings) because of the pain in my back.
_____ 17. I only walk short distances because of my back pain.
_____ 18. I sleep less well because of my back.
_____ 19. Because of my back pain, I get dressed with help from someone else.
_____ 20. I sit down for most of the day because of my back.
_____ 21. I avoid heavy jobs around the house because of my back.
_____ 22. Because of my back pain, I am more irritable and bad tempered with people than usual.
_____ 23. Because of my back, I go upstairs more slowly than usual.
_____ 24. I stay in bed most of the time because of my back.

Figure 11-3

pain intensity, and a section of words describing the temporal nature of pain. A short form of the MPQ is available. The MPQ is widely used and has been shown to be valid and reliable.

Back Pain Disability

The Roland-Morris Disability Questionnaire (RMDQ) (Figure 11-3) and the Oswestry Disability Index (ODI) (Figure 11-4) are measures of back pain disability commonly used in clinical research.[7] The RMDQ measures physical disability caused by low-back pain. It is a short, simple, easy-to-understand 24-item questionnaire that assesses common functions, including sitting, standing, bending, lying down, sleeping, and self-care. Respondents place a check mark beside the statements that apply to them on that day. The RMDQ score is calculated by adding up the number of checked items. Zero indicates no disability, whereas 24 reflects maximum disability. RMDQ scores correlate with other measures of physical function, reflecting a high level of validity. According to the authors of the questionnaire, changes in scores of 2 to 3 points should be regarded as clinically significant. The RMDQ has been translated into 11 languages.

The ODI is a 10-section questionnaire consisting of statements describing pain intensity, personal care, lifting, walking, sitting, standing, sleeping, sex life, social life, and travel ability. Respondents are asked to mark the box that is most descriptive of their experience that day. It can be completed in 5 minutes and scored in less than 1 minute.

Following a thorough review of the RMDQ and ODI, Roland and Fairbank conclude that both instruments are suitable for use with back pain patients.[7] They note that at high levels of disability, the ODI may continue to show change, whereas RMDQ scores plateau. At lower levels of disability, the RMDQ may continue to reveal change, whereas the ODI may be limited to discern change. Therefore, the RMDQ may be slightly better suited for patients with mild to moderate disability and the ODI better suited for patients with severe disability caused by back pain.

Fitness Tests

As with other assessment instruments, fitness tests must be simple to administer, feasible for participants to complete without undue distress, and easy to analyze. Measures of fitness identify cardiovascular capacity, flexibility, and strength. Cardiovascular fitness can be assessed through an exercise tolerance test on the treadmill or by determining the distance walked in a given time period, which is less costly and more convenient. The 6-minute walk test has been shown to be reliable and valid.[8-10] Flexibility and strength are components of fitness commonly measured by physical and occupational therapists through range-of-motion measurement and manual muscle testing.

Balance

Clinicians offering wellness programs for seniors may want to include a balance assessment in any fitness measure. The Berg Balance Test (BBT) (Figure 11-5) was developed to assess balance in seniors.[11] It consists of 14 mobility tasks scored on a 0 to 4 scale. A person who is unable to perform a task is scored 0, whereas a person

Oswestry Low Back Pain Disability Questionnaire

(The Robert Jones and Agnes Hunt Orthopaedic Hospital, Oswestry, Shropshire, Department for Spinal Disorders)

NAME ______________________ PHONE ______________________

DATE __________ TIME __________ SUBJECT CODE ______________________

ADMINISTRATION # ______________ ORDER ______________________

Please read:

This questionnaire has been designed to give the doctor information as to how your back pain has affected your ability to manage in everyday life. Please answer every section, and mark in each section only the one box which applies to you. We realize you may consider that two of the statements in any one section relate to you, but please just mark the box which most closely describes your problem.

Section 1–Pain Intensity
- □ I can tolerate the pain I have without having to use pain killers.
- □ The pain is bad but I manage without taking pain killers.
- □ Pain killers give complete relief from pain.
- □ Pain killers give moderate relief from pain.
- □ Pain killers give very little relief from pain.
- □ Pain killers have no effect on the pain and I do not use them.

Section 2–Personal Care (washing, dressing, etc.)
- □ I can look after myself normally without causing extra pain.
- □ I can look after myself normally but it causes extra pain.
- □ It is painful to look after myself and I am slow and careful.
- □ I need some help but manage most of my personal care.
- □ I need help every day in most aspects of self care.
- □ I do not get dressed, wash with difficulty and stay in bed.

Section 3–Lifting
- □ I can lift heavy weights without extra pain.
- □ I can lift heavy weights but it gives extra pain.
- □ Pain prevents me from lifting heavy weights off the floor, but I can manage if they are conveniently positioned, e.g. on a table.
- □ I can lift only very light weights.
- □ I cannot lift or carry anything at all.

Section 4–Walking
- □ Pain does not prevent me walking any distance.
- □ Pain prevents me walking more than 1 mile.
- □ Pain prevents me from walking more than $\frac{1}{2}$ mile.
- □ Pain prevents me from walking more than $\frac{1}{4}$ mile.
- □ I can only walk using a cane or crutches.
- □ I am in bed most of the time and have to crawl to the toilet.

Section 5–Sitting
- □ I can sit in any chair as long as I like.
- □ I can only sit in my favorite chair as long as I like.
- □ Pain prevents me sitting more than 1 hour.
- □ Pain prevents me from sitting more than $\frac{1}{2}$ hour.
- □ Pain prevents me from sitting more than 10 minutes.
- □ Pain prevents me from sitting at all.

Section 6–Standing
- □ I can stand as long as I want without extra pain.
- □ I can stand as long as I want but it gives me extra pain.
- □ Pain prevents me from standing for more than 1 hour.
- □ Pain prevents me from standing for more than 30 minutes.
- □ Pain prevents me from standing for more than 10 minutes.
- □ Pain prevents me from standing at all.

Figure 11-4

Section 7–Sleeping
- □ Pain does not prevent me from sleeping well.
- □ I can sleep well only by using tablets.
- □ Even when I take pills, I have less than six hours sleep.
- □ Even when I take pills, I have less than four hours sleep.
- □ Even when I take pills, I have less than two hours sleep.
- □ Pain prevents me from sleeping at all.

Section 8–Sex Life
- □ My sex life is normal and causes no extra pain.
- □ My sex life is normal but causes some extra pain.
- □ My sex life is nealy normal but is very painful.
- □ My sex life is severely restricted by pain.
- □ My sex life is nearly absent because of pain.
- □ Pain prevents any sex life at all.

Section 9–Social Life
- □ My social life is normal and gives me no extra pain.
- □ My social life is normal but increases the degree of pain.
- □ Pain has no significant effect on my social life apart from limiting my more energetic interests, e.g., dancing, etc.
- □ Pain has restricted my social life and I do not go out as often.
- □ Pain has restricted my social life to my home.
- □ I have no social life because of pain.

Section 10–Traveling
- □ I can travel anywhere without extra pain.
- □ I can travel anywhere but it gives me extra pain.
- □ Pain is bad but I manage journeys over two hours.
- □ Pain restricts me to journeys of less than one hour.
- □ Pain restricts me to short necessary journeys under 30 minutes.
- □ Pain prevents me from traveling except to the doctor or hospital.

Figure 11-4—Cont'd

who is able to optimally perform a task is scored 4. The BBT has been shown to be reliable and valid. The BBT and scoring instructions can also be found at www.chcr.brown.edu/balance.htm.

Depression

The Center for Epidemiological Studies Depression Scale (CESD) (Figure 11-6) is a 20-item scale of depression symptoms.[12] Respondents rate the frequency with which they experience symptoms on a 0 to 3 scale; 0 indicating rarely and 3 indicating they experience the symptom 6 or 7 days of the week. The sum of the responses comprises the score. The CESD has been determined to be both a valid instrument and sensitive to changes in depression severity.

Patient Satisfaction

A valid and reliable standardized instrument measuring patient satisfaction following participation in a group wellness treatment has not been established. The Wellness Program Satisfaction Questionnaire (WPSQ) (Figure 11-7) was adapted

BALANCE SCALE*

Name ______________________ Date ______________________

Location ______________________ Rater ______________________

ITEM DESCRIPTION	SCORE (0-4)
1. Sitting to standing	____
2. Standing unsupported	____
3. Sitting unsupported	____
4. Standing to sitting	____
5. Transfers	____
6. Standing with eyes closed	____
7. Standing with feet together	____
8. Reaching forward with outstretched arm	____
9. Retrieving object from floor	____
10. Turning to look behind	____
11. Turning 360 degrees	____
12. Placing alternate foot on stool	____
13. Standing with one foot in front	____
14. Standing on one foot	____
TOTAL	____

*references on page 202

GENERAL INSTRUCTIONS

Please demonstrate each task and/or give instructions as written. When scoring, please record the lowest response category that applies for each item.

In most items, the subject is asked to maintain a given position for specific time. Progressively more points are deducted if the time or distance requirements are not met, if the subject's performance warrants supervision, or if the subject touches an external support or receives assistance from the examiner. Subjects should understand that they must maintain their balance while attempting the tasks. The choices of which leg to stand on or how far to reach are left to the subject. Poor judgment will adversely influence the performance and the scoring.

Equipment required for testing are a stopwatch or watch with a second hand, and a ruler or other indicator of 2, 5 and 10 inches (5, 12.5 and 25 cm). Chairs used during testing should be of reasonable height. Either a step or a stool (of average step height) may be used for item #12.

1. **SITTING TO STANDING**
INSTRUCTIONS: Please stand up. Try not to use your hands for support.
( ) 4 able to stand without using hands and stabilize independently
( ) 3 able to stand independently using hands
( ) 2 able to stand using hands after several tries
( ) 1 needs minimal aid to stand or to stabilize
( ) 0 needs moderate or maximal assist to stand

2. **STANDING UNSUPPORTED**
INSTRUCTIONS: Please stand for two minutes without holding.
( ) 4 able to stand safely 2 minutes
( ) 3 able to stand 2 minutes with supervision
( ) 2 able to stand 30 seconds unsupported
( ) 1 needs several tries to stand 30 seconds unsupported
( ) 0 unable to stand 30 seconds unassisted

If a subject is able to stand 2 minutes unsupported, score full points for sitting unsupported. Proceed to item #4

Figure 11-5 Berg Balance Test. *(From Berg K, Wood-Dauphinee S, Williams JI, Maki B. Measuring balance in the elderly: Validation of an instrument. Can J Pub Health July/Aug. Supp 2:S7-11, 1992; and Berg K, Wood-Dauphinee S, Williams JI, Gayton D. Measuring imbalance in the elderly: Preliminary development of an instrument. Physiotherapy Can 41:304-311, 1989.)*

3. **SITTING WITH BACK UNSUPPORTED BUT FEET SUPPORTED ON FLOOR OR ON A STOOL**
INSTRUCTIONS: Please sit with arms folded for 2 minutes.
( ) 4 able to sit safely and securely 2 minutes
( ) 3 able to sit 2 minutes under supervision
( ) 2 able to sit 30 seconds
( ) 1 able to sit 10 seconds
( ) 0 unable to sit without support 10 seconds

4. **STANDING TO SITTING**
INSTRUCTIONS: Please sit down.
( ) 4 sits safely with minimal use of hands
( ) 3 controls descent by using hands
( ) 2 uses back of legs against chair to control descent
( ) 1 sits independently but has uncontrolled descent
( ) 0 needs assistance to sit

5. **TRANSFERS**
INSTRUCTIONS: Arrange chairs(s) for a pivot transfer. Ask subject to transfer one way toward a seat with armrests and one way toward a seat without armrests. You may use two chairs (one with and one without armrests) or a bed and a chair.
( ) 4 able to transfer safely with minor use of hands
( ) 3 able to transfer safely definite need of hands
( ) 2 able to transfer with verbal cueing and/or supervision
( ) 1 needs one person to assist
( ) 0 needs two people to assist or supervise to be safe

6. **STANDING UNSUPPORTED WITH EYES CLOSED**
INSTRUCTIONS: Please close your eyes and stand still for 10 seconds.
( ) 4 able to stand 10 seconds safely
( ) 3 able to stand 10 seconds with supervision
( ) 2 able to stand 3 seconds
( ) 1 unable to keep eyes closed 3 seconds but stays steady
( ) 0 needs help to keep from falling

7. **STANDING UNSUPPORTED WITH FEET TOGETHER**
INSTRUCTIONS: Place your feet together and stand without holding.
( ) 4 able to place feet together independently and stand 1 minute safely
( ) 3 able to place feet together independently and stand for 1 minute with supervision
( ) 2 able to place feet together independently and to hold for 30 seconds
( ) 1 needs help to attain position but able to stand 15 seconds feet together
( ) 0 needs help to attain position and unable to hold for 15 seconds

8. **REACHING FORWARD WITH OUTSTRETCHED ARM WHILE STANDING**
INSTRUCTIONS: Lift arm to 90 degrees. Stretch out your fingers and reach forward as far as you can. (Examiner places a ruler at end of fingertips when arm is at 90 degrees. Fingers should not touch the ruler while reaching forward. The recorded measure is the distance forward that the finger reach while the subject is in the most forward lean position. When possible, ask subject to use both arms when reaching to avoid rotation of the trunk.)
( ) 4 can reach forward confidently >25 cm (10 inches)
( ) 3 can reach forward >12.5 cm safely (5 inches)
( ) 2 can reach forward >5 cm safely (2 inches)
( ) 1 reaches forward but needs supervision
( ) 0 loses balance while trying/requires external support

9. **PICK UP OBJECT FROM THE FLOOR FROM A STANDING POSITION**
INSTRUCTIONS: Pick up the shoe/slipper which is placed in front of your feet.
( ) 4 able to pick up slipper safely and easily
( ) 3 able to pick up slipper but needs supervision
( ) 2 unable to pick up but reaches 2-5cm (1-2 inches) from slipper and keeps balance independently
( ) 1 unable to pick up and needs supervision while trying
( ) 0 unable to try/needs assist to keep from losing balance or falling

Figure 11-5—Cont'd (See opposite page for legend).

10. **TURNING TO LOOK BEHIND OVER LEFT AND RIGHT SHOULDERS WHILE STANDING**
INSTRUCTIONS: Turn to look **directly** behind you over toward left shoulder. Repeat to the right. Examiner may pick an object to look at directly behind the subject to encourage a better twist turn.
( ) 4 looks behind from both sides and weight shifts well
( ) 3 looks behind one side only other side shows less weight shift
( ) 2 turns sideways only but maintains balance
( ) 1 needs supervision when turning
( ) 0 needs assistance to keep from losing balance or falling

11. **TURN 360 DEGREES**
INSTRUCTIONS: Turn completely around in a full circle. Pause. Then turn a full circle in the other direction.
( ) 4 able to turn 360 degrees safely in 4 seconds or less
( ) 3 able to turn 360 degrees safely one side only in 4 seconds or less
( ) 2 able to turn 360 degrees safely but slowly
( ) 1 needs close supervision or verbal cueing
( ) 0 needs assistance while turning

12. **PLACING ALTERNATE FOOT ON STEP OR STOOL WHILE STANDING UNSUPPORTED**
INSTRUCTIONS: Place each foot alternately on the step/stool. Continue until each foot has touched the step/stool four times.
( ) 4 able to stand independently and safely and complete 8 steps in 20 seconds
( ) 3 able to stand independently and complete 8 steps >20 seconds
( ) 2 able to complete 4 steps without aid with supervision
( ) 1 able to complete >2 steps needs minimal assistance
( ) 0 needs assistance to keep from falling/unable to try

13. **STANDING UNSUPPORTED ONE FOOT IN FRONT**
INSTRUCTIONS: (DEMONSTRATE TO SUBJECT)
Place one foot directly in front of the other. If you feel that you cannot place your foot directly in front, try to step far enough ahead that the heel of your forward foot is ahead of the toes of the other foot. (To score 3 points, the length of the step should exceed the length of the other foot and the width of the stance should approximate the subject's normal stride width)
( ) 4 able to place foot tandem independently and hold 30 seconds
( ) 3 able to place foot ahead of other independently and hold 30 seconds
( ) 2 able to take small step independently and hold 30 seconds
( ) 1 needs help to step but can hold 15 seconds
( ) 0 loses balance while stepping or standing

14. **STANDING ON ONE LEG**
INSTRUCTIONS: Stand on one leg as long as you can without holding.
( ) 4 able to lift leg independently and hold >10 seconds
( ) 3 able to lift leg independently and hold 5-10 seconds
( ) 2 able to lift leg independently and hold = or >3 seconds
( ) 1 tries to lift leg unable to hold 3 seconds but remains standing independently
( ) 0 unable to try or needs assist to prevent fall
( ) **TOTAL SCORE (Maximum = 56)**

***References**

Wood-Dauphinee S, Berg K, Bravo G, Williams JI: The Balance Scale: Responding to clinically meaningful changes. Canadian Journal of Rehabilitation 10: 35-50, 1997

Berg K, Wood-Dauphinee S, Williams JI: The Balance Scale: Reliability assessment for elderly residents and patients with an acute stroke. Scand J Rehab Med 27:27-36, 1995

Berg K, Maki B, Williams JI, Holliday P, Wood-Dauphinee S: A comparison of clinical and laboratory measures of postural balance in an elderly population. Arch Phys Med Rehabil 73: 1073-1083, 1992

Berg K, Wood-Dauphinee S, Williams JI, Maki B: Measuring balance in the elderly: validation of an instrument. Can. J. Pub. Health July/August supplement 2:S7-11, 1992

Berg K, Wood-Dauphinee S, Williams JI, Gayton D: Measuring balance in the elderly: preliminary development of an instrument. Physiotherapy Canada 41:304-311, 1989

Figure 11-5—Cont'd (For legend see page 200).

MEASURES OF DEPRESSION

Center for Epidemiologic Studies Depression (CES-D)

Below is a list of some of the ways you may have felt or behaved. Please indicate how often you have felt this way during the **past week** by checking (✓) the appropriate space.

Rarely or none of the time (less than 1 day)	*Some or a little of the time (1-2 days)*	*Occasionally or a moderate amount of time (3-4 days)*	*All of the time (5-7 days)*
______	______	______	______

1. I was bothered by things that usually don't bother me.
2. I did not feel like eating; my appetite was poor.
3. I felt that I could not shake off the blues even with help from my family.
4. I felt that I was just as good as other people.
5. I had trouble keeping my mind on what I was doing.
6. I felt depressed.
7. I felt that everything I did was an effort.
8. I felt hopeful about the future.
9. I thought my life had been a failure.
10. I felt fearful.
11. My sleep was restless.
12. I was happy.
13. I talked less than usual.
14. I felt lonely.
15. People were unfriendly.
16. I enjoyed life.
17. I had crying spells.
18. I felt sad.
19. I felt that people disliked me.
20. I could not get "going."

Scoring

Item Weights	*Rarely or none of the time (less than 1 day)*	*Some or a little of the time (1-2 days)*	*Occasionally or a moderate amount of time (3-4 days)*	*All of the time (5-7 days)*
Items 4, 8, 12, and 16:	3	2	1	0
All other items:	0	1	2	3

Score is the sum of 20 item weights. Possible range is 0 to 60. If more than four questions are missing answers, do not score the CES-D. A score of 16 or more is considered depressed.

Bibliography

Radloff, L. S. (1977). The CES-D scale: A self-report depression scale for research in the general population. *Applied Psychological Measurement,* I, 385-401.

Figure 11-6 Center for Epidemiological Studies Depression Scale. *(Copyright 1977, West Publishing Company/Applied Psychological Measurement Inc. Reproduced by permission.)*

Wellness Program Satisfaction Questionnaire

Dear Wellness Program Participant,

Because we strive to deliver the best possible service, we are interested in learning from you how we might improve or enhance our program. Please take a few moments to complete and return this questionnaire. Please place an X in the appropriate box to indicate your rating or answer the descriptive questions on the appropriate line. Any additional comments you wish to make are welcome. You can include them in the "Comments" section at the end of the questionnaire or attach additional pages if you require more space. Please return the questionnaire to us at your earliest convenience. Thank you very much for your feedback!

Descriptive Questions

1. Your age ______ years
2. Your sex ______male ______female
3. How did you learn about The Wellness Program?

_____	physician	_____	website listing
_____	friend	_____	health newsletter
_____	former participant	_____	other, please indicate __________

4. Please identify the main diagnosis for which you sought self-management strategies through The Wellness Program:

_____	arm pain	_____	fibromyalgia	_____	headache
_____	leg pain	_____	arthritis	_____	high blood pressure
_____	back pain	_____	multiple sclerosis	_____	heart disease
_____	neck pain	_____	cancer	_____	other, please indicate _____

Please rate your degree of satisfaction with each of the following statements. *(1=strongly disagree, 2=disagree, 3=neither agree nor disagree, 4=agree, 5=strongly agree. Please check 9 if you have no opinion on the subject.)*

Strongly disagree	Disagree	Neither agree nor disagree	Agree	Strongly agree	No opinion
1	2	3	4	5	9

5. I was treated with respect throughout the program.
6. All staff members were courteous.
7. The program instructor understood my problem or condition.
8. The program instructor was knowledgeable.
9. The program instructor effectively presented the course material.
10. The program provided me with valuable information that helped improve my well-being.
11. I learned specific skills that helped improve my well-being.
12. The program handouts were helpful to me.
13. The group discussions were helpful to me.
14. The location of the facility was convenient for me.
15. The program was offered at a convenient time.
16. Parking was convenient and available.
17. The cost of the program was reasonable.
18. My bills were accurate.
19. I would recommend The Wellness Program to family and friends.
20. Overall, I was satisfied with my experience in The Wellness Program.

Comments ____

Figure 11-7 Wellness Program Patient Satisfaction Questionnaire. *(Modified with permission of Goldstein and the American Physical Therapy Association.)*

from the Physical Therapy Patient Satisfaction Questionnaire (PTPSQ), which was developed by Goldstein et al.[13] Although the PTPSQ has been determined to be valid and reliable, the WPSQ has not undergone psychometric analysis.

A patient satisfaction survey can include questions measuring both satisfaction with care and with treatment outcome. Both global measures, identifying general satisfaction, and multidimensional measures, identifying satisfaction with specific program components, can be included.

Patient satisfaction questionnaires are usually completed at the end of a program. Because dissatisfied patients may drop out early in a program, a clinician must make the extra effort to include people who drop out of a program in any survey of patient satisfaction.

Summary

Valid and reliable assessment instruments provide a useful resource for clinicians to determine the effectiveness of a wellness program. Any assessment instrument must be easy to administer and analyze. The appropriate qualitative and/or quantitative tools selected by clinicians for use depends on a program's patient population, goals, and questions of clinical interest.

References

1. Lorig K. *Patient Education: a Practical Approach.* Thousand Oaks, Calif: SAGE Publications, 1996, pp. 25-26.
2. Polgar S, Thomas SA. *Introduction to Research in the Health Sciences* 4th ed. Philadelphia: Harcourt Publishers, 2000.
3. Ware JE. SF-36 Health Survey update. *Spine* 2000;25(24):3130-3139.
4. Ware JE, Sherbourne CD. The MOS 36-item short-form health survey (SF-36): conceptual framework and item selection. *Med Care* 1992;30(6):473-483.
5. Von Korff M, Jensen MP, Karoly P. Assessing global pain severity by self-report in clinical and health services research. *Spine* 2000;25(24):3140-3151.
6. Melzack R, Katz J. The McGill Pain Questionnaire: appraisal and current. In Turk DC, Melzack R (eds), *Handbook of Pain Assessment.* New York: Guilford Press, 1992, pp. 152-168.
7. Roland M, Fairbank J. The Roland-Morris Disability Questionnaire and the Oswestry Disability Questionnaire. *Spine* 2000;25(24):3115-3124.
8. Hamilton DM, Haennel RG. Validity and reliability of the 6-minute walk test in a cardiac rehabilitation population. *J Cardiopulm Rehabil* 2000;20(3):156-164.
9. King S, Wessel J, Bhanbhani Y et al. Validity and reliability in the 6-minute walk in persons with fibromyalgia. *J Rheumatol* 1999;26(10):2233-2337.
10. Steffen TM, Hacker TA, Mollinger L. Age- and gender-related test performance in community-dwelling elderly people: six-minute walk test, Berg balance scale, timed up and go test and gait speeds. *Phys Ther* 2002;82:128-137.

11. Berg KO, Maki BE, Williams JI. Clinical and laboratory measures of postural balance in an elderly population. *Arch Phys Med Rehabil* 1992;73:1073-1080.
12. Geisser ME, Roth RS, Robinson ME: Asssessing depression among persons with chronic pain using the Center for Epidemiological Studies Depression Scale and the Beck Depression Inventory: a comparative analysis. *Clin J Pain* 13:163-170, 1997.
13. Goldstein MS, Elliott SD, Guccione AA. The development of an instrument to measure satisfaction with physical therapy. *Phys Ther* 2000;80(9):853-863.

Annotated Bibliography

Cohen S, Kessler RC, Gordon LU (eds). *Measuring Stress: a Guide for Health and Social Scientists.* New York: Oxford University Press, 1997. Sheldon Cohen from Carnegie Mellon University, Ron Kessler from Harvard Medical School, and Lynn Gordon from the Fetzer Institute combine their expertise to provide an authoritative resource for state-of-the-art definition, evaluation, and measurement of stress and stress-reducing interventions. This text examines measures of stressful events, stress appraisal and affective response, and biological indices of stress, including stress hormone, cardiovascular, and immune responses. The wealth of information presented in this text leaves the reader with a rich understanding and appreciation of the multiple and complex factors that contribute to defining and measuring stress. This text provides researchers and clinicians with information needed to choose appropriate measures for specific programs and studies.

Lorig K, Stewart A, Retter P et al. *Outcome Measures for Health Education and Other Health Care Interventions.* Thousand Oaks, Calif: SAGE Publications, 1996. The authors of this text are associated with the Stanford Patient Education Research Center and The Chronic Disease Self-Management Program, a collaborative research effort by Stanford University and the Kaiser Permanente Medical Care Program. They combine their expertise to offer a practical resource for outcome measures that assess health behaviors, health status, self-efficacy, and health care utilization. This text identifies several psychometrically sound instruments, along with providing instructions for administering the measures and scoring the results. It is an outstanding and invaluable resource for the clinician who is in search of outcome measures appropriate for assessing a group wellness intervention.

Turk DC, Melzack R (eds). *Handbook of Pain Assessment.* New York, Guilford Publications, 2001. Dennis C. Turk, Ph.D., from the University of Washington, and Ronald Melzack, Ph.D., from McGill University, are leaders in the field of pain assessment and research. This text is the gold standard in the field of pain assessment. It offers a thorough and authoritative examination of the multiple dimensions of pain assessment. The medical and physical evaluation of pain patients, the measurement of pain, the psychological evaluation of patients with pain, and the assessment of the behavioral expression of pain are among the topics covered. The authors identify the limitations and advantages of available assessment instruments and provide guidelines for selecting measures appropriate to diverse populations. This text is a valuable resource for the health care practitioner who is measuring treatment outcomes in patients with chronic pain.

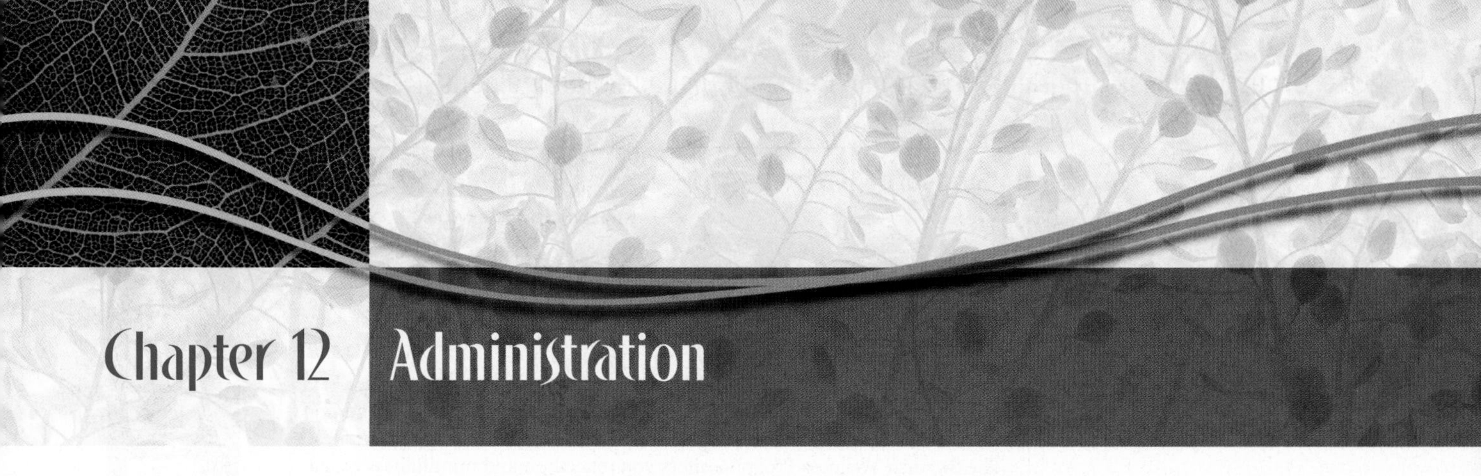

Chapter 12 Administration

This chapter examines two aspects of program administration: marketing and finances. Practical marketing suggestions are offered to build relationships with health care providers, patients, and the public that lead to program referrals. An introductory overview of the financial considerations involved in offering a group program is presented.

Marketing

A great program is of little value without participants. Successful marketing strategies are required to ensure successful program enrollment. Clinicians who are passionate about patient care often have a negative attitude toward marketing. Interested in serving people, not selling something, they often drag their heels when it comes to developing a marketing plan. To dispel my own hesitancy about marketing, I define marketing as building relationships. Relationships with other health care providers, previous program participants, and the general public result in referrals to a program.

Printed Materials

Before approaching potential referral sources, written material describing a program is needed. Develop a flier, brochure, and/or poster that offer a simple, straightforward description of the program (Figure 12-1). You may wish to include testimonies from other health care providers or program participants. Include a telephone number and, if appropriate, Web site address where people can receive additional information.

Relationship Building

Positive relationships with other health care professionals, previous group participants, and the general public are the key to building a successful referral base.

Health Care Professionals

The opportunity to work with respected and skilled colleagues is one of the joys and privileges of being a health care practitioner. The relationships that develop in the course of providing health care services can be drawn on to create a program referral base. Identify those physicians who care for the population your program serves and who already refer patients to your services. In many settings, physician assistants and nurse practitioners provide primary care services and should be

Rehabilitation Services

SWEDISH

The Wellness Program

If you live with chronic pain, illness or a stress-related medical condition, you may be interested in learning skills that will help you to help yourself. The Swedish Wellness Program offers you relaxation and mindfulness-based stress-reduction strategies in an eight-week class designed to complement your medical care. Join instructors Carolyn McManus, P.T., M.A., and Peggy Maas, P.T., as they provide you with:

- Effective ways to manage stress, pain and illness
- Instruction in relaxation and mindfulness meditation
- Gentle stretching exercises that enhance mobility and build mind-body awareness
- Specific tools to integrate class material into daily life
- A supportive group for sharing experiences and feelings about illness and healing

The Wellness Program is appropriate for individuals with medical conditions such as:

- Anxiety
- Arthritis
- Back pain
- Cancer
- Chronic pain
- Cumulative trauma disorder
- Fatigue
- Fibromyalgia
- Gastrointestinal distress
- Headache
- Heart disease
- Hypertension
- Insomnia
- Multiple sclerosis
- Muscle disorders
- Neurological disorders
- Rheumatological conditions

"This program gave me the tools I needed to cope with my disease. Even on bad days, I don't have to leave work. I can take a few minutes, practice what I've learned and help myself feel better." — Cynthia R.

"This program has helped me decrease my anxiety, and has provided me with practical ways to respond to pain. By relaxing and keeping a clear head rather than get all tensed up, I have felt a decrease in the intensity of my pain. If I do flare up, these skills keep the flare short. It has been a very helpful part of my treatment program." — Sue T.

This program is modeled on the class series outlined in "Full Catastrophe Living" by Jon Kabat-Zinn.

Classes are offered throughout the year. For this self-pay program, the fee is $375. Additionally, if you are not an outpatient rehabilitation patient, a referral from a physician is necessary for a one-time screening evaluation by a class instructor. This visit can be billed to an insurance company.

For program information, class dates and to register, call (000) 000-0000.

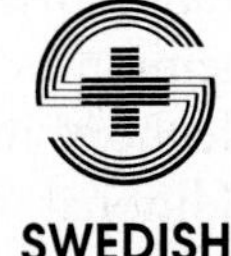

SWEDISH

Figure 12-1 The Wellness Program flier.

identified as main referral sources. Begin a process of educating these groups about the benefits of your program. This can occur in the following ways:

1. Send a letter describing the program along with fliers (Figure 12-2) to potential referral sources. Follow up the letter with a phone call or arrange to have an individual meeting to describe the program in more detail and answer any questions. When a referral is received, send an additional thank-you letter (Figure 12-3). On program completion, send a discharge summary highlighting the program themes and the participant's progress (Figure 12-4).
2. Referring practitioners are often willing to have program fliers posted in their waiting area or treatment rooms. These posted fliers often trigger

```
August 1, 2002

Dear Physician,

The diagnosis of a chronic medical condition often
presents people with a range of life challenges from
decreased physical activity to emotional isolation.
The Wellness Program helps people face these challenges
skillfully in a program designed to complement their
medical care. Through the application of specific
physical and cognitive strategies, participants learn
to maximize what they can do for themselves to heal,
manage symptoms and live fully. These strategies
include relaxation, mindfulness meditation, gentle
stretching and strengthening exercises and principles
of cognitive restructuring. Upon completing the
program, participants are independent on a comprehensive
home program. Many describe a decrease in symptom
severity or an improved ability to cope with their
symptoms.

The next classes begin September 24th. Both daytime and
evening programs will be available. Thank you for
considering The Wellness Program as a resource for your
patients with chronic pain, illness and stress-related
medical conditions. If you have further questions or
would like to speak with me personally,
I can be reached at (000) 000-0000.

Sincerely,
Instructor's name
```

Figure 12-2 A sample letter introducing a wellness program to a potential referral source.

patient interest and stimulate a discussion of the program initiated by a patient.

3. Referral pads for referring physician use are a common practice among physical therapists. A wellness program service can easily be added to a list of rehabilitation services on a standard referral form.
4. If you practice in or near a major medical center, attend or present at professional conferences that concern the population served by your program. Bring fliers and business cards and actively introduce yourself to other attendees and educate them about your program.
5. Initiate a special interest group of health care providers. This can increase referrals and prove to be a professionally enhancing experience on many levels. In the spring of 2000, I invited nine physicians, nurses, and physical therapists who were interested in mind-body medicine to dinner. This evening discussion led to the formation of a group of a dozen health care providers who meet once a month for a discussion of topics of professional interest. Not only is this group a natural source of referrals among all involved, but it is also a source of professional support, learning, and friendship.
6. If you find a physician, physician's assistant, or nurse practitioner who is an enthusiastic supporter of your services, ask if he or she knows of other

September 4, 2002

Dear Dr. Smith,

Thank you for referring Jane Jones to The Wellness Program. This program provides participants with instruction in effective self-management strategies including relaxation, mindfulness meditation, gentle stretching and strengthening exercises and principles of cognitive restructuring. Upon completing the program, you will receive a discharge summary describing Ms. Jones's progress with this course of care.

Thank you again for referring Ms. Jones to The Wellness Program.

Sincerely,
Instructor's name

Figure 12-3 A sample letter thanking a physician for a referral.

providers who would be interested in your program. A recommendation from a colleague is often a wonderful introduction to a provider who is new to your services.

7. Send a quarterly wellness newsletter to physicians and other health care providers that highlights recent medical journal publications on wellness-related topics and includes a brief description of your program. A newsletter summarizing relevant research reinforces your credibility and authority in the field.

When I began my program, I found it invaluable to have the strong and consistent support of four physicians: a physiatrist, rheumatologist, and two pain specialists. With this in mind, you may want to identify four to six physicians or other referral sources who you believe may be especially receptive to your program and spend additional time and effort building your relationships with them. Ultimately, a broad referral base of multiple providers is needed for the long-term success of a program.

In addition to physicians, physician assistants, and nurse practitioners, building relationships with other nurses, physical therapists, occupational therapists, dieticians, exercise physiologists, and medical social workers increases referrals. Letters, fliers, wellness newsletters, and personal contacts can also be used to reach these groups.

Previous Participants

Once you have a program up and running, maintain an e-mail address list of participants. One month before starting a program, send program information to past participants. Sending information electronically is a simple process requiring minimal time and effort and can be a source of referrals.

The General Public

Informing the public directly about a wellness program is as important as building a network of referring health care professionals. Because our present medical system focuses primarily on disease treatment, strategies for the self-management

Figure 12-4 A sample letter to a physician highlighting wellness program themes and a patient's progress.

November 20, 2002

Dear Dr. Smith,

Thank you for referring Jane Jones to The Wellness Program for the treatment of chronic back pain. Ms. Jones successfully completed the 8-week group program and demonstrated very high motivation throughout the class series. Jane was introduced to mindfulness and mindfulness meditation, diaphragmatic breathing, relaxation and gentle stretching and strengthening exercises emphasizing body awareness. Pain management strategies and cognitive restructuring were also presented. Ms. Jones experienced a decrease in pain severity. She felt the variety of self-management skills improved her attitude and ability to manage pain and stress more effectively. This was verified by pre- and post-program responses to a pain assessment questionnaire:

	9/20/02	11/18/02
On average, how severe has your pain been during the last week? 0 = not at all severe, 6 = extremely severe	6	4
During the past week, how much do you feel you've been able to deal with your problems? 0 = not at all, 6 = extremely well	3	5
During the past week, how successful were you in coping with stressful situations? 0 = not at all, 6 = extremely successful	2	5

Ms. Jones also demonstrated a decrease in symptoms of depression on the Center for Epidemiology Depression Scale. She described increasing functional activities in her home. She had difficulty performing some of the class stretching exercises and it is my general impression that a community pool exercise program remains the most suitable exercise program for her continued rehabilitation.

Ms. Jones described the group sharing and support as playing an important role in her overall positive experience. She especially benefited from the group's open discussions about coping with pain.

Thank you again for referring Jane Jones to The Wellness Program. It was a pleasure to have her in the class.

Sincerely,
Instructor's name

of chronic problems may not be high on the list of treatment options in the mind of a medical provider. A patient, however, may be very interested.

In my experience, being part of a major medical center greatly enhances the ability to reach the general public directly. Major medical centers often have ongoing community education services that are perfectly suited to introducing and promoting wellness programs. Many facilities send health newsletters quarterly with health-related stories and a description and dates of upcoming programs. They often sponsor health fairs and health conferences that promote medical center services as well as educate the public.

A one-evening introductory session that presents a basic theme or component of your program can be an effective strategy to generate interest. For example, preliminary skills and concepts for pain management can be presented in a one-evening class entitled "Managing Chronic Pain: Self-Help Strategies." Enticed with initial skills for managing pain, attendees may be inspired to enroll in a more comprehensive program.

Do not be discouraged if enrollment in the first year of a program is low. My first classes had six to eight participants. Recognize that it takes time to build a program. Once a program has an established track record and favorable reputation, word of mouth contributes significantly to enrollment. Even once a program is successful, marketing remains an ongoing process. High enrollment in one group does not automatically ensure high enrollment in the next. Once relationships are established with referral sources, they must be maintained through ongoing and frequent contacts. In my experience, what is out of sight is out of mind. A provider who sends people to one group can easily forget to refer anyone to the next. Repeated contacts through letters, phone calls, presentations, and personal meetings are necessary to secure a steady referral base for your program.

Financial Considerations

A wellness program must be shown to be financially sound to receive approval and support from health care facility administrators and to survive in today's cost-conscious health care climate. A program budget, identifying expenses and revenue, needs to be developed.

Expenses

A capital budget allocates for major expenses such as renovations, furniture, and equipment. Capital expenses are those expenses that run generally over $1000. The only capital allocation that might be incurred for a wellness program would be for renovating space to create a classroom.

An operating budget identifies the expected revenue collected and expenses incurred during the month-to-month operation of a program. Components of an operating expense budget include instructor salary, marketing, educational materials and supplies such as mats, and refreshments. Rental space costs are also operating expenses. Some clinicians may provide programs in facilities with classroom space already available and incur no rental expense. Other clinicians may need to rent space. The cost of renting space can vary widely depending on location.

Revenue

Revenue can be collected through private pay, insurance billing, or some combination of both. The simplest of these revenue collection procedures is the private-pay method in which participants personally pay a set fee. In addition to being simple to administer, personally paying for a service may create added incentive for participants to regularly attend and actively participate in a program.

Alternately, a group treatment charge can be billed to an insurance carrier. Reimbursement for group treatment can vary widely among insurance plans and, in some instances, group treatment is not a covered benefit. Consequently, billing group treatment alone may result in inconsistent revenue that is inadequate to cover expenses. If a group treatment charge is billed, individual state Medicare and insurance guidelines need to be reviewed to determine the specific parameters for billing this service.

A combination of private pay and insurance billing is a third model of revenue collection. If this method is chosen, the portion of the service billed as group treatment must be clearly separate from a nonbillable private-pay component of the service. For example, a physical therapist offering a wellness program that includes one hour of exercise can bill the exercise component of the program as a group physical therapy service. In addition, if the physical therapist also facilitates one hour of group support, that component of the program is not covered by insurance and can be billed directly to the participants as an out-of-pocket fee for the program.

An efficient system for billing and collection should be in place for processing financial transactions. The ability to monitor the rate of reimbursement by different insurance carriers, denial of payments, and documentation requests is needed to ensure the financial solvency of a program.

Sample Operating Budget

Figure 12-5 outlines a budget for a private-pay group program for 15 participants meeting once a week for 2 hours for 8 consecutive weeks at a medical center with free classroom space.

Operating Expenses:		
Instructor salary (3 hr./class x 8 classes)		
$31.25/hr (salary) x 24 hrs =		$ 750
$750 x 0.25 (benefits expense)=		$ 250
	Total	$ 1000
Marketing		$ 150
Supplies		
1/2" binders ($ 2 ea. x 15)		$ 30
paper		$ 5
exercise cassettes/CDs		$ 180
Refreshments		$ 160
	Total expenses	$ 1525
Revenues:		
Program fee: private pay		
$40/class x 8 classes x 15 participants		$ 4800
Materials fee		
$30 x 15 participants		$ 450
	Total revenues	$ 5250
Total revenues – total expenses = net revenue		
$5250 – $1525 = $3725		

Figure 12-5 Sample budget for an eight-session wellness program.

For a program to achieve financial success, revenue must exceed expenses; however, in the early months of a program, enrollment may be small, and financial losses may occur. The length of time a clinician and facility willingly incur losses depends on the unique circumstances of the facility and program. As a program grows, enrollment fees should cover program expenses.

Summary

A successful marketing strategy is necessary to achieve program enrollment goals. Marketing requires building and maintaining relationships with health care professionals, patients, and the general public. Attractive, informative, and easy-to-read written materials describing a program are needed. Letters, newsletters, phone calls, individual meetings, and participation in professional conferences and community health fairs are among the avenues available to promote your program.

A clinician must develop a program budget that identifies expenses and revenue and that demonstrates the financial viability of a wellness program. The major operating expense in a group wellness program in most cases will be the instructor's salary. Revenue collection can occur through private-pay charges and/or insurance billing. Although in the initial months of a program financial losses may occur, a wellness program must be financially successful to receive support from administrators and thrive in today's cost-conscious health care environment.

Annotated Bibliography

Roitman J (ed). *ASCM's Resource Manual for Guidelines for Exercise Testing and Prescription* 4th ed. Philadelphia: Lippincott Williams & Wilkins, 2001. This text is an authoritative manual on exercise guidelines, procedures, and protocols. It is a resource for fitness professionals who are candidates for certification by the American College of Sports Medicine and a companion to the *ACSM's Guidelines for Exercise Testing and Prescription.* In addition to offering a comprehensive examination of exercise physiology and principles of fitness, it offers a detailed discussion of fitness program management and administration in clinical, corporate, or community settings. Topics covered include developing policies and procedures, operations management, personnel issues, financial management, and legal considerations. This comprehensive manual is a practical and informative resource for a health care professional.

Complete Listing of Books Noted in Annotated Bibliographies

Chapter 1: Wellness

Edelman CL, Mandle CL (eds). *Health Promotion Throughout the Lifespan* 5th ed. St. Louis: Mosby, 2002.

Gorin SS, Arnold J. *Health Promotion Handbook.* St. Louis: Mosby, 1998.

Kabat-Zinn J. *Full Catastrophe Living: Using the Wisdom of Your Body and Mind to Face Stress, Pain and Illness.* New York: Delacorte Press, 1990.

Ornish D. *Love & Survival.* New York: HarperCollins, 1998.

Remen RN. *My Grandfather's Blessings: Stories of Strength, Refuge and Belonging.* New York: Riverhead Books, 2000.

Chapter 2: Group Leadership

Corey MS, Corey G. *Groups: Process and Practice.* Pacific Grove, Calif: Brooks/Cole Publishing, 2002.

Lee RJ, King SN. *Discovering the Leader in You: A Guide to Realizing Your Personal Leadership Potential.* San Francisco: Josey-Bass, 2001.

Lorig K. *Patient Education: A Practical Approach.* Thousand Oaks, Calif: SAGE Publications, 1996.

Santorelli S. *Heal Thy Self: Lessons on Mindfulness in Medicine.* New York. Bell Tower, 1999.

Chapter 3: Mindfulness

Farhi D. *The Breathing Book: Good Health and Vitality Through Essential Breath Work.* New York: Henry Holt, 1996.

Gunaratana H. *Mindfulness in Plain English.* Boston: Wisdom Publications, 1994.

Kabat-Zinn J. *Full Catastrophe Living: Using the Wisdom of Your Body and Mind to Face Stress, Pain and Illness.* New York: Delacorte Press, 1990.

Kabat-Zinn J. *Wherever You Go, There You Are: Mindfulness Meditation in Everyday Life.* New York: Hyperion, 1994.

Langer EJ. *Mindfulness.* Cambridge, Mass: Perseus Books, 1989.

Nhat Hanh T. *Peace is Every Step: The Path of Mindfulness in Everyday Life.* New York: Bantam Books, 1991.

Chapter 4: Stress and Relaxation

Payne RA. *Relaxation Techniques: A Practical Handbook for the Health Care Professional* 2nd ed. New York: Churchill Livingston, 2000.

Rabin BS. *Stress, Immune Function and Health: The Connection.* New York: Wiley, John & Sons, 1999.

Sapolsky RM. *Why Zebras Don't Get Ulcers: An Updated Guide to Stress, Stress-Related Diseases and Coping.* New York: Henry Holt, 1998.

Sternberg E. *The Balance Within: The Science Connecting Health and Emotions.* New York: WH Freeman and Co., 2000.

Chapter 5: Attitudes and Beliefs

Burns D. *Feeling Good: The New Mood Therapy.* New York, William Morrow and Co, 1999.

Foster R, Hicks G. *How We Choose to be Happy.* New York: Berkley Publishing Group, 1999.

Greenberger D, Padesky C. *Mind Over Mood.* New York: Guilford Publications, 1995.

Segal ZV, Williams MG, Teasdale JD. *Mindfulness-Based Cognitive Therapy for Depression: A New Approach to Preventing Relapse.* New York: Guilford Publications, 2001.

Chapter 6: Nutrition

Tribole E, Resch E. *Intuitive Eating.* New York: St Martin's Press, 1996.

Duyff RL. *The American Dietitic Association's Complete Food & Nutrition Guide.* Minneapolis: Chronimed Publishing, 1998.

Chapter 7: Exercise

Durstine LJ (ed). *ASCM's Exercise Management for Person's with Chronic Diseases and Disabilities.* New York: Human Kinetics, 1998.

Franklin B. *ASCM's Guidelines for Exercise Testing and Prescription* 4th ed. Philadelphia: Lippincott Williams & Wilkins, 2001.

National Heart, Lung and Blood Institute, National Institutes of Health. *Clinical Guidelines on the Identification, Evaluation and Treatment of Overweight and Obesity in Adults: The Evidence Report.* Washington, DC: 1998. NIH Publication No. 98-4083.

Roitman J (ed). *ASCM's Resource Manual for Guidelines for Exercise Testing and Prescription* 4th ed. Philadelphia: Lippincott, 2001.

Ruderman N, Devlin JT. *Health Professional's Guide to Diabetes and Exercise.* Alexandria, Va: American Diabetes Association, 1995.

Chapter 8: Mindful Movement

Carrico M. *Yoga Journal's Yoga Basics: The Essential Beginner's Guide to Yoga for a Lifetime of Health and Fitness.* New York: Henry Holt and Co., 1997.

Cohen KS. *The Way of Qigong: The Art and Science of Chinese Energy Healing.* New York: Random House, 1999.

Huang CA. *Essential T'ai Ji.* Berkeley, Calif: Ten Speed Press, 2001.

MacDonald G, MacDonald G. *The Complete Illustrated Guide to the Alexander Technique: A Practical Program for Health, Poise and Fitness.* Rockport, Mass: Element Books, 1998.

Shafarman S. *Awareness Heals: The Feldenkrais Method for Dynamic Health.* Reading, Mass: Perseus Books 1997.

Chapter 11: Assessment Tools

Cohen S, Kessler RC, Gordon LU (eds). *Measuring Stress: A Guide for Health and Social Scientists.* New York: Oxford University Press, 1997.

Lorig K, Stewart A, Retter P et al. *Outcome Measures for Health Education and Other Health Care Interventions.* Thousand Oaks, Calif: SAGE Publications, 1996.

Turk DC and Melzack R (eds). *Handbook of Pain Assessment.* New York: Guilford Publications, 2001.

Chapter 12: Administrative Functions

Roitman J (ed). *ASCM's Resource Manual for Guidelines for Exercise Testing and Prescription* 4th ed. Philadelphia: Lippincott, 2001.

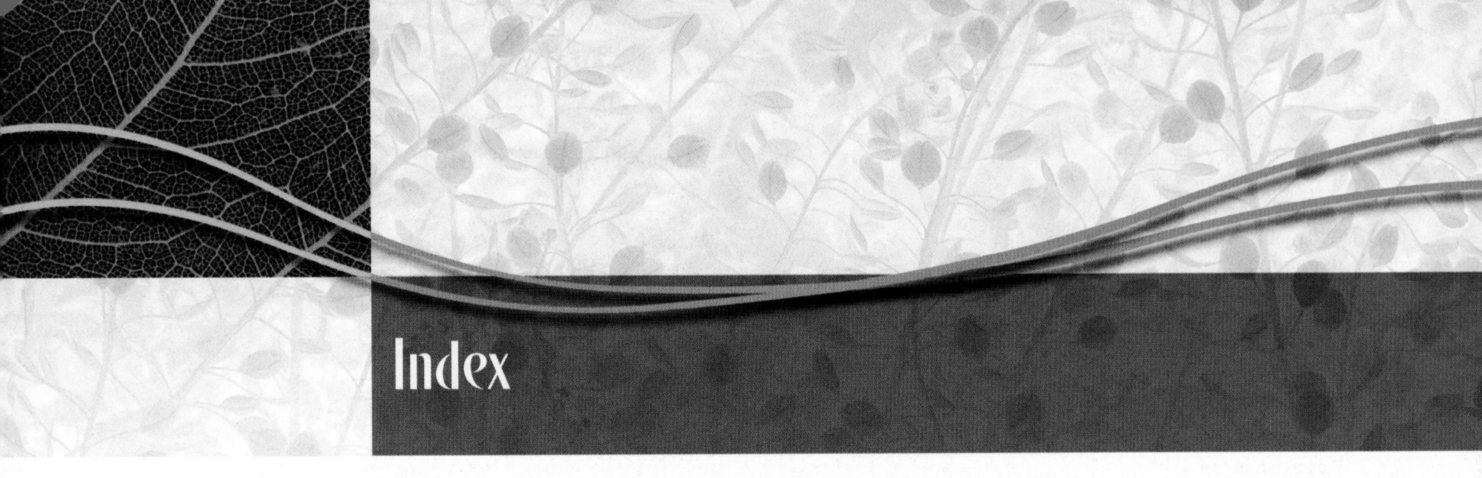

Index